Contemporary Diabetes

Series Editor: Aristidis Veves, MD, DSc

For further volumes:
http://www.springer.com/series/7679

Anders A.F. Sima
Editor

Diabetes & C-Peptide

Scientific and Clinical Aspects

Humana Press

Editor
Anders A.F. Sima, MD, PhD, FRCP(C)
Professor, Departments of Pathology and Neurology
Wayne State University
Detroit, MI, USA
asima@med.wayne.edu

ISBN 978-1-4939-5957-0 ISBN 978-1-61779-391-2 (eBook)
DOI 10.1007/978-1-61779-391-2
Springer New York Dordrecht Heidelberg London

Printed on acid-free paper

Humana Press is part of Springer Science+Business Media (www.springer.com)

Foreword

Type 1 diabetes has in recent years shown an alarming increase in incidence, particularly in heavily populated regions of the globe, occurring at steadily younger ages. This increase in incidence of type 1 diabetes will likely be paralleled by a similar increase in the frequency of the disorder's debilitating secondary complications.

Since its discovery, C-peptide has evolved from a non-bioactive marker of β-cell function to a highly significant multifunctional hormone in the pathobiology of diabetes and its complications. The wealth of information that has appeared over the last decade and a half is reviewed in depth in this volume. This review provides current insights into the multiple physiological functions of C-peptide, its pathophysiological role in the development of chronic complications and ultimately the significance of its replacement in the prevention and treatment of these complications in patients with type 1 diabetes. The chapters are authored by the leading investigators in the field. This volume of *Contemporary Diabetes* provides the first comprehensive collection of current, detailed and critical reviews on C-peptide biology. It is highly recommended to clinicians, diabetologists, residents, basic scientists, and students who are seeking insights into C-peptide and the rapidly growing biology surrounding this versatile and highly relevant hormone.

Ann Arbor, MI, USA

Eva L. Feldman, MD, PhD

Preface

It is well known that C-peptide, the connecting peptide of the proinsulin molecule, is an important part in the biosynthesis of insulin in that it facilitates its correct folding. Following the cleavage of proinsulin into insulin and C-peptide, both peptides are stored in the secretory granules of pancreatic b-cells and are released into the circulation in equimolar concentrations. After its discovery in 1967 by Steiner et al, C-peptide was anticipated to have physiological effects similar to those of insulin. Disappointingly, no effects could be documented with respect to glucose or lipid metabolism, and C-peptide was written off as a non-bioactive peptide. It was not until the 1990s that C-peptide was revisited in a clinical setting. A series of studies were performed on type 1 diabetic patients to whom C-peptide was administered. These studies demonstrated that replacement of physiological levels of C-peptide led to improvements in kidney function and nerve conduction velocities in type 1 diabetic patients. C-peptide also augmented capillary blood flow in skeletal muscle, skin, and the kidney. These findings led to a renewed interest in the physiological function of C-peptide and possible pathophysiologic roles of its deficiency in type 1 diabetes. During the last decade and a half there has been a steadily increasing number of reports on C-peptide, its physiology, as well as the effects of its replacement on type 1 diabetic complications. The information to date includes, in vitro studies pertaining to its interaction with cell membranes, internalization into endosomes and nucleoli, its function in red blood cells, its interaction with insulin signaling mechanisms as well as direct interaction between insulin and C-peptide. However, a remaining obstacle in the characterization of the physiological role of C-peptide is the existence of a specific C-peptide receptor, which remains elusive. Instead it has been suggested that the effects are mediated via G-protein coupled receptor mechanisms and/or by enhancing insulin signaling via its direct interaction with insulin signaling and with oligomeric insulin.

The revealed actions of C-peptide result in a myriad of cellular effects, including anti-inflammatory effects on the vasculature and the central nervous system, anti-apoptotic and anti-oxidative effects, gene regulatory effects pertaining to trophic factors, and cell-adhesive molecules perturbed in type 1 diabetes. In vivo animal studies of type 1 diabetes have described functional and structural benefits on complications affecting the vasculature, kidney, and peripheral and central nervous systems. Several clinical studies have appeared recently, confirming the benefits of C-peptide replacement on peripheral nerve and kidney function. Therefore, there exists today a wealth of information attesting to a multitude of sometimes contradictory physiological effects in different tissue systems mediated by C-peptide. The data to date strongly support the notion that together with regular insulin therapy in type 1 diabetes, replacement of C-peptide will have additional beneficial effects on the prevention and treatment of complications accompanying type 1 diabetes.

This volume of *Contemporary Diabetes* provides an update of the current knowledge of C-peptide's physiological function and the role of its deficiency in the development of type 1 diabetic complications. This rapidly moving field is dealt with in detail by the most prominent investigators in the field. The evidence summarized in this volume will hopefully convey the urgency with which both continuing mechanistic studies and clinical trials are needed. In reflection, it is nearly 100 years since the discovery of insulin and yet we have no causal and effective therapy for the complications accompanying type 1 diabetes.

I wish to thank Professor Aristides Veves, Harvard Medical School for inviting me to put together this volume of the *Contemporary Diabetes* series. Also, I thank Richard Lansing and Maureen Alexander of Springer Verlag for their help, encouragement, and support. I am grateful to Professor John Wahren for his support. Finally, I wish to sincerely thank all the authors for their relentless efforts and their invaluable contributions to this volume.

Detroit, MI, USA Anders A.F. Sima, MD, PhD, FRCP(C)

Contents

Donald F. Steiner
Department of Medicine, Section of Adult and Pediatric Endocrinology, Diabetes and Metabolism, The University of Chicago, Chicago, IL, USA

Sara Stridh
Department of Medical Cell Biology, Division of Integrative Physiology, Uppsala University, Uppsala, Sweden

Massimo Trucco
Division of Immunogenetics, Children's Hospital of Pittsburgh of UPMC, Rango's Research Center, Pittsburgh, PA, USA

John Wahren
Department of Molecular Medicine and Surgery, Karolinska Institutet, Stockholm, Sweden

Daniel Walcher
Department of Cardiology, University of Ulm, Ulm, Germany

Matthias M. Weber
Department of Endocrinology and Metabolism, Johannes Gutenberg University, Mainz, Germany

Wei-Xian Zhang
Department of Pathology, Wayne State University, Detroit, MI, USA

C-Peptide and Insulin: A Happy Marriage

1

Donald F. Steiner

Keywords
Proinsulin • Convertases • Insulin genes • Mutations • Biosynthesis

One of the most important outgrowths of the discovery of proinsulin was the finding that the 31-residue connecting segment, or C-peptide, that joins the insulin chains in the prohormone is excised intact and secreted in equal amounts along with insulin. This finding allowed the development of the human C-peptide radioimmunoassay which has become indispensable as an accurate measure of insulin production in vivo in various forms of diabetes [1].

In a recent study, it has been shown that 67% of individuals (Joslin Medalists) who have lived more than 50 years after the diagnosis of type 1 diabetes at a mean age of 11.0 ± 6.4 years still retain detectable levels of C-peptide, indicating the survival of some beta-cells [2]. However, most of these patients showed little or no rise in C-peptide in response to a test meal, while a few (~2.6%) showed a small response that was about 11% of normal control values. Although the presence of detectable C-peptide levels correlated with slightly improved hemoglobin A1c levels, the small C-peptide responsive group did not have significantly better A1c levels. Perhaps more significantly, their age at onset was about 5 years later than the mean and they showed a higher frequency of the HLA DR3 genotype, while the DR4 genotype was more common in the group with undetectable C-peptide levels. The C-peptide responsive group, however, exhibited a lower level of proliferative retinopathy, but a higher level of microalbuminuria and comparable levels of neuropathy. These findings obviously have little bearing on the question as to whether the C-peptide helps to prevent diabetic complications. However, it encourages the view that beta-cells are capable of some regeneration even in the face of autoimmune destruction.

This volume contains a number of new reports of research indicating possible biological actions of the C-peptide. This new evidence certainly adds a further impetus to the desirability of designing clinical studies to evaluate the potential value of C-peptide therapy, either at replacement levels along with insulin in type 1 diabetes or at pharmacological levels in patients with diabetic complications.

In addition to its possible roles in physiology, information has continued to accumulate bearing on the role of the C-peptide in the biosynthesis of insulin [1]. Proinsulin is the founding member of a large and diverse group of prohormones and

D.F. Steiner (✉)
Department of Medicine, Section of Adult and Pediatric Endocrinology, Diabetes and Metabolism, The University of Chicago, 5841 S. Maryland Avenue, MC1027, Chicago, IL 60637, USA
e-mail: dfsteine@uchicago.edu

A.A.F. Sima (ed.), *Diabetes & C-Peptide: Scientific and Clinical Aspects*, Contemporary Diabetes, DOI 10.1007/978-1-61779-391-2_1, © Springer Science+Business Media, LLC 2012

proneuropeptides that continues to slowly enlarge. All of these precursor forms obviously share the common purpose of ensuring the synthesis and controlled secretion of the large number of small regulatory peptides that act to help maintain homeostasis in our bodies. These peptides are mainly neuroendocrine (metabolic and/or neural) in function and are processed proteolytically from precursors by PC1/3 and PC2, members of a large ten-member family of specially adapted calcium-dependent subtilisin-like endoproteases, or "convertases," that act mainly within the secretory pathway of neuroendocrine cells. Since their action creates new C-terminal basic residues by cleaving at sites usually containing two or more lysine or arginine residues, specialized carboxypeptidases such as CPE and CPD must remove these amino acids to facilitate further maturation steps such as amidation [3, 4]. The convertases must have a high degree of cleavage site selectivity and accuracy in order to avoid making promiscuous cleavages in the large number of proteins that normally traverse the secretory pathway [1, 5]. Thus, polypeptide hormone precursors must be designed in a way that allows them to move relatively quickly through the secretory pathway from the initial site of their biosynthesis and folding in the endoplasmic reticulum (ER) to and through the Golgi apparatus and on into newly formed secretory vesicles or "granules" where they are acidified and processed at specific recognition sequences, resulting in the storage and release mainly of the mature peptide products along with any other retained fragments of their "pro" regions and only low percentages of unprocessed or partly-processed precursor forms.

Recent structural studies on proinsulin in solution using NMR [6] indicate that while the insulin moiety has a highly defined structure closely similar to that defined by X-ray crystallography, the C-peptide has minimal secondary structure and is not spatially well defined (i.e., lacks tertiary structure). Its presence also blocks the interaction of proinsulin with the insulin receptor to a considerable extent, such that its receptor binding affinity is only 3% of that for insulin [7].

Despite its lack of complete structural organization, proinsulin rapidly exits the ER and moves on through the Golgi apparatus into newly forming secretory granules within 30–40 min, faster than many larger proteins. However, recent studies of dominant-negative mutations in the proinsulin molecule that inhibit its folding and the correct formation of its disulfide bonds have shown that these mutations greatly slow the progress of the mutant proinsulin in the secretory pathway, preventing its secretion and also negatively impacting the folding and transport of the normal proinsulin chains, leading to ER stress and eventual beta-cell death [1, 8, 9]. Very few of these pathogenic substitutions occur within the C-peptide, indicating that its role in folding is mainly confined to that of a flexible spacer that allows the B and A chain regions to freely interact to efficiently assemble the insulin molecule (see Fig. 1.1).

Most C-peptides in vertebrate proinsulins have a conserved length of approximately 30 amino acids, although various studies have shown that shorter C-peptides of only a few amino acids enable correct and efficient proinsulin folding [10]. However, they are more difficult to remove by the convertases to produce the finished active insulin molecule. In other words, it appears that the entirety of the C-peptide is required for efficiently making insulin, but it must also be structured in a way that prevents it from interfering with the A and B chains as they interact during folding. It must also be easily and efficiently cleavable by the prohormone convertases PC1/3 and PC2 which coexist in the insulin secretory granules with proinsulin and are responsible, along with CPE, for its efficient processing into active insulin [11, 12].

The C-peptides usually lack basic residues, such as lysine, histidine, and arginine. Instead they usually contain four or five acidic residues, such as glutamic or aspartic acid. These give the C-peptide a relatively strong negative charge and may contribute to its tendency to bind bivalent cations such as zinc and perhaps others such as calcium. Thus, porcine proinsulin binds considerably more zinc than does insulin, although with a lower affinity than the zinc binding involved in hexamerization [13]. A still unresolved issue is whether the hexameric form of proinsulin can be cleaved efficiently by the convertases. Recently, it has been shown that ablation of the beta-cell zinc transporter ZnT8 prevents uptake of zinc into secretory granules, dramatically altering their

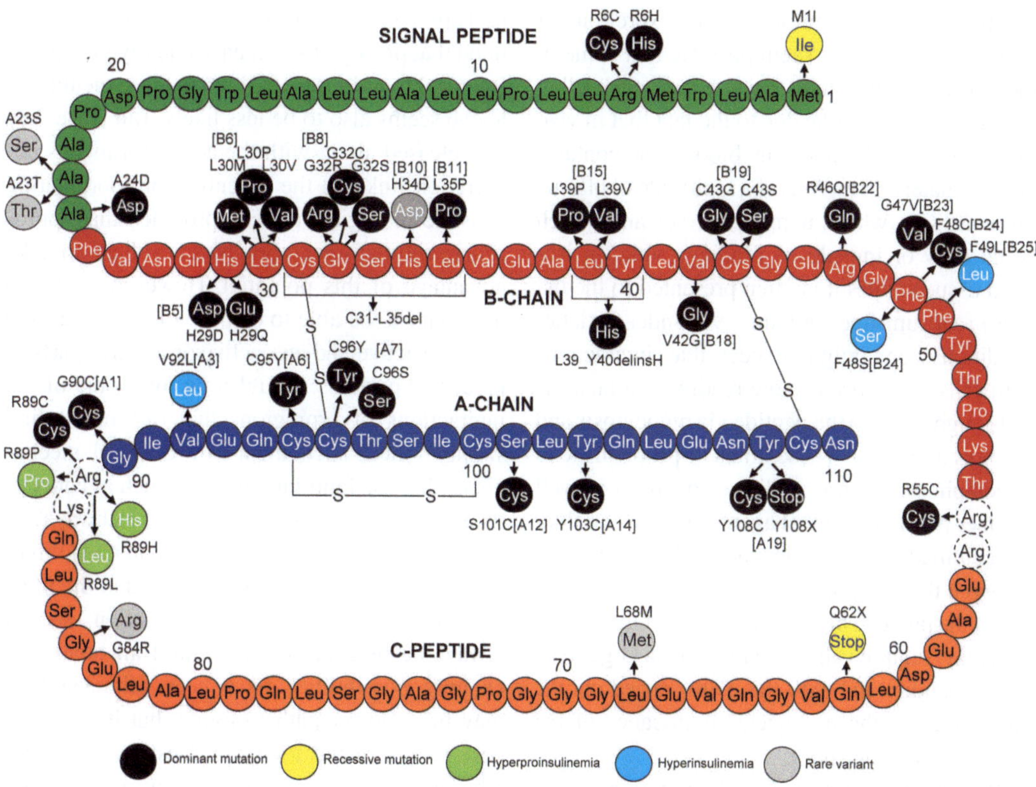

Fig. 1.1 Summary of mutations affecting the primary structure of human preproinsulin. Those associated with dominant and recessive forms of diabetes are shown in *black* and *yellow circles*, respectively, and those associated with hyperproinsulinemia and hyperinsulinemia in *green* and *blue circles*. Several rare variants that are probably not associated with disease have also been identified and they are shown in *gray circles*. Note the relative absence of functionally significant mutations within the C-peptide, consistent with its role in insulin biosynthesis (see text for details and refs. [1, 8] for sources – figure kindly provided by Honggang Ye and Graeme I. Bell)

structure and appearance in electron micrographs [14, 15]. However, this absence of zinc has little, if any, effect on the rate of conversion of proinsulin to insulin, supporting the idea that hexamerization exists mainly as an efficient storage mechanism of insulin as crystalline inclusions. Some impairment in insulin secretion has been noted under conditions that increase insulin demand in ZnT8-deficient mice, suggesting that zinc may assist in granule exocytosis in some way [15]. Clearly, perturbation of the ionic environment of the secretory granule does have important consequences that need to be further explored. It has been claimed that zinc released along with insulin may inhibit glucagon secretion from the alpha-cell [16]. A related question might be whether zinc binding by the C-peptide might also tend to modulate such an action. It also seems probable that the acidic nature of the C-peptide and its possible cation binding properties are related to its binding to vascular or other cell surfaces, as well as its putative interactions to assist in the dispersal of insulin hexamers [17] on the one hand, or with cell surface "receptors" which might mediate either its uptake and/or some of its biological actions in vivo [18].

One puzzling question raised by the studies that demonstrate C-peptide binding and uptake into cells and even nuclei is why this seems to have such a small effect on its clearance from the blood which is unusually slow for a biologically active peptide. In contrast to insulin, which is well known to be rapidly metabolized via receptor-mediated endocytosis, and has a half-life of about 3 min in the circulation, C-peptide disappearance rates are about 1/10 that of insulin – about 30 min. Moreover, much less is known about the pathways involved in degradation and/or excretion of C-peptide, but it does seem possible that some of the recent studies may have given misleading answers. This might be due to the fact that in vivo the C-peptide circulates in blood that contains approximately 50 mg/mL of a multitude of plasma proteins with which it may interact and which could slow or impede its binding, while in isolated tissue studies it is often presented to the tissues in a serum-free medium [19]. Under the latter conditions, one might expect that interactions with cells might occur more readily – in fact, the cells might take up the peptide via pinocytosis and use it as a nutrient. These kinds of problems tend to complicate in vitro studies of peptides as well as other pharmacological agents and are certainly not confined to C-peptide studies. However, they do argue that the potential therapeutic efficacy of any of the putative biological actions of the human C-peptide require validation in vivo via large scale clinical studies and until these are carried out the question as to the biological significance of the C-peptide remains moot.

Progress in understanding the functions of the C-peptide has been accelerating in recent years and many interesting new properties have been revealed [20]. A report recently described the localization in the brain and possible activity of the C-peptide of C-INSL7, a relaxin related insulin-like peptide [21]. It should be pointed out that there is a much greater dearth of definitive information about the possible biological effects of the proregions of many other precursor proteins, such as are also found in pro-opiomelanocortin (POMC), proglucagon, prosomatostatin, and many other neuropeptide precursors. The issue is whether it is likely that many other bioactive peptides may be masquerading as throw-away proregions. I think that here we have to assume that function of some kind is invariably the main driver of evolutionary conservation of the sequences of related proteins. Since proregions of precursor proteins have important biosynthetic functions enabling physiologically important domains to be successfully synthesized, folded, targeted to granules, processed to yield the biologically active peptides, and then stored and secreted, they are also likely to be conserved, but perhaps less stringently. Accordingly, the likelihood that proregions will have equally vital physiological functions in addition to those mentioned above seems also to be less likely. But since they are released along with the active forms this co-secretion link has the potential for coordinating possible biological effects, provided that appropriate cellular receptors have evolved to take advantage of this potential. However, it is also necessary to be able to dispose of and/or recycle both the active and less active or inactive parts of precursor proteins. Could it be that some of the interactions of proregions that one might find simply reflect such metabolic disposal mechanisms that use familiar pathways such as endocytosis coupled with degradative pathways? I believe it is important to maintain an open mind, coupled with a healthy skepticism, that the most exciting and attractive interpretation should always be held in abeyance until all other less exciting possibilities have been eliminated. It may be a slower path to follow but it gives the best results in the long run. Best wishes to all who are searching for useful new roles for the proinsulin C-peptide, as represented by the contributions that follow.

Conflict of Interest

The author declares no conflict of interest.

References

1. Steiner DF, Park SY, Støy J, et al. A brief perspective on insulin production. Diabetes Obes Metab. 2009;11 Suppl 4:189–96.
2. Keenan HA, Sun JK, Levine J, et al. Residual insulin production and pancreatic β-cell turnover after 50 years of diabetes: Joslin Medalist Study. Diabetes. 2010;59:2846–53.
3. Rouillé Y, Duguay SJ, Lund K, et al. Proteolytic processing mechanisms in the biosynthesis of neuroendocrine peptides: the subtilisin-like proprotein convertases. Front Neuroendocrinol. 1995;16:322–61.
4. Zhou A, Webb G, Zhu X, et al. Proteolytic processing in the secretory pathway. J Biol Chem. 1999;274:20745–8.
5. Remacle AG, Shiryaev SA, Oh ES, et al. Substrate cleavage analysis of furin and related proprotein convertases. A comparative study. J Biol Chem. 2008;283: 20897–906.
6. Yang Y, Hua QX, Liu J, et al. Solution structure of proinsulin: connecting domain flexibility and prohormone processing. J Biol Chem. 2010;285:7847–51.

7. Gliemann J, Sorensen HH. Assay of insulin-like activity by the isolated fat cell method. IV. The biological activity of proinsulin. Diabetologia. 1970;6: 499–504.
8. Støy J, Edghill EL, Flanagan SE, et al. Insulin gene mutations as a cause of permanent neonatal diabetes. Proc Natl Acad Sci U S A. 2007;104:15040–4.
9. Hodish I, Liu M, Rajpal G, et al. Misfolded proinsulin affects bystander proinsulin in neonatal diabetes. J Biol Chem. 2010;285:685–94.
10. Rajpal G, Liu M, Zhang Y, et al. Single-chain insulins as receptor agonists. Mol Endocrinol. 2009;23:679–88.
11. Steiner DF. The proinsulin C-peptide A multirole model. Exp Diabesity Res. 2004;5:7–14.
12. Zhu X, Orci L, Carroll R, et al. Severe block in processing of proinsulin to insulin accompanied by elevation of des-64,65 proinsulin intermediates in islets of mice lacking prohormone convertase 1/3. Proc Natl Acad Sci U S A. 2002;99:10299–304.
13. Grant PT, Coombs TL, Frank BH. Differences in the nature of the interaction of insulin and proinsulin with zinc. Biochem J. 1972;126:433–40.
14. Rajpal G, Liu M, Zhang Y, et al. Insulin crystallization depends on zinc transporter ZnT8 expression, but is not required for normal glucose homeostasis in mice. Proc Natl Acad Sci U S A. 2009;106:14872–7.
15. Nicolson TJ, Bellomo EA, Wijesekara N, et al. Insulin storage and glucose homeostasis in mice null for the granule zinc transporter ZnT8 and studies of the type 2 diabetes-associated variants. Diabetes. 2009;58: 2070–83.
16. Robertson RP. The welcome resurgence of the α-cell: a pro glucagon commentary. Diabetes. 2010;59:2735–6.
17. Shafqat J, Melles E, Sigmundsson K, et al. Proinsulin C-peptide elicits disaggregation of insulin resulting in enhanced physiological insulin effects. Cell Mol Life Sci. 2006;63:1805–11.
18. Hills CE, Brunskill NJ. C-peptide and its intracellular signaling. Rev Diabet Stud. 2009;6:138–47.
19. Lindahl E, Nyman U, Zaman F, et al. Proinsulin C-peptide regulates ribosomal RNA expression. J Biol Chem. 2010;285:3462–9.
20. Lind J, Lindahl E, Perálvarez-Marín A, et al. Structural features of proinsulin C-peptide oligomeric and amyloid states. FEBS J. 2010;277:3759–68.
21. Brailoiu E, Dun SL, Gao X, et al. C-peptide of preproinsulin-like peptide 7: localization in the rat brain and activity in vitro. Neuroscience. 2009;159:492–500.

Peptide Interactions of Proinsulin C-Peptide

2

Charlotte Nerelius, Emma Lindahl, Michael Landreh, and Hans Jörnvall

Keywords
Proinsulin C-peptide • Insulin • Surface plasmon resonance • Mass spectrometry • Gel electrophoresis • Oligomerization • Chaperone • Amyloid-like

Introduction

This review summarizes results on peptide interactions of proinsulin C-peptide. As we see it, knowledge on functional interactions of C-peptide has passed through several stages of research, now with at least three modes of postulated molecular explanations for the beneficial effects of C-peptide in diabetes. Here, we first summarize the stages and then concentrate on the subject of C-peptide interaction studies. The latter should not be interpreted to contradict other modes of action, but rather to reflect our present emphasis and interest.

C-peptide functions in insulin synthesis and secretion. The first era of C-peptide research established the existence of C-peptide, its structure, proforms, cosecretion with insulin into blood, and its basic function in insulin synthesis and secretion, all largely started and led by Steiner and coworkers [1, 2]. It now constitutes textbook material in biochemistry, endocrinology, and molecular medicine and is a lifetime achievement of great importance to our understanding of diabetes.

C-peptide in receptor-like cellular binding. The second era, derived from the discovery of the C-peptide cosecretion with insulin into blood, initiated studies to find a hormonal role for C-peptide. Johansson, Wahren, and collaborators showed clinically observable effects of C-peptide [3, 4]. They also initiated molecular studies, including those in our laboratory [5]. This phase led to the discovery of a specific cellular binding of C-peptide, sensitive to pertussis toxin, probably related to a G-protein-coupled receptor [6]. The C-terminal pentapeptide of C-peptide was able to compete with this binding, suggesting that this part of C-peptide constitutes an "active site." The binding constant determined suggested receptor saturation at normal, nanomolar C-peptide concentrations in vivo and a functional loss of this activity in type 1 diabetes. Gradually,

C. Nerelius • E. Lindahl • M. Landreh • H. Jörnvall (✉)
Department of Medical Biochemistry
and Biophysics (MBB), Karolinska Institutet,
SE-171 77, Stockholm, Sweden
e-mail: Hans.Jornvall@ki.se

A.A.F. Sima (ed.), *Diabetes & C-Peptide: Scientific and Clinical Aspects*, Contemporary Diabetes,
DOI 10.1007/978-1-61779-391-2_2, © Springer Science+Business Media, LLC 2012

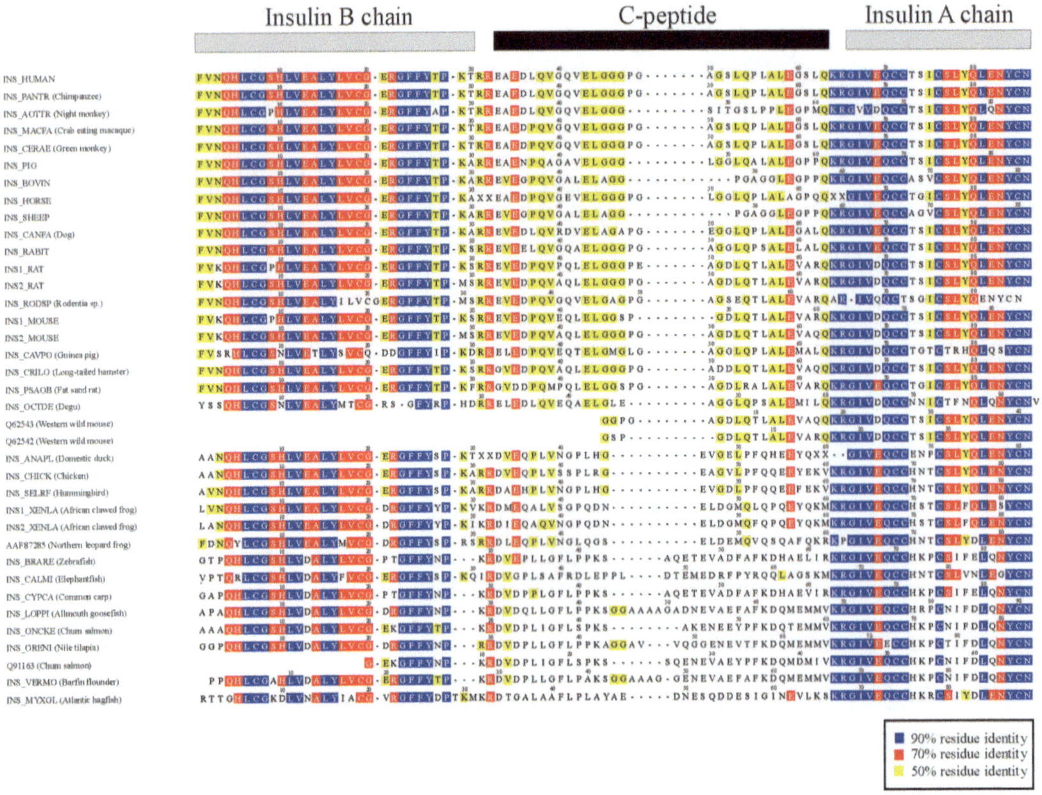

Fig. 2.1 Conservation pattern for the residues of proinsulin in 37 species variants, from the human (*top*) to Atlantic Hagfish (*bottom*). Color code: *Blue*, 90% conservation; *red*, 70%; *yellow*, 50%. As is obvious from the figure, insulin is extremely well-conserved, which is typical for a peptide hormone in defined receptor interactions and functions, while C-peptide has a completely different pattern, not promoting the concept of tight, conserved C-peptide receptor interactions like for insulin. Original figure from ref. [40] now (reproduced with permission)

this led to the concept of type 1 diabetes being a double-hormone deficiency disorder and its late complications as possibly derived from chronic lack of C-peptide [7]. Additional findings from many groups (reviewed in [7]) supported the concept of a receptor-mediated C-peptide signaling pathway, and clinical studies with C-peptide treatment confirmed beneficial influences on deteriorating functions in type 1 diabetes [8, 9]. However, a receptor-mediated role of C-peptide is still unresolved and does not appear to have caught the attention of the insulin-producing pharmaceutical industry. The enigmas include: (1) a receptor has not been found or characterized; (2) the homology pattern of C-peptide is markedly different from that of insulin (Fig. 2.1) and other traditional signaling peptides; (3) the long time to life-threatening late complications in diabetes type 1 is at least not typical of the type of immediate withdrawal effects noticed upon lack of insulin and many other signaling peptides; and (4) a definite disease link between the late complications and C-peptide hormonal effects is yet indirect, at most.

C-peptide cellular internalization. The third era showed C-peptide to be rapidly internalized into several cell types [10], and into the nucleoli, where it binds to histones and promotes histone acetylation and rRNA transcription as an intracrine factor via epigenetic mechanisms [11]. This finding opened a new approach and may blur interpretations previously ascribed to receptor-activated signaling, since intracrine effects could also lead to protein inductions. In fact, recent follow-up studies by mRNA microarrays of early

C-peptide influences on renal tubular cells suggest multiple effects on expression levels [12]. This research is complex and requires further work, although our results on C-peptide internalization have been confirmed by others [13] and noticed in the field of intracrine peptides [14].

In other attempts, we found intra- and extracellular proteins binding to Biacore chip-attached C-peptide, as briefly reported [15], and have used a specific interactive labeling to establish an association of C-peptide with yet another protein, protein tyrosine phosphatase [16], earlier implied in insulin-like signaling effects of C-peptide via scaffolding on insulin signaling ([17], reviewed in [18]). In conclusion, C-peptide can interact with several extra- and intracellular proteins. This is not surprising, considering the extreme negative charge of C-peptide, facilitating interactions with other charged proteins in the complexity of tissues.

C-peptide in oligomeric peptide interactions. The early, chip-based screenings for binding interactions also led to a further mode of possible C-peptide peripheral action, via oligomeric peptide binding and its effects on hetero- and homopeptide interactions of C-peptide [19]. This field is reviewed below. We therefore now appear to have three separate modes and localizations of C-peptide interactions, in addition to its role in insulin synthesis and secretion: surface-mediated receptor binding, intracrine effects, and oligomeric peptide interactions. This multiplicity of measurable effects was unexpected of a peptide that was long regarded as having no bioactivity beyond that in insulin synthesis and secretion.

Peptide Interactions

C-peptide desaggregation of insulin oligomers in a chaperone-like manner. In our early attempts with affinity assays in Biacore experiments, we tested for C-peptide interactions with insulin, but never noticed a strong binding between a chip with one of the peptides and an eluent with the other. However, under some conditions binding appeared to be observable in assays with insulin on the chip and insulin plus C-peptide in the eluent. This was interpreted to mean that insulin oligomers first formed on the chip and then bound C-peptide in an apparently specific manner, since replacement of C-peptide with scrambled C-peptide (i.e., C-peptide with the same composition but random sequence) did not elicit the same binding [19]. It appeared as if the best fit of the binding curves was that of a model where an insulin dimer bound a C-peptide monomer [19]. However, these binding estimates are sensitive to many variables, and their exact stoichiometry should not necessarily be interpreted to be as initially estimated. Nevertheless, the binding analyses indicated that C-peptide/insulin interactions may involve peptide oligomers, at least of insulin, and that specific interactions between C-peptide and insulin may play a role.

This was unexpected and led to further mass spectrometric analyses of solutions with C-peptide, insulin, and insulin/C-peptide mixtures which revealed two findings (Fig. 2.2).

One, mass spectrometry analysis of peptide solutions clearly shows oligomers of both peptides, but with different patterns. The insulin oligomers are easily detectable and are already well-known in the literature [20, 21]. They appeared to reach the hexameric stage, while the C-peptide oligomers were somewhat less abundant and appeared to approach lower stages, like trimers. Initially, we did not fully believe in the C-peptide oligomers and did not emphasize their presence, since C-peptide is highly charged (including six negatively charged residues) and was considered to be self-repulsive.

Two, the oligomers were largely nondetectable in the peptide mixtures, and especially the strong insulin oligomers appeared to vanish upon addition of C-peptide [19, 22]. This suggested that C-peptide disintegrated insulin oligomers, forcing insulin into the monomeric state, thus acting on it in a chaperone-like manner.

These findings initiated further in vivo studies of diabetic patients receiving C-peptide in addition to their regular insulin injections [19]. Simultaneous injection of insulin and C-peptide was then found to lead to a more rapid increase in plasma insulin, suggesting that C-peptide also in vivo has an insulin-desaggregating effect (Fig. 2.3 [19]). Thus, our concept of a chaperoning effect of C-peptide on insulin oligomers appeared to be valid also in vivo. In fact, this

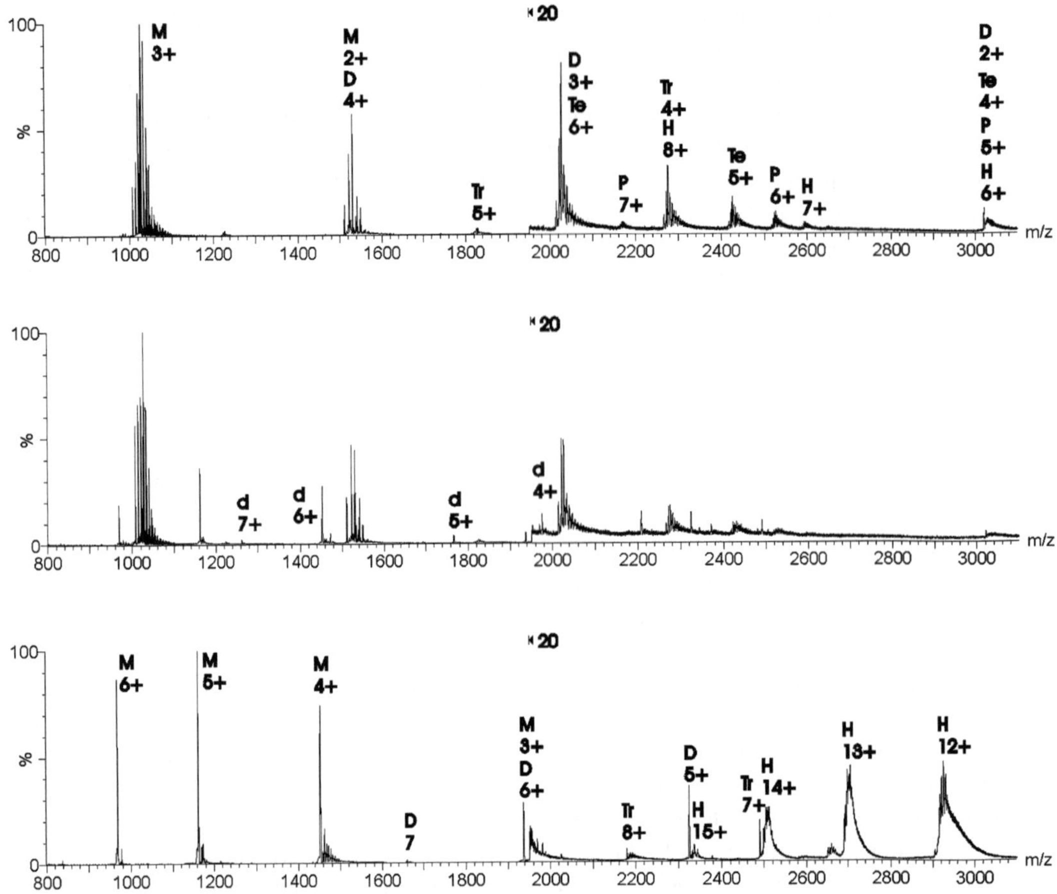

Fig. 2.2 Mass spectra centring on the part showing the maximal oligomers, with only C-peptide (*top*) and only insulin (*bottom*), but desaggregated oligomers in the C-peptide/insulin mixture (*middle*). Original figure from ref. [22] now (reproduced with permission)

direct link between insulin plasma increase and C-peptide injection still appears to be a direct link between a clinically observable effect of C-peptide and the observed molecular interaction.

Oligomer formations of C-peptide itself. The findings regarding insulin-C-peptide interactions led us to further analyses of the possible oligomeric nature of C-peptide itself by additional mass spectrometric and gel electrophoretic studies.

Regarding the mass spectrometric analyses, we confirmed the previously not emphasized observation that C-peptide itself is in equilibrium with a family of homooligomers and is observable by electrospray analysis [22]. It showed that much like C-peptide desaggregates insulin oligomers, insulin has a similar effect on C-peptide oligomers (Fig. 2.2), either through desoligomerization or because C-peptide interaction with insulin is stronger than C-peptide homooligomerization. In any event, both insulin and C-peptide alone exhibit an oligomerization tendency. Similarly, gel electrophoretic analyses also established the ability of C-peptide to form oligomers in many solutions [22, 23]. This was initially observed when we set up Western blots of C-peptide in order to detect the peptide in cellular internalization studies [10]. The combined results from mass spectrometry and gel electrophoresis made us draw several conclusions regarding the interactions of C-peptide and insulin oligomers.

Homooligomers. The two peptides can individually form homooligomers in solution, discernable

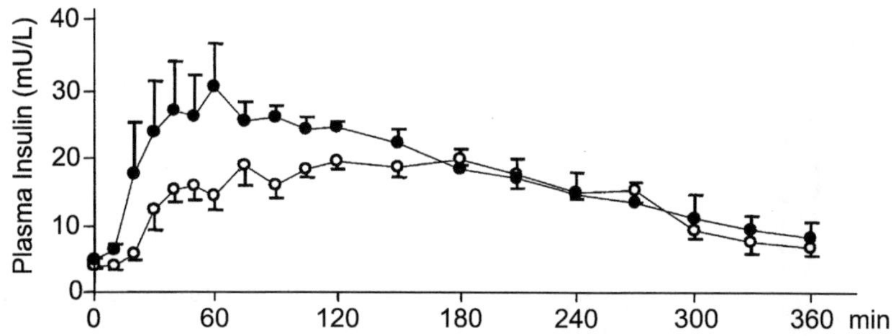

Fig. 2.3 Plasma insulin after injection of insulin (*unfilled circles*) or the same amount insulin with C-peptide also added (*filled circles*). As shown, the latter increases blood glucose to higher levels and thus a more rapid early phase, compatible with C-peptide desaggregation of insulin oligomers in vivo in diabetic patients. Original figure from ref. [19] now (reproduced with permission)

with several methods. Monomers are by far the major components, at least in fresh solutions, and the oligomeric patterns differ, involving several types of multiplicity, but with hexamers being strong oligomers of insulin and trimers of C-peptide. Simple monitoring showed concentration to be important, and less intense mass spectrometric oligomer peaks were observed upon dilution. However, the relative patterns between different oligomeric components appeared unaffected by dilution, with similar peak ratios for 300 and 30 μM C-peptide at weakly acidic conditions [22]. Upon maximal amplification, oligomers could be mass spectrometrically detectable in the sub-μM range. Although pH had an effect (oligomers were not detectable in nanospray analysis of weakly basic solutions), the patterns visible with sufficient amplification in the electrospray analyses appeared to have surprisingly similar peak ratios upon spraying from pH 5 (with weak HCl) and pH 8 (with 10 mM ammonium bicarbonate [22]). Temperature, time, and metal ions all increased the C-peptide oligomerization tendency. We concluded that C-peptide in solution is by far largely monomeric, but can form an equilibrium with oligomers present in low yield.

Heterointeractions. The two peptides can interact. Heterooligomers are mass spectrometrically noticeable in the peptide mixtures, but to a low extent, below that of the homooligomers. The major homooligomers of either peptide literally vanish with the presence of also the other peptide (Fig. 2.2) [19, 22]. Hence, monomerization especially of insulin is promoted in the mixture, which is consistent with the interpretation of the rapid plasma rise upon coinjection in diabetic patients (Fig. 2.3) [19].

Reaction-like transitions. Combined, these two observations suggest a complex pattern for the heterointeractions between the two peptides. Obviously, they must first bind each other in order to interact, causing the surface plasmon resonance binding signals. However, binding is apparently transient, causing an effect (desoligomerization). The apparent reaction resembles chaperone-like actions, where desaggregation results and where interactions involve polymers. Hence, C-peptide appears to have a chaperone-like activity for oligomerized/aggregated insulin.

Aggregation and possible fibrillation of C-peptide. Continuing the interactive studies, an obvious next step was to evaluate to what extent C-peptide might oligomerize further, polymerize, aggregate, and even perhaps fibrillate, having amyloid-like properties.

Already gel electrophoretic analyses revealed the presence of higher aggregates (Fig. 2.4 [22]), and with time, positive staining with thioflavin T [22], which is often considered indicative of fibrillat β-sheet structures. Together with Lind et al. [23], the behavior of C-peptide in the presence of sodium dodecyl sulfate (SDS) as a catalyst for structural transitions was therefore monitored. It then became obvious that C-peptide can form large oligomers and aggregates in

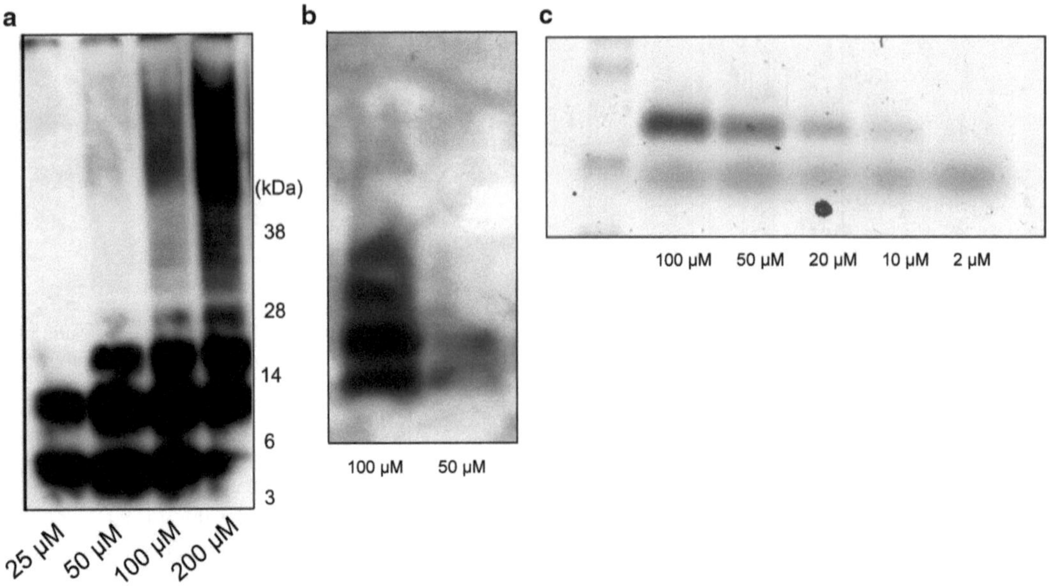

Fig. 2.4 C-peptide oligomer formations as observed in nondenaturing gel electrophoresis and Western blotting (**a**), denaturing gel electrophoresis, blotting, and double antibody detection (**b**) or direct photography of rhodamine-labeled C-peptide (**c**). Original figure from ref. [22] now (reproduced with permission)

complex transitions that can be monitored by NMR spectroscopy and dynamic light scattering. Monomers were initially the major component, but with time and increasing concentrations, C-peptide became stainable with thioflavin T [23] in a manner resembling that observed for amyloidogenic proteins [24].

We therefore concluded that C-peptide is capable of oligomerization in multiple steps under suitable conditions, and that this can be modeled in the presence of SDS. The end result can apparently lead to aggregation and amyloid-like, presumably β-sheet aggregates. Therefore, solutions of C-peptide, like those of insulin, appear to be in equilibrium with a small population of oligomers that potentially can aggregate further. In the early stages of this equilibrium pathway, C-peptide can in addition interact with oligomeric insulin and desaggregate such oligomers. The two peptides therefore have a complicated biophysical behavior, which suggests that both their absolute amounts and ratios may be of importance. Undoubtedly, this whole series of observations opens one further mode of possible pathways in which C-peptide could constitute a bioactive peptide. If the amyloid-like properties turn out to be of importance, links to depository diseases and other conditions may also apply. As initially noted here, we therefore now know of three modes of postsecretion, C-peptide activity, and possible role in diabetes: through receptor-mediated cell surface pathways, intracrine pathways, and peptide interaction pathways. Before trying to evaluate which of these activities may explain the observed beneficial effects of C-peptide replacement in type 1 diabetes, it appears motivated to reflect on the possible relevance of peptide interactions in vivo.

Precaution. We are aware that objections can be raised against attempts at in vivo conclusions regarding consequences of the C-peptide oligomerizations. First, most of the biophysical studies were performed at nonphysiological peptide concentrations and nonphysiological environmental conditions. In vivo, SDS does not occur, circulating C-peptide is present at nM concentrations, and insulin is present at a considerably lower concentration. Before dismissing the peptide results on such objections, however, one should consider also the following facts.

First, SDS is not necessary for the observed effects. The gel patterns (Fig. 2.4) and the mass spectrometry (Fig. 2.2) show oligomerizations also in nonextreme, aqueous solutions and surface plasmon resonance studies suggest binding of peptide oligomers in ordinary solvents. SDS in the biophysical study [23] was used as a catalyst to promote transitions, much like trifluoroethanol is frequently used in NMR spectroscopy studies to promote detection of helix tendencies.

Second, the very nature of the structural transitions to β-sheet fibril conformation, as in the already known amyloidogenic diseases, is profound and involves large rearrangements of the proteins involved. Hence, rough tools for study of these phenomena need not be irrelevant.

Third, regarding peptide concentrations, maximal amplification in the mass spectrometric studies detected oligomers down to sub-μM C-peptide levels [22]. In the prediabetic type 2 diabetes stage, there is hyperpeptidism, as well as locally at injection sites in type 1 diabetics where deposits have been found [25], making the span between the in vivo and experimental conditions about two orders of magnitude for C-peptide, a range that is often considered sufficient for chemical cross-interpretations. Initial transitions are in apparent equilibrium, which makes rapid shifts towards further transitions possible, should the conditions change.

In conclusion, the objections suggested above constitute only relative concerns, making further proof for a link between in vitro observed oligomerizations and in vivo diabetic disease desirable. Hence, these objections are not excluding a relevance of peptide interactions in vivo, especially not under special conditions such as hyperpeptidism or peptide ratio imbalances.

A second precaution concerns the fact that biophysical phenomena are complex and difficult to study; mass spectrometry involves transitions to gas-phase measurements and surface plasmon resonance surface attachments and model curve fittings. Additional studies are therefore desirable. However, the present agreements between interpretations from mass spectra, surface plasmon resonance, and gel electrophoresis appear relevant and are known to be so in many other systems.

A third precaution concerns the link between C-peptide molecular effects and observed beneficial clinical effects. Before dismissal of peptide interactions on that issue, one should consider also the following two facts.

There is, as mentioned above, a direct experimental result that indicates a link between peptide interactions and clinical effects. Thus, in vivo coinjection of insulin and C-peptide appears to enhance the plasma insulin level obtained [19]. It is hard to visualize any other mechanism to explain that observable curve (Fig. 2.3) than direct peptide interaction. We initially probably underestimated the strength of this fact and should have emphasized it further.

The only concern with the depository model that is difficult to answer at present is which deposit and where that may be critical for diabetes. Reports exist of deposits of several peptides (including of insulin [26] and C-peptide [27]), but they still appear few and difficult to consistently interpret regarding size and organ. Perhaps, though, microdeposits or deposits in special organs, like the pancreas, anyway loaded with insulin, C-peptide, and other peptides, may have escaped detection or proper attention.

In conclusion, considering the clinical beneficial effects of C-peptide, which to us seems reasonable, based on the amelioration of kidney and nerve dysfunctions, organs commonly affected in diabetes, all three hypotheses on how the molecular mechanisms may work appear feasible. None can be excluded, but the peptide interactions as explanation appear equally valid or even more so than the other alternatives at the present stage.

Perspectives and Future Work

With the precautions and reservations thus considered, which are the most attractive consequences of homo- and heteropeptide interactions as a molecular explanation for the clinical effects of C-peptide?

- First, of the several attractive consequences, two enigmas of C-peptide actions (the lack of strict sequence conservation and the slow onset of type 1 complications), which constitute problems with the receptor-mediated explanation, are no problems with the peptide interactive model. A slow onset of the chronic complications could be consistent with the depository model, thus suggesting that amyloid-like properties of insulin would be a factor in the late complications of type 1 diabetes. Notably, the only drug all type 1 diabetics have got for decades is insulin, so if the insulin desaggregation power of C-peptide is of relevance, the implication is that insulin is its target in the beneficial effect on the late complications. Similarly, the lack of C-peptide sequence conservation would be less important in the peptide interactive model, since charge (which is conserved in C-peptide) rather than sequence is important in oligomerization [23]. Indeed, relationships have been demonstrated also between diabetes and Alzheimer's disease [28–30].

- Second, the peptide interaction model would also be consistent with the onset of type 2 diabetes, in which increased levels of insulin and/or C-peptide rather than hyperglycemia have been claimed as disease-promoting factors [31, 32]. Hence, not only would type 1 late complications, but also those of type 2 diabetes onset be consistent with the peptide interactive model. The implication is then that in type 2 diabetes, it is the absolute amount of peptides rather than their ratio (as in type 1 diabetes) that is wrong and that the depository tendency would derive from either of insulin, C-peptide, or other peptides, alone or in mixtures.
- Third, also metabolically, a depository tendency of C-peptide and insulin could fit known facts. Thus, peptide deposits in general may derive not only from increased synthesis, but also from decreased breakdown. In this regard, it is of interest that insulin and C-peptide appear to depend on similar enzyme activities for degradation [33]. This enzyme activity, in the case of insulin-degrading enzyme, is sensitive to inhibition by alkylation of a critical Cys residue through lipid peroxidation products [34], hence compatible with the fact that increased abdominal fat is a risk factor for type 2 diabetes [35].
- Finally, there is a tantalizing theoretical parallel in the model of C-peptide as a chaperone for reversal of insulin depository tendencies, in the fact that several depository diseases recently have been ascribed to peptide deposits derived from proforms biosynthetically equipped with an autospecific chaperone (a BRICHOS domain protein [36]). Lung surfactant peptide C is such a depository peptide derived from a proform (prosurfactant protein C) equipped with a C-terminal autospecific chaperone [37, 38]. Hence, nature has apparently not evolutionarily eliminated these structures although potentially dangerous, but may equip their proforms with a "rucksack" of a specific chaperone reducing the depository tendency. Perhaps, proinsulin is another such type of proform, with an inbuilt C-peptide "rucksack" for the active hormone function of insulin. Hence, both types of diabetes may reflect imbalances, where the insulin/C-peptide pair illustrates general principles for regulatory peptides in nature.

The question then arises, how do we proceed to expand our knowledge as to how C-peptide ameliorates diabetic renal and neural disorders? Of course, one mode of approach is to continue investigations of all three molecular explanations, including a search for specific deposits in the endocrine pancreas, nerves, and kidneys, which are the organs ultimately affected. However, such broad approaches may be difficult, and our latest results appear to offer a further opening.

Thus, using C-peptide fragments we recently found additional evidence for particular fragments of C-peptide having separate activities in relation to the three molecular explanation modes. The N-terminal fragment (residues 1–11) appears to be ascribable to an insulin interaction of C-peptide and is not identical to the site for the homo-C-peptide oligomerization [39]. Previously, we have found the C-terminal pentapeptide of C-peptide to be associated with the receptor-mediated actions [5, 6], and the whole C-peptide to be tripartite (Fig. 2.5 [40]). Hence, further work with definitions of the C-peptide fragment activities may define shorter segments with just one activity rather than the intact C-peptide with all three

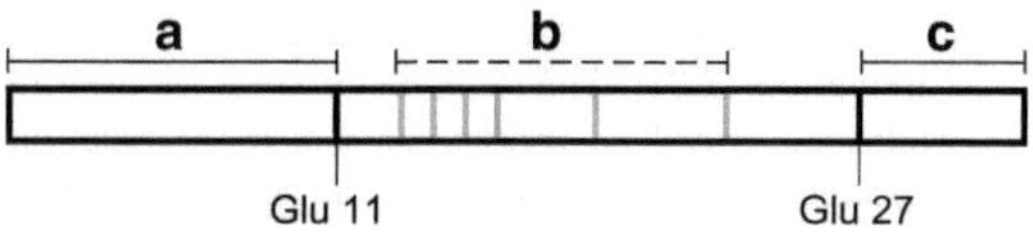

Fig. 2.5 Schematic representation of C-peptide into a tripartite correlation with different properties. (**a**) the N-terminal segment with Glu11 (*black vertical line*) apparently important in insulin binding [39]; (**c**) the C-terminal part with Glu27 (*black vertical line*) ascribed importance in the receptor-mediated capacity [5, 6], and (**b**) the intervening part with many Gly and Pro (*gray vertical lines*) and resulting separate structural properties, possibly a part of the homo-oligomerizations [39]

activities. If so, C-peptide fragments or analogs with just one of the three alternative effects may allow for treatment with only the beneficial part, eliminating even the possibility of a risk of depository tendencies derived from other segments.

In summary, recent results have given further complexity and unexpected multiplicity in functional interpretations of C-peptide molecular interactions, but also offer an approach to continue with fragment research that may finally give a both efficient (chaperone-like) and in all circumstances safe (nondepository) C-peptide derivative.

Acknowledgments We thank John Wahren, Jan Johansson, Jawed Shafqat, Lena Mäler, Michael Henriksson, Ermias Melles, Juan Astorga-Wells, Gunvor Alvelius, and coworkers in several other laboratories for valuable collaborative efforts. Grant support from the Swedish Research Council (03X-3532) and the Knut and Alice Wallenberg Foundation is gratefully acknowledged.

References

1. Steiner DF, Oyer PE. The biosynthesis of insulin and a probable precursor of insulin by a human islet cell adenoma. Proc Natl Acad Sci U S A. 1967;57:473–80.
2. Steiner DF, Cunningham D, Spigelman L, et al. Insulin biosynthesis: evidence for a precursor. Science. 1967;157:697–700.
3. Johansson BL, Sjöberg S, Wahren J. The influence of human C-peptide on renal function and glucose utilization in type1 (insulin-dependent) diabetic patients. Diabetologia. 1992;35:121–8.
4. Johansson BL, Linde B, Wahren J. Effects of C-peptide on blood flow, capillary diffusion capacity and glucose utilization in the exercising forearm of type1 (insulin-dependent) diabetic patients. Diabetologia. 1992;35:1151–8.
5. Ohtomo Y, Bergman T, Johansson B-L, et al. Differential effects of proinsulin C-peptide on Na+, K+-ATPase activity of renal tubule segments. Diabetologia. 1998;41:287–91.
6. Rigler R, Pramanik A, Jonasson P, et al. Specific binding of proinsulin C-peptide to human cell membranes. Proc Natl Acad Sci U S A. 1999;96:13318–23.
7. Wahren J, Ekberg K, Jörnvall H. C-peptide is a bioactive peptide. Diabetologia. 2007;50:503–9.
8. Ekberg K, Brismar T, Johansson B-L, et al. C-peptide replacement therapy and sensory nerve function in type 1 diabetes neuropathy. Diabetes Care. 2007;30:71–6.
9. Ekberg K, Johansson B-L. Effect of C-peptide in diabetic neuropathy in patients with type 1 diabetes. Exp Diabetes Res. 2008;2008:457912.
10. Lindahl E, Nyman U, Melles E, et al. Cellular internalization of proinsulin C-peptide. Cell Mol Life Sci. 2007;64:479–86.
11. Lindahl E, Nyman U, Zaman F, et al. Proinsulin C-peptide regulates ribosomal RNA expression. J Biol Chem. 2010;285:3462–9.
12. Lindahl E, Nordquist L, Müller P, et al. Early transcriptional regulation by C-peptide in freshly isolated rat proximal tubular cells. Diabetes Metab Res Rev. 2011, epub doi:10.1002/dmrr.1220.
13. Luppi P, Geng X, Cifarelli V, et al. C-peptide is internalised in human endothelial and vascular smooth muscle cells via endosomes. Diabetologia. 2009;52:2218–28.
14. Re RN, Cook JL. Mechanisms of disease: intracrine physiology in the cardiovascular system. Nat Clin Pract Cardiovasc Med. 2007;4:549–57.
15. Shafqat J, Melles E, Wiberg D, et al. Proinsulin C-peptide elicits disaggregation of insulin resulting in enhanced physiological insulin effects. In: Melles E. C-peptide structural and functional relationships studied by biosensor technology and mass spectrometry. Thesis, Karolinska Institutet, Stockholm, Sweden; 2005.
16. Jägerbrink T, Lindahl E, Shafqat J, et al. Proinsulin C-peptide interaction with protein tyrosine phosphatase 1B demonstrated with a labeling reaction. Biochem Biophys Res Commun. 2009;387:31–5.
17. Li Z-G, Qiang X, Sima AAF, et al. C-peptide attenuates protein tyrosine phosphatase activity and enhances glycogen synthesis in L6 myoblasts. Biochem Biophys Res Commun. 2001;280:615–9.
18. Sima AAF. Diabetic encephalopathies – the emerging complications. Acta Diabetol. 2010;47:279–93.
19. Shafqat J, Melles E, Sigmundsson K, et al. Proinsulin C-peptide elicits disaggregation of insulin resulting in enhanced physiological insulin effects. Cell Mol Life Sci. 2006;63:1805–11.
20. Brange J, Andersen L, Laursen ED, et al. Towards understanding insulin fibrillation. J Pharm Sci. 1997;86:517–25.
21. Nettleton EJ, Tito P, Sunde M, et al. Characterization of the oligomeric states of insulin in self-assembly and amyloid fibril formation by mass spectrometry. Biophys J. 2000;79:1053–65.

22. Jörnvall H, Lindahl E, Astorga-Wells J, et al. Oligomerization and insulin interactions of proinsulin C-peptide: threefold relationships to properties of insulin. Biochem Biophys Res Commun. 2010;391: 1561–6.
23. Lind J, Lindahl E, Perálvarez-Marín A, et al. Structural features of proinsulin C-peptide oligomeric and amyloid states. FEBS J. 2010;277:3759–68.
24. Khurana R, Coleman C, Ionescu-Zanetti C, et al. Mechanism of thioflavin T binding to amyloid fibrils. J Struct Biol. 2005;151:229–38.
25. Dische FE, Wernstedt C, Westermark GT, et al. Insulin as an amyloid-fibril protein at sites of repeated insulin injections in a diabetic patient. Diabetologia. 1988;31:158–61.
26. Furuta T, Seino J, Saito T, et al. Insulin deposits in membranous nephropathy associated with diabetes mellitus. Clin Nephrol. 1992;37:65–9.
27. Marx N, Walcher D, Raichle C. C-peptide colocalizes with macrophages in early arteriosclerotic lesions of diabetic subjects and induces monocyte chemotaxis in vitro. Arterioscler Thromb Vasc Biol. 2004;24:540–5.
28. Janson J, Laedtke T, Parisi JE, et al. Increased risk of type 2 diabetes in Alzheimer disease. Diabetes. 2004;53:474–81.
29. Li Z-G, Zhang W, Sima AAF. Alzheimer-like changes in rat models of spontaneous diabetes. Diabetes. 2007;56:1817–24.
30. Sima AAF, Li Z-G. Diabetes and Alzheimer's disease – is there a connection? Rev Diabet Stud. 2007;4:161–8.
31. Rosselin G, Rathery M, Assan R, et al. Hyperinsulinism in moderate diabetes and prediabetes. Rein Foie. 1966;9:47–62.
32. Park SH, Marso SP, Zhou Z, et al. Neointimal hyperplasia after arterial injury is increased in a rat model of non-insulin-dependent diabetes mellitus. Circulation. 2001;104:815–9.
33. Melles E, Jörnvall H, Tryggvason S, et al. Degradation of proinsulin C-peptide in kidney and placenta extracts by a specific endoprotease activity. Cell Mol Life Sci. 2004;61:2979–82.
34. Neant-Fery M, Garcia-Ordonez RD, Logan TP, et al. Molecular basis for the thiol sensitivity of insulin-degrading enzyme. Proc Natl Acad Sci U S A. 2008;105:9582–7.
35. Carey DG, Jenkins AB, Campbell LV, et al. Abdominal fat and insulin resistance in normal and overweight women: direct measurements reveal a strong relationship in subjects at both low and high risk of NIDDM. Diabetes. 1996;45:633–8.
36. Sánchez-Pulido L, Devos D, Valencia A. BRICHOS: a conserved domain in proteins associated with dementia, respiratory distress and cancer. Trends Biochem Sci. 2002;27:329–32.
37. Nerelius C, Gustafsson M, Nordling K, et al. Anti-amyloid activity of the C-terminal domain of proSP-C against amyloid β-peptide and medin. Biochemistry. 2009;48:3778–86.
38. Fitzen M, Alvelius G, Nordling K, et al. Peptide binding specificity of the prosurfactant protein C Brichos domain analyzed by electrospray mass spectrometry. Rapid Commun Mass Spectrom. 2009;23: 3591–8.
39. Nerelius C, Alvelius G, Jörnvall H. N-terminal segment of proinsulin C-peptide active in insulin interaction/desaggregation. Biochem Biophys Res Commun. 2010;403:462–7.
40. Henriksson M, Nordling E, Melles E, et al. Separate functional features of proinsulin C-peptide. Cell Mol Life Sci. 2005;62:1772–8.

The Effect of Combined C-Peptide and Zinc on Cellular Function

3

Dana M. Spence

Keywords
C-peptide • Zinc • Red cells • ATP • Metals

Introduction to the RBC and Its Role as a Determinant of Blood Flow

The average adult human has approximately 5 L of blood, of which, nearly 40–45% is comprised of the red blood cell (RBC). The physiological significance of the RBC, its ability to carry and deliver oxygen to organs and tissues that may be hypoxic, is without question. Indeed, the idea of the RBC playing a role in such an important and complex mechanism may seem difficult to understand given that this cell has no nucleus or mitochondria. In fact, to some, this 7 or 8 μm-sized cell, whose life span in a healthy human is about 110–120 days, is nothing more than a simple cell with minimal machinery whose function is solely that of oxygen delivery. However, since the early 1990s, there has been a significant increase in the number of reports providing strong evidence that the RBC, in addition to its role as a deliverer of oxygen, is also a participant in overall blood flow itself [1, 2]. Currently, there are two main mechanisms describing the RBC as a possible determinant in blood flow, specifically, its ability to release nitric oxide (NO) directly into the bloodstream resulting in subsequent relaxation of the smooth muscle cells and vessel dilation [3, 4] and its ability to release ATP [5, 6]. Both of these mechanisms are important in relation to C-peptide, as this 31 amino acid molecule is reported to stimulate the production of NO in the endothelium [7] and ATP release from the RBC [8, 9]. Accordingly, further information pertinent to both of these possible mechanisms is provided, followed by the significant effects that C-peptide may play in both mechanisms.

D.M. Spence (✉)
Department of Chemistry, Michigan State University, East Lansing, MI 48824, USA
e-mail: dspence@chemistry.msu.edu

The Importance of C-Peptide in the Cellular Production and Release of Molecules Affecting the Vasculature

C-peptide stimulates many cellular reactions and biochemical pathways [10–14] and in doing so, is able to stimulate the production and release of certain molecules [7–9]. In order to have a clear understanding of the overwhelming potential of C-peptide replacement therapy, it is first necessary to understand how important these secreted molecules, namely RBC-derived ATP and endothelium-derived NO, are in the vasculature.

A.A.F. Sima (ed.), *Diabetes & C-Peptide: Scientific and Clinical Aspects*, Contemporary Diabetes, DOI 10.1007/978-1-61779-391-2_3, © Springer Science+Business Media, LLC 2012

It is well established that the endothelium-derived relaxing factor, NO, is produced by endothelial cells and, when released, is capable of relaxing vascular smooth muscle [15–17]. Physiologically, an alteration in shear stress to which the endothelial lining of blood vessels is subjected has been suggested to be a major stimulus for NO release [18, 19]. A reappraisal of this viewpoint was required, however, when it was reported that, in the rabbit pulmonary circulation, in the absence of RBCs, alterations in shear stress *alone* did not evoke release of NO in the pulmonary circulation [20]. In contrast, in lungs perfused with rabbit blood, NO was a determinant of vascular resistance. Importantly, the component of blood responsible for the stimulation of endogenous NO synthesis was determined to be the RBC [21]. Importantly, in the absence of RBCs, the addition of dextran to the perfusate of isolated lungs to increase viscosity and perfusion pressure to that of blood-perfused lungs did not stimulate NO synthesis. Taken collectively, these studies demonstrate that a property of the RBC not related to effects on viscosity or pressure contributes to endogenous NO synthesis.

There is debate in the current literature over the mechanism of vasodilation under hypoxic conditions. Each mechanism concludes with NO reaching the smooth muscle of the vessel, but they disagree in the source of the NO and the role of the RBC. One proposed mechanism states that NO_2^- present in the bloodstream is reduced under hypoxic conditions by hemoglobin to NO, which then participates in vasodilation [4]. Supporting information for this hypothesis includes physiological nitrite concentrations from 500 to 100 nM in plasma and as high as 10 μM in tissues [22]. While this hypothesis benefits from the bioavailability of nitrite in the bloodstream in a stable form, there is some debate over how quickly hemoglobin can act as a nitrite reductase, and how much NO_2^- it can convert.

A second proposed mechanism states that NO is transported as S-nitrosothiols, the two most common being nitrosylated glutathione and nitrosylation of the highly-conserved cysteine 63 on hemoglobin [3]. This mechanism allows for the bioactive NO to be protected from the short half-life of NO [23], and the mechanism was developed utilizing bioassays involving extracted vessels [24]. These studies suggest that the endothelium is not a major factor in vasodilation because when the endothelium layer is removed from the vessel, vasodilation still occurs; this suggests that RBC derived NO is the source of the vasodilation.

Each of these discussed mechanisms require the unstable NO molecule to originate in the RBC and then diffuse through the endothelial layer where it can interact with the smooth muscle to participate in vasodilation. A third mechanism, which does not require this diffusional path of an unstable molecule, proposed by Sprague et al. [21], Ellsworth et al. [2] and others [25] is that vasodilation is ATP-mediated, requiring endothelial nitric oxide synthase (eNOS) to produce NO in the endothelium; an overview of this mechanism is shown in Fig. 3.1.

Indeed, the application of ATP to endothelial cells results in increases in NO synthesis [26, 27]. ATP is of particular interest because it is present in millimolar amounts in RBCs [20, 21, 28, 29]. Multiple receptors for ATP have been identified and partially characterized [30–34]. In the vasculature, the P_{2x} purinergic receptor is present primarily on vascular smooth muscle cells and its activation results in contraction of that cell [32, 35, 36]. In contrast, the P_{2y} receptor is found primarily on the endothelium [30, 31, 33, 35]. The binding of ATP to the endothelial P_{2y} receptor results in the synthesis of NO [26, 28] and/or vasodilator arachidonic acid metabolites [37, 38]. Thus, ATP applied directly to the vascular smooth muscle of an intact vessel, e.g., that are released from nerve terminals, would be expected to produce vasoconstriction via activation of P_{2x} receptors. In contrast, ATP applied to the luminal side of a vessel, e.g., that released within the circulation from RBCs, would be expected to produce endothelium-dependent vasodilation through interaction with the P_{2y} receptor present on the endothelial cell and the subsequent release of NO [31, 36].

If ATP is an important regulator of pulmonary NO synthesis and, thereby, vascular resistance in vivo, a hemodynamic response to ATP should be demonstrable in the intact circulation. Hassessian

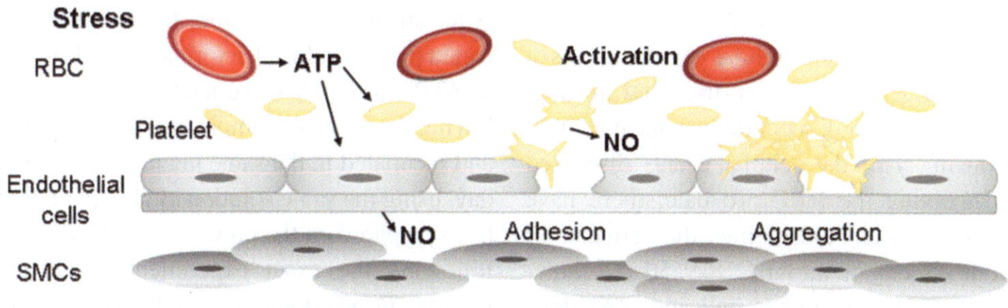

Fig. 3.1 Proposed mechanism for ATP effects in the bloodstream. Various stimuli, such as hypoxia or flow-induced shear, result in the release of ATP from RBCs, which may participate in vessel dilation by stimulating NO production in the endothelium through purinergic receptor signaling. Furthermore, this ATP may stimulate NO production in platelets, inhibiting their ability to readily activate under normal conditions

and Burnstock [38] reported that, in isolated physiological salt solution (PSS)-perfused rat lungs, the addition of ATP to the perfusate resulted in a decrease in perfusion pressure. In addition, McCullough et al. [39] reported that the application of ATP into the lumen of microvessels of striated muscle (hamster cheek pouch retractor muscle) resulted in vasodilation. In both circulations, the effect of ATP was prevented by an inhibitor of endogenous NO synthesis [38, 39]. These results suggest that intraluminal ATP produces vasodilation via stimulation of endothelial P_{2y} receptors resulting in NO synthesis [38]. Although these studies demonstrate that ATP administered into the lumen of the pulmonary blood vessels results in vasodilation and that NO may mediate this response, an endogenous source of ATP was not defined. Sprague et al. postulated that ATP was released from the RBC in response to mechanical deformation, as would occur in association with vasoconstriction or increased velocity of blood flow. This RBC-derived ATP can then act on the endothelial cell to stimulate endogenous NO synthesis and enable the RBC to participate in local regulation of vascular caliber [20, 21, 40, 41].

In support of this hypothesis, it was reported that ATP is released from RBCs in response to decreases in oxygen tension [2, 28, 39, 40], acidosis [28] and, mechanical deformation [41, 42]. The release of ATP from RBCs in response to mechanical deformation was determined by measuring ATP in the effluent of filters with pores of known diameter through which RBCs were passed (filtration). Thus, it was reported that passage of RBCs of rabbits and healthy humans through filters with average pore sizes of 12, 8 or 5 μm resulted in ATP release [41, 43, 44]. Indeed, amounts of ATP release increased *pari passu* with decreases in average pore size. These species were chosen because in both rabbits and humans, NO is a determinant of pulmonary vascular resistance. In contrast, in the dog, NO does not subserve this role in the pulmonary circulation [1, 45, 46]. Dog RBCs passed through identical filters did not release ATP [21]. To demonstrate that the ability to release ATP in response to mechanical deformation was associated with the stimulation of endogenous NO synthesis in the pulmonary circulation, experiments were performed in which RBCs of either rabbits, healthy humans or dogs were added to the perfusate (PSS) of isolated rabbit lungs to achieve a minimum hematocrit of 20%. These studies demonstrated that NO is a determinant of endogenous NO synthesis solely in the presence of RBCs that release ATP in response to mechanical deformation (rabbits and humans) [21].

There have now been a number of studies reporting the release of RBC-derived ATP using in vitro systems that employed resistance-vessel sized capillary tubing [47, 48] and microfluidic devices [25, 49] whose channels approximate larger arterioles, in vivo. These same in vitro, flow-based systems have demonstrated that the RBC-derived ATP has a direct effect on the ability of endothelial cells to produce NO [6, 25]. In summary, it is now clear that the RBC has the ability to release ATP when subjected to various stimuli and, importantly, this ATP is able to participate in downstream cellular signaling. As a modulator of ATP release, as discussed in more detail in this chapter, C-peptide may have a direct effect on many of the cellular events discussed above involving the RBC. To date, there have been few groups examining the effects of C-peptide directly on the RBC [8, 9, 50–52]; however, to date, our group has only measured biological activity when the RBCs are subjected to C-peptide that is bound to certain metals [8, 9].

The Discovery of Metal Binding to C-Peptide

In 2006, within about 5 months of each other, two manuscripts were published describing the reduced release of ATP from RBCs obtained from people with type 2 diabetes [47, 53]. In continuance with these studies, an examination of the ATP release from the RBCs obtained from subjects with type 1 diabetes was planned. Importantly, it was also during this time that we first learned about the many exciting results from numerous research groups involving C-peptide replacement therapy to humans and animal models of type 1 diabetes. Of particular interest was the work describing the improvements in RBC deformability when these cells were incubated with C-peptide [52]. As mentioned earlier in this chapter, ATP release from the RBC increases with enhanced deformability of the cell. This report on improvements in RBC deformability in the presence of C-peptide, coupled with other reports involving improvements in blood flow with C-peptide replacement therapy [50, 51, 54], was motivation for a study involving the ability of C-peptide to stimulate an increase in the release of ATP from RBCs incubated with C-peptide.

Our first attempts to quantitatively determine an increase in the release of ATP from RBCs incubated with C-peptide were partially successful. That is, a sample of a commercially available, synthetic form of human C-peptide was initially dissolved in deionized water. An aliquot of this C-peptide was then moved to a physiological saline solution, followed by the addition of RBCs. After an incubation period, the RBCs were subjected to flow-induced deformation and an increase in ATP was easily discernable. However, the following day, another sample of RBCs was obtained and incubated in the same manner as the previous day, using the same solution of C-peptide that had been prepared on the previous day. Unfortunately, following the exact experimental protocol, no increase in ATP release from the RBCs incubated with the C-peptide was measured. Another sample of the C-peptide was prepared from powder (as on day 1 where the increase in ATP release was measured) and incubated with fresh RBCs and, once again, an increase in ATP release was found. At this point, it was speculated that either the C-peptide was being cleaved in solution after a period of time had elapsed or, there was some type of covalent modification to C-peptide (e.g., phosphorylation, methylation, glycation or glycosylation) that was contributing to its inactivity.

A mass spectrometric analysis was performed and it was determined that, upon dissolution, the C-peptide was modified with a substance; however, it was not a covalent modification. Rather, it was determined that there was a metal bound to C-peptide that was subsequently disassociated upon dissolution in aqueous environments. This metal, which was suspected to have been introduced during the purification of the synthetically-prepared C-peptide, was initially determined to be either Fe^{2+} or Cr^{3+}. In the subsequent weeks, high-resolution mass spectrometric analysis proved that the metal bound to the C-peptide was Fe^{2+}. However, prior to these results, our group, based on a wealth of literature involving Cr^{3+} and glucose control [55–58], initially decided to try Cr^{3+} additions to C-peptide.

To begin, older samples of C-peptide that we had deemed "nonactive" based on experiments performed in the laboratory and stored for future investigations, were re-evaluated for activity upon small additions of a Cr^{3+} salt. When added in equimolar amounts, the Cr^{3+} addition to our "inactive" C-peptide restored activities to levels near that seen upon initial dissolution. Subsequently, the first manuscript reporting the necessity of metal binding to C-peptide for certain biological effects on the RBC utilized both Cr^{3+} and Fe^{2+} [8].

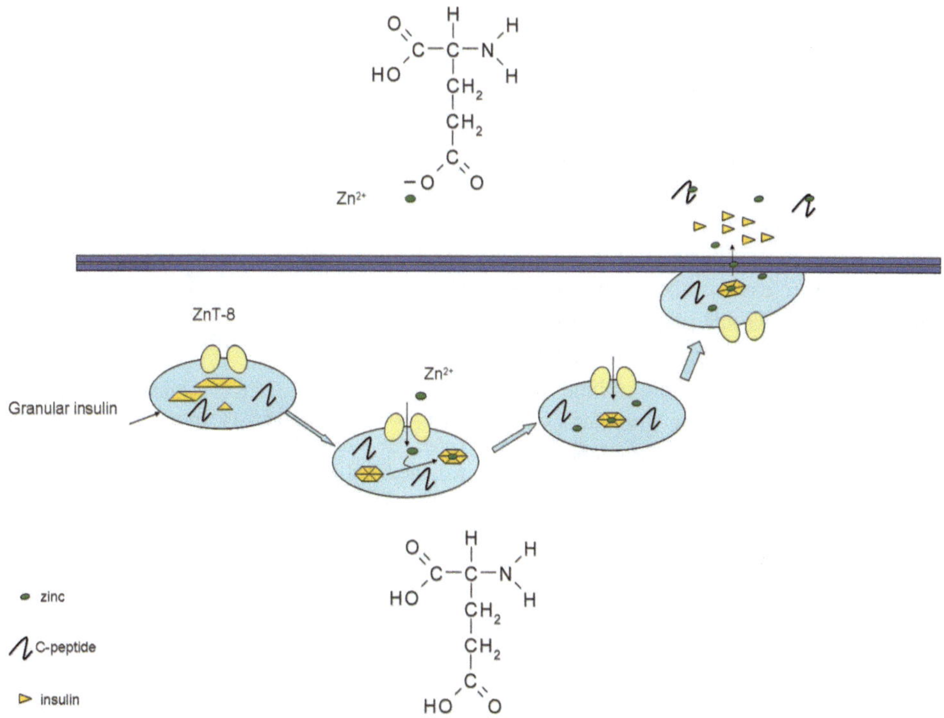

Fig. 3.2 A possible mechanism for the origin of C-peptide interacting with Zn^{2+} upon secretion from the pancreatic beta cell granules. In the granules (depicted as *light blue circles*), Zn^{2+} transporter proteins (ZnT8) shuttle Zn^{2+} into the granules where it participates in the packaging of insulin as a crystalline hexamer. Also depicted in the granules is C-peptide; the pH inside the granules is estimated to be ca. 5. Upon secretion from the granules into the islets, the pH raises rapidly, resulting in the breakdown of the insulin hexamer into individual monomer units. The role of C-peptide in this breakdown remains incomplete, although studies have shown that C-peptide does participate in the breakdown process. One possible mechanism is that the low pH of the granules keeps glutamic acid residues (structure shown *below* in the beta cell) protonated until secretion where it changes to glutamate (structure shown *above* beta cell), a substance capable of binding Zn^{2+}

The use of these aforementioned metals was placed under scrutiny when one considers possible mechanisms for the metal-C-peptide interaction under in vivo conditions. Specifically, it is known that the physiological level of C-peptide (in nondiabetic subjects) is typically in the single-digit nanomolar range. When one considers that the concentration of other metals in the bloodstream (e.g., Na^{+}, K^{+}, etc.) are in the millimolar range, it becomes highly unlikely that Fe^{2+} or Cr^{3+}, two species that have bioavailable concentrations well below that of even C-peptide, would ever be able to compete for binding sites on C-peptide. However, there is one metal that has both the requisite concentration and physiological location to actively compete for binding sites on C-peptide: and that is zinc.

While zinc exists in vivo, the concentration of free, bioavailable zinc in the bloodstream is also sub-nanomolar. Moreover, as mentioned above, the concentrations of other metals are so much more concentrated than zinc that the addition of C-peptide to the bloodstream directly would have minimal opportunities to interact with a metal such as zinc; it would simply be outcompeted by the other metals in the bloodstream. Of course, this idea of "metal competition" during C-peptide replacement therapy then begs the question of how C-peptide becomes activated at all in vivo.

An examination of the unique features of the beta cells suggests that the concept of zinc activation of C-peptide is plausible at the molecular level. Consider the following scenario, shown in Fig. 3.2; in the pancreatic beta cell granules, insulin is in a crystalline hexameric form comprised of six insulin molecules and two zinc atoms. Also present in these granules is C-peptide, which contains four glutamic acid residues and one aspartic acid residue. The C-peptide and the hexameric insulin coexist waiting for secretion from the slightly acidic environment [59] of the beta cell granules into the islets. Upon secretion, the hexameric insulin and C-peptide are now released into an environment where the pH is ~7.4. At this pH, the C-peptide's glutamic and aspartic acid residues would be negatively charged and readily available to bind to the zinc atoms that were also in the granules as free zinc, or those that were released upon dehexamerization of insulin. Thus, the hexamer disaggregates, resulting in monomeric insulin and C-peptide capable of binding to zinc atoms.

In previous work, Kennedy et al. [60] show that a pH change (towards physiological pH) is a requirement for proper disaggregation of the insulin hexamer. In separate studies, Shafqat et al. [61] show that C-peptide has the ability to enhance the disaggregation of hexameric insulin into monomeric form. In the work by Shafqat et al. [61], in vitro studies reveal an approximate 10–20% increase in monomeric insulin in the presence of C-peptide at pH 5; moreover, when insulin and C-peptide are added subcutaneously at the same depot to humans with type 1 diabetes, the increase in plasma insulin is approximately doubled between 10 and 60 min after injection in comparison to when the C-peptide and insulin were administered at different ports. Therefore, the studies by Kennedy and Shafqat suggest that, while there may be a reliance on pH for the breakdown of hexameric insulin, there also appears to be a clear role for C-peptide in that process as well. One possibility is that the increase in pH deprotonates the glutamic acid and aspartic acid residues, rendering them ionized and more capable of binding Zn^{2+} and facilitating the breakdown of the insulin hexamer.

If C-peptide binding to Zn^{2+} was involved in the breakdown of the insulin hexamer, it would also be expected that insulin containing Zn^{2+} would be able to activate C-peptide induced release of ATP from RBCs. In an in vitro study, we have been able to demonstrate that insulin containing 0.5% (w/w) Zn^{2+} added to C-peptide prior to incubation with RBCs did indeed elicit a response from these cells in the form of ATP release [62]. However, similar studies in which insulin was purified by HPLC to contain no Zn^{2+} prior to adding it to C-peptide resulted in an ATP release value that was not statistically different from RBCs incubated in buffer or purified C-peptide alone (i.e., C-peptide with no exogenous metal added). The data shown in Fig. 3.3 suggest that C-peptide may be obtaining Zn^{2+} during the insulin secretion from the beta cell granulae.

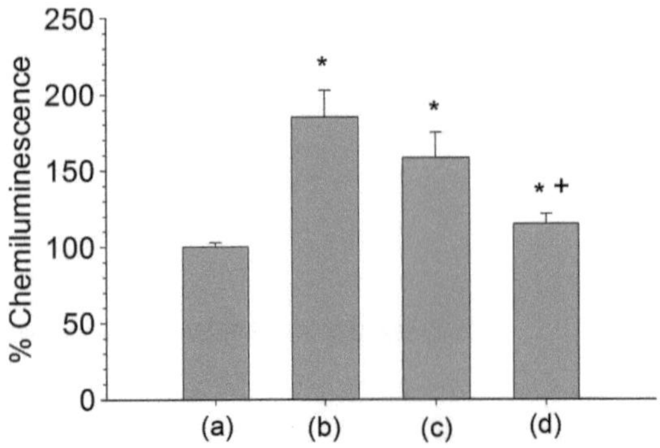

Fig. 3.3 The effect of Zn-C-peptide and the source of the zinc on the release of ATP from RBCs. ATP was measured via the luciferase assay (chemiluminescence). In (*a*), the basal levels of extracellular ATP were measured for an aliquot of RBCs. In (*b*) another aliquot of these cells that had incubated with Zn-C-peptide for 2 h was assayed for ATP and, as shown, the emission due to ATP release increased. Next, another aliquot of RBCs was assayed (*c*) that had been subjected to C-peptide and insulin that contained Zn and again an increase over basal levels was recorded. Finally, in (*d*) RBCs incubated with C-peptide in the presence of Zn-free insulin were determined. Although, a slight increase was measured, this increase was significantly less than that in (*b*) and (*c*). These data suggest that C-peptide's efficacy, at least with regard to ATP release from the RBC, is significantly enhanced in the presence of a zinc source

Effects of C-Peptide on Cells in the Bloodstream

The preceding sections have described the role of the RBC in the vasoregulation via its ability to release ATP (an NO stimulus) and the importance of NO itself as the endothelium-derived relaxing factor. Moreover, the importance of C-peptide is evident based on its ability to stimulate the release of RBC-derived ATP when bound to a metal such as zinc. Here, the effect of Zn-activated C-peptide on the RBC's ability to release ATP is described in greater detail. In addition, the downstream effect of this ATP release on other cell types is also considered, thus demonstrating the far-reaching effects of C-peptide.

Previous reports showing beneficial effects of C-peptide involving such complications as nephropathy [63], neuropathy [64], vascular [65], and inflammatory functions [66] suggest that C-peptide is a multitasking molecule. For example, previous studies have demonstrated that C-peptide has the ability to improve blood flow in skin [50] and in the microvasculature [65]. Although no mechanism for this improved blood flow has been reported, there was a concomitant increase in the Na^+ K^+ ATPase pump activity. In a recent publication [8], it was demonstrated that, when incubated with C-peptide at physiological concentrations (1–10 nM), the ability of RBC's obtained from healthy rabbits to release ATP more than doubled over an 8 h incubation period. The discovery that C-peptide induces an increase in the release of ATP from RBCs may help explain the blood flow improvements measured with C-peptide, if one considers the discussion of the RBC as a mediator of blood flow in vivo.

In addition to the effects on RBCs obtained from nondiabetic animals (both rabbits and rats), C-peptide has also been shown to have a positive effect on RBCs obtained from rat models of both type 1 and type 2 diabetes, albeit with varying activities. Specifically, in a small scale study involving RBCs obtained from a rat model of type 1 diabetes, it was found that the overall percentage increase in ATP release was not statistically different than the release measured from RBCs obtained from control rats [9]. However, in a study involving RBCs from a rat model of type 2 diabetes, it was reported that the ATP release from these cells was significantly less, approximately 50%, than the ATP release from RBCs harvested from healthy controls [9]. Subsequent studies suggested that exogenously added C-peptide was interacting with the RBCs obtained from the type 2 rat models to a much lesser extent than the control RBCs.

In addition to its apparent differential effects on the RBC depending upon the RBC source (healthy subject, type 1 subject, or a type 2 subject), we have determined that multiple mechanisms may exist to explain C-peptide's stimulatory effects on the RBC. Specifically, initial efforts focused on deformation-induced release of ATP from the RBC based on the work describing improvements in RBC deformability after these cells were incubated with C-peptide [8]. However, during the course of control experiments, it was also discovered that C-peptide, when metal activated, is able to increase the release of ATP from RBCs even in the absence of any flow-induced deformation. Although a mechanism for this release has not been completely elucidated, it seems apparent that glucose uptake into the RBC must occur before the ATP release from the cell can occur. This is in agreement with a recent finding suggesting that increased glycolytic metabolism by the RBC facilitates an increase of ATP release from these cells [67]. Therefore, in addition to stimulating ATP release in the absence of any physical external stimuli, the ability of C-peptide to improve the deformability of the RBC may coincide with a mechanism proposed by Sprague et al. [41, 68, 69]. In this mechanism, Sprague describes a deformation-induced activation of a G-protein coupled receptor that subsequently leads to the release of ATP release from the RBC.

In summary, C-peptide may have more than one way of effecting RBC-derived ATP release, namely, through improvement in cell deformability prior to being subjected to flow-induced shear or through an increase of glycolytic activity due to C-peptide's ability to stimulate glucose uptake into the RBC. Independent of the mechanism, the released ATP now becomes a possible determinant in the function of other such cell types in the bloodstream as the endothelial cell and the platelet.

In addition to effects on the RBC, C-peptide affects function in the endothelium, in particular the production of NO via stimulation of eNOS in these cells. By sampling the supernatant above endothelial cells and applying it to smooth muscle fibroblasts, Wallerath et al. [7] measured an increase in c-GMP via immunoassay, which was attributed to stimulation by NO in the supernatant. Other studies have shown that people with type 2 diabetes with good residual C-peptide secretion are better protected from endothelial dysfunction than those with poor C-peptide secretion [70].

C-peptide's effects on the endothelium are also important to other cell types as C-peptide decreases leukocyte adhesion [71]. When C-peptide was administered to rats previously administered L-NAME to inhibit NO production, a significant increase in leukocyte rolling and adhered leukocytes were measured. However, in the presence of C-peptide, these measured leukocyte effects were attenuated. It was concluded that these effects were related to the ability of C-peptide to affect endothelial cell adhesion molecules and maintenance of NO release from the endothelium.

We have found that C-peptide may also have an effect on the platelet, although indirectly mediated through the RBC or endothelium. The identification of C-peptide as a mediator of platelet function would be important clinically as people with diabetes have a higher occurrence of hyperactive platelets, resulting in increased platelet adhesion [72–74], and therefore higher rates of stroke and associated complications. Previously, it was shown that C-peptide had no direct effect on platelet behavior [75], and studies performed in our laboratory have agreed with this prior report, even when the C-peptide was activated with zinc. However, although there was no direct effect on the platelets due to treatment with C-peptide, there was an indirect effect due to C-peptide's ability to stimulate ATP release from erythrocytes, which subsequently affected platelet behavior and the stimulation of NO by the platelet [62]. Once produced by the platelet, NO acts as a platelet inhibitor, reducing the hyperactivation and aggregation of platelets. Therefore, even NO that is produced by the endothelium as a function of C-peptide directly or RBC-derived ATP would be a determinant in reducing platelet activation.

Previously, C-peptide has been shown to have a possible effect on platelet adhesion to the endothelium via its ability to stimulate ATP release from the RBC [62]. Using an in vitro flow model, the number of platelets adhering to the endothelium was reduced when the platelets were pumped over the endothelial cells in the presence of RBCs (Fig. 3.4). Interestingly, the platelet adhesion was lowered even further when the platelets were pumped in the presence of RBCs that had been incubated in Zn-activated C-peptide. When the RBC's ability to release ATP was inhibited, the platelet adhesion to the endothelium significantly increased. These results suggest that the ATP being released from the RBCs incubated with zinc-activated C-peptide is resulting in an increase in NO production in the platelet, or the endothelium, which leads to a decrease in platelet adherence to the endothelium.

Based on the above discussion, Zn-activated C-peptide has the ability to affect the platelet via stimulation of ATP from the RBC. Therefore, due to the decreased release of ATP release from the

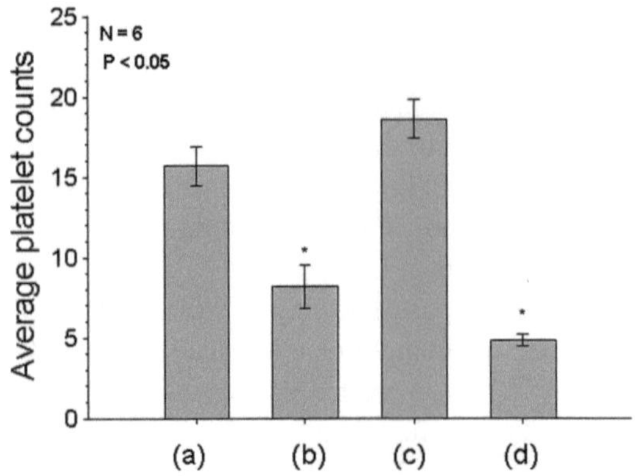

Fig. 3.4 Determination of platelet adhesion to an immobilized endothelium under various conditions. The *first bar* represents platelets alone adhering to an endothelium under conditions of flow. The *second bar* is another aliquot of those platelets flowing across the endothelium, but in the presence of RBCs; note the decrease in platelets adhering to the endothelium. However, in the *third bar*, the ATP release from the RBCs was inhibited with glybenclamide and the platelet adhesion number increased. The *final bar* is the platelets flowing over the endothelium in the presence of RBCs that had been incubated with Zn^{2+}-activated C-peptide. C-peptide alone or Zn^{2+} alone had no effect on platelet adhesion. These data suggest that C-peptide-induced ATP release from RBCs may have a beneficial effect on the reduction of platelet adhesion in vivo. The *asterisks* indicate statistically significant differences from adhesion of platelets alone

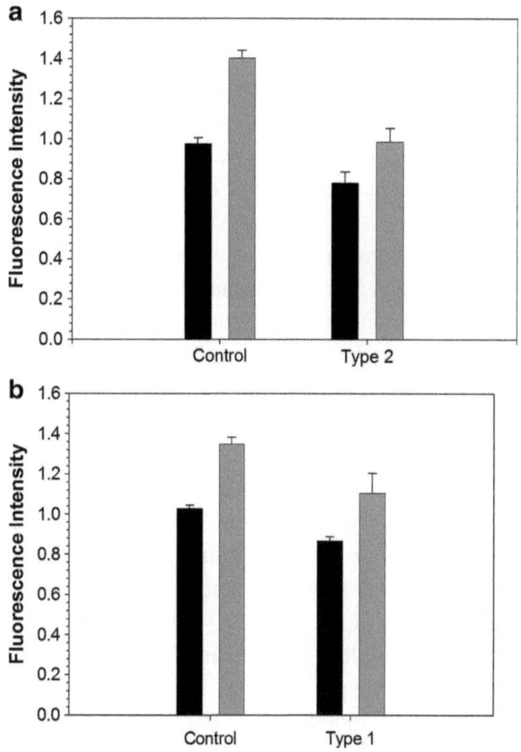

Fig. 3.5 In (**a**), the effect of metal-activated C-peptide on the NO production by platelets from type 2 (BB/ZDB) and control rats. *Black bars* represent the fluorescence intensity from platelet NO production incubated with supernatant from rat RBCs and *gray bars* represent the fluorescence intensity from platelet NO production incubated with supernatant from rat RBCs incubated with metal-activated C-peptide. Error bars are ±SE. In (**b**), the effect of metal-activated C-peptide on the platelet NO production from type 1 and control rats. *Black bars* show the platelet NO production incubated with supernatant from rat RBCs and *gray bars* shoe the platelet NO production incubated with supernatant from rat RBCs incubated with metal-activated C-peptide. Error bars are ±SE

RBCs of type 2 diabetic rats, one may expect a decrease in response for platelets incubated with such RBCs. We have performed experiments in which platelets obtained from rat models of type 1 and type 2 diabetes were incubated with supernatant above RBCs incubated with Zn-activated C-peptide. The resultant NO production from these platelets after incubation with the supernatant was then determined using fluorescence spectrophotometry. As shown in Fig. 3.5a, the NO production from platelets obtained from type 2 rat models increased 30.2±6.6%, while the NO production from control platelets was 53.5±4.6%. The type 1 rat model, however, demonstrated an NO production increase of 31.9±3.4% compared to platelets alone while the control increased similarly (27.8±5.9%) as shown in Fig. 3.5b. While platelet NO production appear similar for the RBCs obtained from the rat models of type 1 and type 2 diabetes, it is important to note that these experiments were performed at different times. The important feature to note is that the NO production for the type 1 rats was very similar to controls run on the same day, while the increase using RBCs from type 2 rat models was significantly different in comparison to controls run on that day. This data suggests that ATP derived from zinc-activated C-peptide treated RBCs may play an important role in platelet hyperactivity and aggregation and, importantly, that the source of the RBC (diabetes type) is a determinant in their response to C-peptide.

People with diabetes often suffer cardiovascular complications as a result of poor circulation of the blood. Interestingly, RBCs from people with diabetes release less ATP than healthy individuals [8, 9, 53, 76]. Because ATP is a primary stimulus for NO production in platelets, then recent reports involving ATP release from RBCs of patients with diabetes becomes important to platelet physiology. The significant decrease in concentrations of RBC-derived ATP from diabetic RBCs may contribute to decreased levels of NO production by platelets and endothelium.

Other studies have also examined the role of C-peptide in platelet behavior. Previously, it has been shown that administration of C-peptide caused a significant delay in arteriolar and venular thrombus growth in normal and diabetic mice [77]. However, subsequent perfusion with insulin (100 μU/mL) reversed these effects leading us to believe that C-peptide may not be beneficial as an anti-thrombotic treatment option. In contrast to these studies demonstrating a beneficial effect of C-peptide on platelet activation, the work by Hu et al. [75], in which insulin or C-peptide, or a combination thereof, was administered to whole blood, show that insulin results in an increase in fibrinogen binding; however, C-peptide demonstrates no ability to reverse this trend.

Moving C-Peptide Forward Towards Acceptance as a Biologically-Active Substance

While it is clear from the literature that C-peptide displays biological activity using both in vivo and in vitro models, there is still a negative connotation surrounding its use as a replacement therapy. Some of these concerns, described by Luzi et al. [78], include the lack of large scale clinical trials, the lack of an identified cell receptor for C-peptide, and the fact that people with type 2 diabetes often have C-peptide levels above that of controls. The first concern, that of the clinical trial, may be attributed to the lack of necessary funds to carry out such large-scale studies by individual academic institutions. Moreover, although a receptor for C-peptide has never been identified, studies have shown that C-peptide does interact with cellular membranes [79–81]. Finally, the argument against C-peptide and its apparent noneffects in type 2 diabetes should not preclude its current use in type 1 diabetes, especially in light of the fact that people with type 2 diabetes still produce insulin and C-peptide. Of course, the role of insulin as a beneficial substance is without question.

Nevertheless, there are some issues with C-peptide that could emerge in the very near future that may eventually slow the momentum that has been gained involving studies with C-peptide. For example, C-peptide has beneficial effects on many complications associated with diabetes, and some of these complications have very different origins. C-peptide improves metrics associated with neuropathy and nephropathy; it has been shown to play a role in cellular function, insulin-induced neointima [82], and physical characteristics. It affects different types of enzymes. In fact, C-peptide, in some instances, doesn't even need to be "C-peptide" as fragments of the molecule have been shown to demonstrate activity [83]. To a C-peptide novice, it may appear that this biomolecule is approaching the "magic bullet" status and can help reduce or ameliorate many different complications on its own. Unfortunately, to the skeptic, it may appear that investigations involving C-peptide is an unorganized mess in need of explanations for its efficacy.

In the near future, studies involving C-peptide must begin to have more detailed mechanistic information to explain the results. For example, all we know about C-peptide and its ability to stimulate ATP release from the RBC is that it needs zinc. We hypothesize that this zinc comes from the beta cells and we also hypothesize that the ATP release is due to an increase in glucose uptake by the RBC. Unfortunately, an exact mechanism is incomplete. Thus, studies are currently underway to validate the source of the zinc and to determine exactly how Zn-activated C-peptide is stimulating glucose uptake into the RBC.

Also, users of C-peptide should slowly come to a consensus on some type of standard operating protocols that go beyond "concentration" of the peptide. For example, rather than concentration added to a sample, all studies should involve the moles or molecules of C-peptide added per cell in the sample. The number of C-peptide molecules binding per cell has been reported for human renal tubular cells [81] and a similar number has been found for RBCs. In addition to the amount of C-peptide added to a sample, the form of the C-peptide must also be confirmed. If C-peptide has certain biological effects that are only measured in the presence of a metal, then mass spectrometric validation of peptide's content must be performed prior to use. As described earlier, there is significant evidence from our group and others (indirectly) that metal-activation of C-peptide changes the activity of the molecule. Perhaps C-peptide works on some cells independent of zinc, but to date, the author has found that both RBCs and endothelial cells only respond to the metal-bound form of C-peptide.

If standard protocols are designed and mechanistic studies are performed, the result may be a unifying hypothesis for C-peptide efficacy that would then thwart any doubt of its biological efficacy. The author has already made such attempts to assemble C-peptide results from his own lab, and those from other labs, into various groups based on events that are more global in vivo. For example, if one considers the importance of purinergic receptor signaling, and how widespread it is in vivo, one could envision that the ability of C-peptide to stimulate ATP release from the RBC to have far-reaching effects. In the kidneys, purinergic receptor signaling is an important determinant in vascular resistance; because ATP and adenine derivatives are ligands for these receptors, one could speculate importance for a substance such as C-peptide, which stimulates ATP release from the RBC, as a mediator of these nucleotide-receptor interactions. The effect of ATP on NO production, one of the more powerful vasodilators, has already been discussed; however, it is worth restating the importance of NO in overall blood flow and inhibition of platelet and leukocyte adhesion. Finally, C-peptide has been shown to activate various pathways involving increases in kinase activities and phosphorylations in multiple cell types. Of course, kinases use ATP as the phosphate source for phosphorylation. These examples suggest that one potential commonality involving C-peptide's biological effects is related to ATP. This author is not suggesting that all mechanisms involving C-peptide's effects should run through ATP; however, it is an example of how researchers investigating C-peptide could begin to think about the possible mechanism that is key to its efficacy. In doing so, it will provide a platform and guide for future studies involving C-peptide which, at this point in time, seem very promising and exciting.

References

1. Ellsworth ML. The red blood cell as an oxygen sensor: what is the evidence. Acta Physiol Scand. 2000;168:551–9.
2. Ellsworth ML, Forrester T, Ellis CG, et al. The erythrocyte as a regulator of vascular tone. Am J Physiol. 1995;269:H2155–61.
3. Allen BW, Stamler JS, Piantadosi CA. Hemoglobin, nitric oxide and molecular mechanisms of hypoxic vasodilation. Trends Mol Med. 2009;15(10):452–60.
4. van Faassen EE, Bahrami S, Feelisch M, et al. Nitrite as regulator of hypoxic signaling in mammalian physiology. Med Res Rev. 2009;29(5):683–741.
5. Sprague RS, Stephenson AH, Ellsworth ML. Red not dead: signaling in and from erythrocytes. Trends Endocrinol Metab. 2007;18(9):350–5.
6. Tolan NV, Meyer JA, Ku C-J, et al. Use of the red blood cell as a simple drug target and diagnostic by manipulating and monitoring its ability to release adenosine triphosphate (ATP). Pure Appl Chem. 2010;82(8):1623–34.
7. Wallerath T, Kunt T, Forst T, et al. Stimulation of endothelial nitric oxide synthase by proinsulin C-peptide. Nitric Oxide. 2003;9(2):95–102.
8. Meyer JA, Froelich JM, Reid GE, et al. Metal-activated C-peptide facilitates glucose clearance and the release of a nitric oxide stimulus via the GLUT1 transporter. Diabetologia. 2008;51(1):175–82.
9. Meyer JA, Subasinghe W, Sima AAF, et al. Zinc-activated C-peptide resistance to the type 2 diabetic erythrocyte is associated with hyperglycemia-induced phosphatidylserine externalization and reversed by metformin. Mol Biosyst. 2009;5(10):1157–62.
10. Kitamura T, Kimura K, Jung BD, et al. Proinsulin C-peptide rapidly stimulates mitogen-activated protein kinases in Swiss 3T3 fibroblasts: requirement of protein kinase C, phosphoinositide 3-kinase and pertussis toxin-sensitive G-protein. Biochem J. 2001;355:123–9.
11. Kitamura T, Kimura K, Jung BD, et al. Proinsulin C-peptide activates cAMP response element-binding proteins through the p38 mitogen-activated protein kinase pathway in mouse lung capillary endothelial cells. Biochem J. 2002;366:737–44.
12. Kitamura T, Kimura K, Makondo K, et al. Proinsulin C-peptide increases nitric oxide production by enhancing mitogen-activated protein-kinase-dependent transcription of endothelial nitric oxide synthase in aortic endothelial cells of Wistar rats. Diabetologia. 2003;46:1698–705.
13. Zhong Z, Davidescu A, Ehren I, et al. C-peptide stimulates ERK1/2 and JNK MAP kinases via activation of protein kinase C in human renal tubular cells. Diabetologia. 2005;48(1):187–97.
14. Zhong Z, Kotova O, Davidescu A, et al. C-peptide stimulates Na+, K+-ATPase via activation of ERK1/2 MAP kinases in human renal tubular cells. Cell Mol Life Sci. 2004;61(21):2782–90.
15. Furchgott RF, Zawadzki JV. The obligatory role of endothelial cells in the relaxation of arterial smooth muscle by acetylcholine. Nature. 1980;288:373–6.
16. Ignarro LJ, Buga G, Dhaudhuri G. EDRF generation and release from perfused bovine pulmonary artery and vein. Eur J Pharmacol. 1988;149:79–88.
17. Palmer R, Ferrige MJ, Moncada S. Nitric oxide release accounts for the biological activity of endothelium-derived relaxation factor. Nature. 1987;327:524–6.
18. Buga GM, Gold ME, Fukuto JM, et al. Shear stress-induced release of nitric oxide from endothelial cells grown on beads. Hypertension. 1991;17:187–93.
19. Rubanyi GM, Romero JC, Vanhoutte PM. Flow-induced release of endothelium-derived relaxing factor. Am J Physiol. 1986;250:H1145–9.
20. Sprague RS, Stephenson AH, Dimmitt RA, et al. Effect of L-NAME on pressure-flow relationships in isolated rabbit lungs: role of red blood cells. Am J Physiol Heart C. 1995;269(38):H1941–8.
21. Sprague RS, Ellsworth ML, Stephenson AH, et al. ATP: the red blood cell link to NO and local control of the pulmonary circulation. Am J Physiol Heart C. 1996;271(40):H2717–22.
22. Gladwin MT, Shelhamer JH, Schechter AN, et al. Role of circulating nitrite and S-nitrosohemoglobin in

the regulation of regional blood flow in humans. Proc Natl Acad Sci U S A. 2000;97(21):11482–7.
23. Tsoukias NM. Nitric oxide bioavailability in the microcirculation: insights from mathematical models. Microcirculation. 2008;15(8):813–34.
24. Stamler JS, Jia L, Eu JP, et al. Blood flow regulation by S-nitrosohemoglobin: a dynamic activity of blood involved in vascular control. Science. 1997;276: 2034–7.
25. Genes LI, Tolan NV, Hulvey MK, et al. Addressing a vascular endothelium array with blood components using underlying microfluidic channels. Lab Chip. 2007;7(10):1256–9.
26. Bogle RG, Coade SB, Moncada S, et al. Bradykinin and ATP stimulate L-arginine uptake and nitric oxide release in vascular endothelial cells. Biochem Biophys Res Commun. 1991;80:926–32.
27. Dull RO, Tarbell JM, Daves PF. Mechanism of flow-mediated signal transduction in endothelial cells: kinetics of ATP surface concentrations. J Vasc Res. 1992;29:410–9.
28. Bergfeld GR, Forrester T. Release of ATP from human erythrocytes in response to a brief period of hypoxia and hypercapnia. Cardiovasc Res. 1992;26(1):40–7.
29. Miseta A, Bogner P, Berenyi M, et al. Relationship between cellular ATP, potassium, sodium and magnesium concentrations in mammalian and avian erythrocytes. Biochim Biophys Acta. 1993;1175:133–9.
30. Allsup DJ, Boarder MR. Comparison of P2 purinergic receptors of aortic endothelial cell with those of adrenal medulla: evidence for heterogeneity of receptor subtype and of inositol phosphate response. Mol Pharm. 1990;38:84–91.
31. Communi D, Raspe E, Pirotton S, et al. Coexpression of P2y and P2u receptors on aortic endothelial cells: comparison of cell localization and signaling pathways. Circ Res. 1991;76:191–8.
32. Houston DA, Burnstock G, Vanhoutte PM. Different P2-purinergic receptor subtypes of endothelium and smooth muscle in canine blood vessels. J Pharmacol Exp Ther. 1987;241:501–6.
33. Liu SF, McCormack DG, Evans TW, et al. Characterization and distribution of P2-purinoreceptor subtypes in rat pulmonary vessels. J Pharmacol Exp Ther. 1989;251:1204–10.
34. Motte S, Perotton S, Boeynaems JM. Heterogeneity of ATP receptors in aortic endothelial cells: involvement of P2y and P2u receptors in inositol phosphate response. Circ Res. 1993;72:504–10.
35. Dazel HH, Westfall DP. Receptors for adenine nucleotides and nucleosides: subclassification, distribution and molecular characterization. Pharmacol Rev. 1994;46:449–66.
36. KennedyC, DelbroD, BurnstockG. P2-purinoreceptors mediate both vasodilation (via the endothelium) and vasoconstriction of the isolated ret femoral artery. Eur J Pharmacol. 1985;107:161–8.
37. Forsberg E, Feuerstein G, Shohami E, Pollard H. Adenosine triphosphate stimulates inositol phospholipid metabolism and prostacyclin formation in adrenal medullary endothelial cells by means of P2-purinergic receptors. Proc Natl Acad Sci USA. 1987;84: 5630–4.
38. Hassessian H, Burnstock G. Interacting roles of nitric oxide and ATP in the pulmonary circulation of the rat. Br J Pharmacol. 1995;114:846–50.
39. McCullough WT, Collins DM, Ellsworth ML. Arteriolar responses to extracellular ATP in striated muscle. Am J Physiol. 1997;272:H1886–91.
40. Dietrich HH, Ellsworth ML, Sprague RS, Dacey Jr RG. Red blood cell regulation of microvascular tone through adenosine triphosphate. Am J Physiol Heart C. 2000;278:H1294–8.
41. Sprague RS, Ellsworth ML, Stephenson AH, et al. Deformation-induced ATP release from red blood cells requires cystic fibrosis transmembrane conductance regulator activity. Am J Physiol. 1998;275: H1726–32.
42. Fischer DJ, Torrence NJ, Sprung RJ, et al. Determination of erythrocyte deformability and its correlation to cellular ATP release using microbore tubing with diameters that approximate resistance vessels in vivo. Analyst. 2003;128:1163–8.
43. Sprague RS, Ellsworth ML, Stephenson AH, et al. ATP: the red blood cell link to NO and local control of the pulmonary circulation. Am J Physiol. 1996;271:H2717–22.
44. Sprague RS, Ellsworth ML, Stephenson AH, et al. Increases in flow rate stimulate adenosine triphosphate release from red blood cells in isolated rabbit lungs. Exp Clin Cardiol. 1998;3:73–7.
45. Leeman M, de Zegers BV, Delcroix M, Naeije R. Effects of endogenous nitric oxide on pulmonary vascular tone in intact dogs. Am J Physiol. 1994;266: H2343–7.
46. Nishiwaki K, Nyhan PD, Rock P, et al. N-nitro-L-arginine and pulmonary vascular pressure-flow relationship in conscious dogs. Am J Physiol. 1992;262: H1331–7.
47. Carroll JS, Subasinghe W, Raththagala M, et al. An altered erythrocyte pentose phosphate pathway affects the ability of red cells to release ATP, a nitric oxide stimulus. Mol Biosyst. 2006;2:305–11.
48. Sprung RJ, Sprague RS, Spence DM. Determination of ATP release from erythrocytes using microbore tubing as a model of resistance vessels in vivo. Anal Chem. 2002;74:2274–8.
49. Price AK, Fischer DJ, Martin RS, et al. Deformation-induced release of ATP from erythrocytes in a poly(dimethylsiloxane)-based microchip with channels that mimic resistance vessels. Anal Chem. 2004;76(16):4849–55.
50. Forst T, Kunt T, Pohlmann T, et al. Biological activity of C-peptide on the skin microcirculation in patients with insulin-dependent diabetes mellitus. J Clin Invest. 1998;101(10):2036–41.
51. Forst T, De La Tour DD, Kunt T, et al. Effects of proinsulin C-peptide on nitric oxide, microvascular blood

flow and erythrocyte Na+, K+-ATPase activity in diabetes mellitus type I. Clin Sci. 2000;98(3):283–90.
52. Kunt T, Schneider S, Pfutzner A, et al. The effect of human proinsulin C-peptide on erythrocyte deformability in patients with type I diabetes mellitus. Diabetologia. 1999;42(4):465–71.
53. Sprague RS, Stephenson AH, Bowles EA, Stumpf MS, Lonigro AJ. Reduced expression of Gi in erythrocytes of humans with type 2 diabetes is associated with impairment of both cAMP generation and ATP release. Diabetes. 2006;55(12):3588–93.
54. Forst T, Kunt T. Effects of C-peptide on microvascular blood flow and blood hemorheology. Exp Diabesity Res. 2004;5(1):51–64.
55. Chen G, Liu P, Pattar GR, et al. Chromium activates glucose transporter 4 trafficking and enhances insulin-stimulated glucose transport in 3T3-LI adipocytes via a cholesterol-dependent mechanism. Mol Endocrinol. 2006;20(4):857–70.
56. Hatfield MJ, Gillespie S, Chen Y, Li Z, et al. Low-molecular-weight chromium-binding substance from chicken liver and American alligator liver. Comp Biochem Phys B. 2006;144:423–31.
57. Mertz W, Roginski EE, Schwarz K. Effect of trivalent chromium complexes on glucose uptake by epididymal fat tissue of rats. J Biol Chem. 1961;236:318–22.
58. Schwarz K, Mertz W. Chromium(III) and the glucose tolerance factor. Arch Biochem Biophys. 1959;85: 292–5.
59. Orci L, Halban P, Perrelet A, et al. pH-independent and -dependent cleavage of proinsulin in the same secretory vesicle. J Cell Biol. 1994;126:1149–56.
60. Kennedy RT, Huang L, Aspinwall CA. Extracellular pH is required for rapid release of insulin from Zn-insulin precipitates in beta-cell secretory vesicles during exocytosis. J Am Chem Soc. 1996;118(7):1795–6.
61. Shafqat J, Melles E, Sigmundsson K, et al. C-peptide elicits disaggregation of insulin resulting in enhanced physiological insulin effects. Cell Mol Life Sci. 2006;63:1805–11.
62. Medawala W, McCahill P, Giebink A, et al. A molecular level understanding of zinc activation of C-peptide and its effects on cellular communication in the bloodstream. Rev Diabet Stud. 2009;6(3):148–58.
63. Nordquist L, Wahren J. C-Peptide: the missing link in diabetic nephropathy? Rev Diabet Stud. 2009;6(3): 203–10.
64. Kamiya H, Zhang W, Sima AAF. The beneficial effects of C-peptide on diabetic polyneuropathy. Rev Diabet Stud. 2009;6(3):187–202.
65. Forst T, Hach T, Kunt T, et al. Molecular effects of C-peptide in microvascular blood flow regulation. Rev Diabet Stud. 2009;6(3):159–67.
66. Haidet J, Cifarelli V, Trucco M, Luppi P. Anti-inflammatory properties of C-peptide. Rev Diabet Stud. 2009;6(3):168–79.
67. Cao ZL, Bell JB, Mohanty JG, et al. Nitrite enhances RBC hypoxic ATP synthesis and the release of ATP into the vasculature: a new mechanism for nitrite-induced vasodilation. Am J Physiol Heart C. 2009;297(4): H1494–503.
68. Olearczyk JJ, Stephenson AH, Lonigro AJ, et al. Receptor-mediated activation of the heterotrimeric G-protein Gs results in ATP release from erythrocytes. Med Sci Monit. 2001;7(4):669–74.
69. Olearczyk JJ, Stephenson AH, Lonigro AJ, et al. Heterotrimeric G protein Gi is involved in a signal transduction pathway for ATP release from erythrocytes. Am J Physiol. 2004;286(3 Pt 2):H940–5.
70. Manzella D, Ragno E, Abbatecola Angela M, et al. Residual C-peptide secretion and endothelial function in patients with type II diabetes. Clin Sci. 2003;105(1):113–8.
71. Scalia R, Coyle KM, Levine BJ, et al. C-peptide inhibits leukocyte-endothelium interaction in the microcirculation during acute endothelial dysfunction. FASEB J. 2000;14(14):2357–64.
72. Freedman JE, Loscalzo J, Barnard MR, et al. Nitric oxide released from activated platelets inhibits platelet recruitment. J Clin Invest. 1997;100(2):350–6.
73. Sobol AB, Watala C. The role of platelets in diabetes-related vascular complications. Diabetes Res Clin Pract. 2000;50(1):1–16.
74. Vinik AI, Erbas T, Park TS, et al. Platelet dysfunction in type 2 diabetes. Diabetes Care. 2001;24(8): 1476–85.
75. Hu H, Li N, Ekberg K, et al. Insulin, but not proinsulin C-peptide, enhances platelet fibrinogen binding in vitro in type 1 diabetes mellitus patients and healthy subjects. Thromb Res. 2002;106(2):91–5.
76. Carroll J, Raththagala M, Subasinghe W, et al. An altered oxidant defense system in red blood cells affects their ability to release nitric oxide-stimulating ATP. Mol Biosyst. 2006;2(6/7):305–11.
77. Lindenblatt N, Braun B, Menger MD, et al. C-peptide exerts antithrombotic effects that are repressed by insulin in normal and diabetic mice. Diabetologia. 2006;49(4):792–800.
78. Luzi L, Zerbini G, Caumo A. C-peptide: a redundant relative of insulin? Diabetologia. 2007;50:500–2.
79. Lindahl E, Nyman U, Melles E, et al. Cellular internalization of proinsulin C-peptide. Cell Mol Life Sci. 2007;64:479–86.
80. Pramanik A, Ekberg K, Zhong Z, et al. C-peptide binding to human cell membranes: importance of Glu27. Biochem Biophys Res Commun. 2001; 284:94–8.
81. Rigler R, Pramanik A, Jonasson P, et al. Specific binding of proinsulin C-peptide to human cell membranes. Proc Natl Acad Sci U S A. 1999;96:13318–23.
82. Mughal RS, Scragg JL, Lister P, et al. Cellular mechanisms by which proinsulin C-peptide prevents insulin-induced neointima formation in human saphenous vein. Diabetologia. 2010;53(8):1761–71.
83. Hach T, Forst T, Kunt T, et al. C-peptide and its C-terminal fragments improve erythrocyte deformability in type 1 diabetes patients. Exp Diabetes Res. 2008;2008:730594.

C-Peptide Signaling in the Kidney and Protection from Diabetic Nephropathy

4

Nigel J. Brunskill

Keywords
C-peptide • Diabetic nephropathy • Signaling • Fibrosis

Introduction

Cell signaling is a fundamental process that allows cells to respond to their macro- or micro-environment by regulating basic cellular functions and processes. Many cell signaling systems rely on an extracellular messenger derived from distant or surrounding tissues, that binds to a receptor embedded in the plasma membrane of the target cell. Ligation of ligand with receptor then stimulates a downstream signaling cascade that transmits and amplifies the signal, thus altering cell function and phenotype. Study and manipulation of such signaling pathways has been a very fruitful avenue for advancing the understanding of disease pathophysiology and drug discovery.

Historically C-peptide has been regarded as an inert by-product of insulin synthesis and processing. However an enlarging body of evidence has challenged this view by reporting both in vitro and in vivo effects of C-peptide of great relevance to the pathophysiology and treatment of diabetes. Indeed these observations indicate that C-peptide exhibits the signaling characteristics of a peptide hormone, and beneficially affects nerve, renal and microvascular functions in diabetic animals and in patients with type 1 diabetes (T1DM) [1–7]. Dissection of the mechanisms by which circulating C-peptide interacts with individual cells to control and regulate cell processes, and ultimately whole organ function is crucial to the full understanding and clinical development of a molecule that significantly influences the development of diabetic complications.

N.J. Brunskill (✉)
Department of Infection, Immunity and Inflammation, University of Leicester School of Medicine, Leicester, England, UK

Department of Nephrology, Leicester General Hospital, Gwendolen Road, Leicester, LE5 4PW, England, UK
e-mail: njb18@le.ac.uk

C-Peptide Binding to Cells and Structure–Function Relationships

Flatt et al. [8] found specific, displaceable C-peptide binding to a rat islet cell tumor composed predominantly of β-cells. Subsequently, high affinity, specific binding of rhodamine-labeled C-peptide to membranes from several cell types was demonstrated using sensitive fluorescence correlation microscopy [9]. Binding was displaced by excess unlabelled C-peptide but not by insulin or scrambled C-peptide. Pertussis toxin also significantly attenuated C-peptide binding suggesting that binding was occurring to

A.A.F. Sima (ed.), *Diabetes & C-Peptide: Scientific and Clinical Aspects*, Contemporary Diabetes,
DOI 10.1007/978-1-61779-391-2_4, © Springer Science+Business Media, LLC 2012

a G-protein coupled receptor (GPCR). Renal tubular cells expressed the most binding sites. These exhibited a K_D of 0.3 nM C-peptide, a figure in complete agreement with the documented potency of C-peptide in signaling experiments (see below). Furthermore, full receptor saturation was observed with 0.9 nM C-peptide, a physiological concentration. Thus, under normal conditions in health or in the presence of raised C-peptide levels in type 2 diabetes (T2DM), no further response would necessarily follow exogenous administration of C-peptide.

C-peptide structure-function relationships have been studied using Na^+,K^+-ATPase as a functional readout [10, 11]. The C-terminal pentapeptide contains amino acids that are conserved in mammalian species and is able to re-capitulate the majority of C-peptide bioactivity [10]. Taken together these studies demonstrate that the C-terminal pentapeptide of C-peptide possesses properties typical of a peptide ligand interacting with a specific receptor, but that the C-peptide molecule comprises a three-part structure where the N- and C-terminal sections participate in functional interactions, and the mid-region serves as a joining segment [10–12].

Attempts to identify a C-peptide receptor have so far been unsuccessful. Luzi et al. recently briefly reported their inability to isolate a C-peptide receptor either by screening a human lung fibroblast λ phage cDNA expression library or by proteomic analysis of proteins co-immunoprecipitated from C-peptide treated human fibroblasts using anti-C-peptide antibodies [13]. Attempts to isolate a receptor using gene cloning or proteomics may be more fruitful using kidney cells that exhibit more robust responses to C-peptide, and certainly the existing data do not prove that a receptor does not exist. Alternative methodologies may successfully identify a C-peptide receptor in the future and continuing effort in this area is required.

Signaling Effects of C-Peptide

C-peptide-evoked signaling is now an unequivocally established fact. Many cell types respond to C-peptide, and a variety of cell of intracellular signaling pathways are activated (see Table 4.1). Many of these pathways are highly relevant to

Table 4.1 Signaling elements influenced by C-peptide according to cell type studied

Cell type studied								
Signaling element	Kidney tubular	Muscle	Fibroblasts	Endothelial	Erythrocytes	Neuroblastoma	CD4+ T cells/ macrophages	Nerve
Na^+,K^+-ATPase	+				+			+
$[Ca^{2+}]_i$	+			+				
PKC	+		+					
NO release		+		+				
ERK	+	+	+	+				
p38 MAPK				+				
JNK	+							
PLC	+							
p90RSK		+						
GSK3		+						
PI3K	+	+		+		+	+	
CREB				+				
NFκB	+		+			+		
PPARγ	+							
Smads	+							
JAK2/STAT1							+	
Retinoic acid	+							
HGF	+							

Adapted from Hills and Brunskill [64]. For abbreviations see text the pathogenesis and treatment of microvascular complications. The most important are described below.

C-Peptide and Na^+,K^+-ATPase Activity

Impaired activity of Na^+,K^+-ATPase is seen in a variety of cell types in diabetes and contributes to the pathogenesis of diabetic complications [14–17], and initial descriptions of C-peptide signaling activities relate to activation of this enzyme. Kidney tubules are a rich source of Na^+,K^+-ATPase where it is activated by C-peptide at low nanomolar concentrations [18]. This effect is pertussis toxin sensitive, suggesting involvement of a GPCR, and appears dependent on increases in intracellular Ca^{2+} concentration.

Reduced Na^+,K^+-ATPase activity is found in erythrocyte membranes from T1DM patients who lack circulating C-peptide, and this results in impaired red cell deformability, increased blood viscosity [19], and adverse implications for microvascular blood flow and oxygen supply. Infusion of C-peptide into such patients increases plasma levels of cGMP and shifts erythrocyte membrane Na^+,K^+-ATPase activity back towards normal with a maximal observed effect achieved with plasma C-peptide levels of ~3.5 nM [20]. Similar improvements in rat nerve Na^+,K^+-ATPase activity and function have also been observed after exogenous administration of C-peptide [21].

C-peptide treatment at physiological concentrations activates Na^+,K^+-ATPase in rat kidney medullary thick ascending limb tubules with concomitant phosphorylation of the Na^+,K^+-ATPase α-subunit and translocation of the Ca^{2+} dependent protein kinase C (PKC)-α to the membrane [22]. Maestroni et al. [23] found that low nM concentrations of C-peptide increased expression of vasopressin-activated calcium mobilizing receptor (VCAM-1) at both RNA and protein levels in human fibroblasts and mesangial cells. Given that vasopressin also stimulates Na^+,K^+-ATPase activity, enhancement of vasopressin action via up-regulation of VCAM-1 may provide a further mechanism for C-peptide action relating to the Na^+,K^+-ATPase.

Thus overall, C-peptide at physiological concentrations stimulates Na^+,K^+-ATPase dependent on intracellular Ca^{2+} and PKC, and sensitive to pertussis toxin. Replacement of C-peptide in diabetic animals and patients with T1DM has a salutary effect on Na^+,K^+-ATPase activity in a variety of tissues affected by diabetic complications, and is likely to have a substantial effect on renal physiology and vascular function.

C-Peptide and the Endothelial Nitric Oxide Synthase (eNOS)

In vivo administration of C-peptide to patients with T1DM is consistently followed by augmentation of microvascular blood flow to tissues and organs including muscle, skin and kidney [11] and these effects relate to stimulatory effects on nitric oxide (NO) pathways. In addition, C-peptide evoked increases in glucose utilization in streptozotocin diabetic rats [24], and increased glucose transport and metabolism by muscle tissue are also NO dependent [25, 26]. Similarly, C-peptide mediated arteriolar dilatation is also reliant on NO [27, 28]. In a bovine aortic endothelial cell (BAEC) model Wallerath et al. [29] reported that physiological postprandial C-peptide levels stimulated NO release following a rise in intracellular Ca^{2+}, and speculated that C-peptide signaled increased cellular Ca^{2+} influx and activation of Ca^{2+}-sensitive endothelial nitric oxide synthase (eNOS), thus explaining the vasodilatory effects of C-peptide observed in vivo [29]. Confirmation of these findings by other workers has revealed that up-regulation of eNOS gene transcription and NO release are dependent on the upstream phosphorylation and activation of extracellular signal-regulated mitogen activated protein kinase (ERK) [30].

In addition to vasodilatation, activation of the NO system by C-peptide may have other consequences. In C-peptide injected rats, basal levels of aortic eNOS gene expression and NO production are both increased. At the same time, reduced cell surface levels of the adhesion molecules P-selectin and ICAM-1 on the microvascular endothelium are observed, and consequently, leukocyte/endothelial interactions are attenuated [31]. These important observations in nondiabetic rats suggest an immunomodulatory or anti-inflammatory action for C-peptide and mandate further study in diabetic animals. Studies in macrophages also provide support for an immunomodulatory role for C-peptide. In this cell type, application of C-peptide increases nitrite production in association with induction of inducible nitric oxide synthase (iNOS), a prominent marker of macrophage activation [32].

C-Peptide Mediated Stimulation of Mitogen Activated Protein Kinases

The mitogen activated protein kinases (MAPKs) are a family of serine threonine specific kinases that respond to extracellular signals and link cell-surface receptors or chemical and physical stresses to fundamental regulatory targets within cells controlling such critical functions as growth, gene expression, survival and adaptation [33–35]. The MAPK family includes the ERKs 1 and 2, c-Jun N-terminal kinases, p38s and ERK5.

Studies from several groups now clearly describe the ability of C-peptide to activate MAPKs. Encouraged by the finding of synergy between C-peptide and NPY signaling in the activation of Na^+,K^+-ATPase [10], Kitamura et al. studied C-peptide effects on MAPK in Swiss 3T3 cells [36]. Using both immunoblotting to quantify phosphorylated activated ERK1 and ERK2, and an ERK specific in vitro kinase assay to directly measure kinase activity, C-peptide was shown to rapidly and potently activate ERK in Swiss 3T3 cells at concentrations as low as 1 pM and maximally at 1 nM [36]. This stimulatory effect was also seen with NPY, but not with retro-sequenced or all d-amino acid human C peptide. The ERK activation was abolished by pertussis toxin. This C-peptide response was also cell type specific in that no ERK stimulation was seen in 3T3-L1 cells, L_6E_9 muscle cells, HepG2 hepatoma cells, NG108.15 neuroblastoma cells or C6 glioma cells [36].

Activation of ERK participates in the stimulation of eNOS gene transcription, suggesting that C-peptide stimulated eNOS expression may be ERK dependent. In order to clarify the potential link between these phenomena, studies of transcription factor activation were performed in LEII mouse lung capillary endothelial cells [37]. This work revealed that C-peptide stimulated activity of both p38 and ERK, whereas insulin activated only ERK. In addition, C-peptide activated the cAMP response element (CRE)-binding protein (CREB)/activating transcription factor-1 (ATF-1) in a p38 dependent manner, resulting in the binding of these transcription factors to CRE. It was subsequently confirmed that enhanced eNOS transcription in BAECs following C-peptide treatment was also MAPK dependent [30]. Differences in C-peptide responses between various cell types clearly exist so that in BAECs ERK activation is required for eNOS gene transcription, but in LEII cells this transcription factor activation follows stimulation of p38.

The prominent association of renal tubulo-interstitial disease with the development of diabetic nephropathy has resulted in the careful study of C-peptide responses in tubular cells. In the opossum kidney, (OK) proximal tubular cell line C-peptide is a potent activator of ERK (Fig. 4.1). This effect is maximal at a C-peptide concentration of 300 pM and declines thereafter and displays a bell shaped concentration response curve [38]. C-peptide also induced wortmannin-sensitive activation of Akt in OK cells indicative of phosphatidylinositide-3-kinase (PI-3-kinase) activation. In this case, the concentration response curve revealed a maximal effect on Akt stimulation with a C-peptide concentration of 5 nM, remaining constant thereafter up to a C-peptide concentration of 100 nM. This activation pattern is therefore quite distinct from that for ERK activation. Moreover C-peptide stimulated Ca^{2+} influx into OK cells with consequent membrane translocation and activation of PKCα [38]. These findings are concordant with the previous studies of Tsimaratos et al. that described PKC-induced activation of Na^+,K^+-ATPase in C-peptide exposed kidney tubular segments [22].

These signaling events had important phenotypic consequences in OK cells where C-peptide displays properties of a functional mitogen by

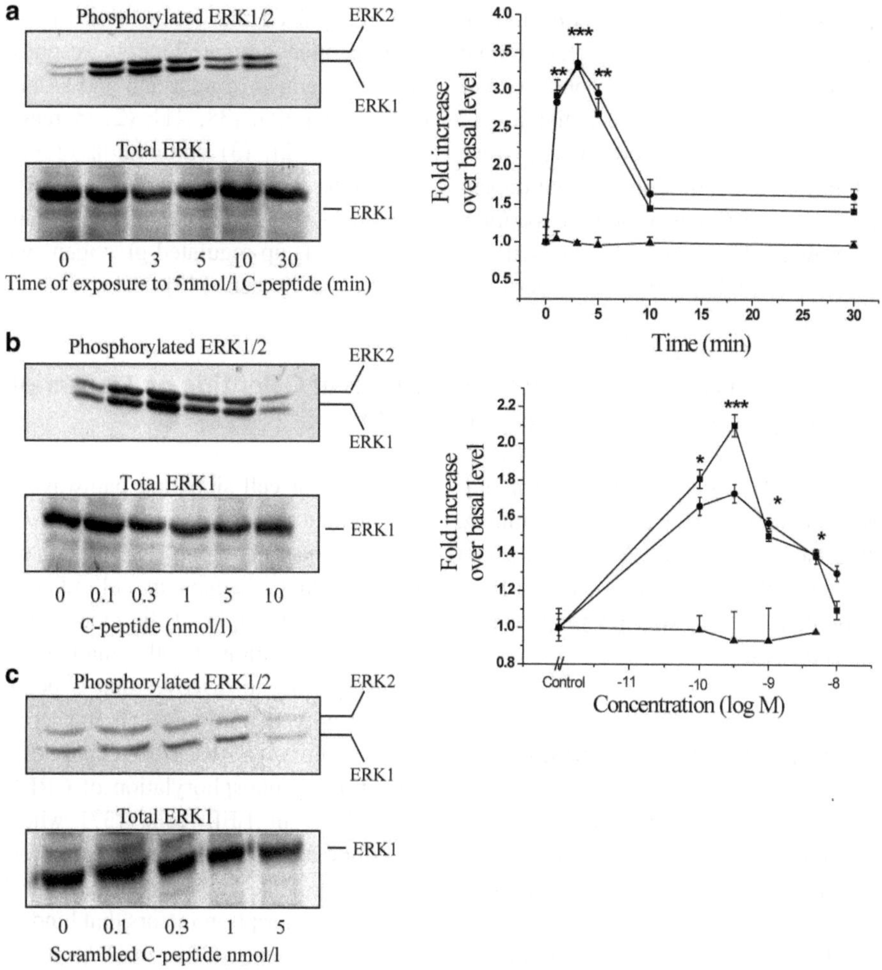

Fig. 4.1 Stimulation of ERK phosphorylation by C-peptide but not scrambled C-peptide in OK cells (adapted from Al-Rasheed et al. [38]). (**a**) Time course of activation. Cells were treated with 5 nM C-peptide for the indicated times and total ERK or pERK detected by immunoblotting. A representative blot is shown (*left*). Phosphorylated bands were quantified and values expressed graphically (*right*). $^{**}p<0.01$, $^{***}p<0.001$, relative to 0 time. (**b**) Concentration-response of activation. Cells were treated with the indicated concentrations of C-peptide for 5 min and total ERK or pERK detected by immunoblotting. A representative blot is shown (*left*). Phosphorylated bands were quantified and values expressed graphically (*right*) revealing a bell shaped concentration response curve. $^{*}p<0.05$,$^{**}p<0.01$,$^{***}p<0.001$, relative to control time. (**c**) Effect of scrambled C-peptide on ERK phosphorylation in OK cells. Cells were treated with the indicated concentrations of scrambled C-peptide for 5 min and total ERK or pERK detected by immunoblotting. A representative blot is shown. Within the graphs data are means ± SEM, $n=3$, and *black triangles* represent total ERK, *black squares* represent phospho-ERK1, and *black circles* represent phospho-ERK2

significantly enhancing cell proliferation [38]. Furthermore, all of these events were sensitive to pertussis toxin providing further evidence of the likely presence of a GPCR for C-peptide. The absence of these C-peptide-mediated growth effects in kidney tubular cells may be of key importance in C-peptide deficient patients with T1DM and diabetic nephropathy, where tubular cell loss and tubular atrophy are prominent.

Very recently, C-peptide has been found promote translocation of the low molecular weight GTP-binding protein, RhoA, from the cytoplasm to the membrane of human kidney proximal tubular cells [39], an effect that was completely reliant on the upstream activation of phospholipase C (PLC). Indeed, in these cells the activation of ERK, JNK and PKC-ε and -δ were each sensitive to PLC inhibition, indicating an obligate dependency on upstream PLC activation by C-peptide. In agreement with other signaling studies all the stimulatory effects of C-peptide were pertussis toxin sensitive [39].

Therefore signal transduction pathways through which C-peptide activates MAPK can now be described in some detail: (1) C-peptide binds to a pertussis toxin sensitive GPCR; (2) PLC is activated; (3) subsequent increases in diacylglycerol and intracellular Ca^{2+} levels stimulate several PKC isoforms; (4) RhoA is translocated to the plasma membrane and activated in a PKC dependent process; and (5) MAPKs are phosphorylated and activated.

C-Peptide Activation of PI-3-Kinase

The PI-3-kinases are a family of enzymes that phosphorylate the hydroxyl group at the 3 position of the inositol ring of phosphatidylinositol and regulate multiple cellular functions such as growth, proliferation, survival, differentiation, motility and intracellular trafficking [40]. Many functions of PI-3-kinases are linked to their ability to activate protein kinase B (Akt). The PI-3-kinases comprise key components of insulin signaling pathways and are of substantial interest in diabetes [40].

Robust activation of PI-3-kinase by physiological concentrations of C-peptide has now been demonstrated in multiple cell types including OK cells [38], Swiss 3T3 fibroblasts [36], SH-SY5Y neuroblastoma cells [41], human $CD4^+$ T cells [42] and L6 myoblasts [43]. In $CD4^+$ lymphocytes PI-3-kinase is activated via Src kinase, and in turn activates several members of the Rho-GTPase family [42, 44]. As a result both Rho and LIM kinases are stimulated which in turn impact on myosin light chain and cofilin respectively to support cell body contraction and migration [44]. As a direct consequence of this signaling it is now recognized that stimulation of PI-3-kinase by C-peptide acting alone is responsible for: (1) enhancement of neuronal and kidney tubular cell proliferation [38, 41]; (2) increased T cell migration [42]; (3) stimulation of peroxisome proliferator activated receptor-γ(PPARγ) in kidney tubule cells and associated gene transcription [45]; and (4) up-regulated glycogen synthesis in skeletal muscle cells [43].

Effects of C-Peptide on Transcription Factors

Activation of cell signaling pathways by bioactive mediators very commonly leads to alterations in gene transcription and protein expression with resultant changes in cell phenotype and function. In the light of the evidence described above for activation of cell signaling cascades, it is unsurprising to discover that C-peptide regulates activity of multiple cell transcription factors. Kitamura et al. described C-peptide mediated activation by phosphorylation of CREB, ATF-1 and ATF-2 in LEII cells [37] where 1 nM C-peptide and the positive control phorbol ester were equipotent. Activated CREB and ATF proteins are transcription factors that bind to specific response elements, CRE, in DNA thereby regulating gene transcription. Although the specific genes subject to regulation were not studied, gel mobility shift assays clearly demonstrated the binding of CREB to CRE in C-peptide treated cells [37]. In the studies of Lee et al. [32] in macrophages, induction of nitrite production and iNOS expression by C-peptide was accompanied by phosphorylation and activation of Janus activated kinase (JAK)/signal transducer and activated transcription pathway (STAT) [32]. These data strongly support a role for C-peptide in regulating gene transcription.

Further to the above evidence derived from endothelial cells, studies in neuroblastoma cells show that incubation with C-peptide enhanced expression and translocation of nuclear factor-κB (NF-κB) and expression of the Bcl_2 protein, a central mediator of NF-κB regulated anti-apoptotic effects [41]. Activity of NF-κB is also modulated by C-peptide in Swiss 3T3 cells where 1 nM C-peptide activates PKC and consequently NF-κB dependent transcription of cyclooxygenase-2 (COX-2) [46]. COX-2 is a cytokine inducible gene and the rate-limiting enzyme in the conversion of arachidonic acid to prostaglandin, although the potential consequences of its up-regulation by C-peptide remain unclear.

We performed detailed studies of transcription factor activation in the immortalized kidney proximal tubule derived OK cell line [45, 47], and compared the effects of C-peptide to those of insulin whilst concentrating on the transcription factors PPARγ and NF-κB. PPARγ is a transcription factor and member of the nuclear hormone receptor family, and is the target for the insulin sensitizing thiazolidinediones drugs currently used as therapeutic agents in T2DM [48]. The cellular expression level of PPARγ may also be dynamically regulated by insulin [49]. Using transient transfection of a peroxisome proliferator response element (PPRE)-luciferase reporter construct we showed that both C-peptide and insulin transactivated PPRE via PPARγ [45]. C-peptide (EC_{50} 4 nM) was more potent than insulin (EC_{50} 10 nM) in this regard, but phosphorylation of PPARγ evoked by both of these agents was dependent on upstream activation of PI-3-kinase. We were particularly interested to confirm that transcriptional factor activation was accompanied by altered expression of relevant gene products. Accordingly, it was observed that a consequence of PPARγ activation by C-peptide and insulin was enhanced transcription of the prototypic PPARγ regulated gene, CD36 [45].

Clearly therefore, there is at least some commonality between insulin and C-peptide signaling, with both agents' effects being directed through PI-3-kinase towards PPARγ. However, only the effects of C-peptide were attenuated by pertussis toxin, whereas the insulin effect was unaffected as would be expected of a mediator acting via a tyrosine kinase receptor system. Therefore, the evidence indicates that C-peptide must be signaling through a receptor system fundamentally distinct from that of insulin, most likely via a GPCR. These data indicate an important novel mechanism whereby C-peptide, at physiologically relevant concentrations, and insulin may interact to regulate glycemia and the expression of PPAR regulated genes such as those involved in metabolic control and inflammation.

C-Peptide Signaling in Kidney Tubular Cells and the Pathophysiology of Diabetic Nephropathy

Given the compelling evidence of C-peptide signaling in kidney cells we postulated that the lack of C-peptide in T1DM may contribute to the cellular pathophysiology of diabetic nephropathy. Therefore, we designed a series of studies to establish proof of principle that C-peptide may act as a protective agent in diabetic nephropathy. To this end we investigated the ability of C-peptide to antagonize the adverse effects of key players in the development of diabetic nephropathy, specifically the effects produced in kidney tubular cells by the administration of TNF-α or TGF-β1.

TNF-α is recognized as a major mediator driving the development of diabetic nephropathy, and may contribute to tubular cell apoptosis and tubular atrophy prominently observed in diabetic nephropathy [50–53]. As a pleiotropic peptide cytokine, TNF-α is capable of eliciting a wide spectrum of cellular responses including differentiation, proliferation, inflammation, and cell death by interacting with two members of the TNF receptor family, TNF-R1 and TNF-R2 [52]. Produced mainly by monocytes/macrophages, but also by T and B-lymphocytes and glomerular mesangial cells [53, 54], TNF-α binding to the TNF-R1 may both trigger pro-apoptotic pathways by recruitment of death effector adaptor molecules and subsequent caspase activation, and anti-apoptotic pathways through a pathway involving TNF receptor-associated factor2 (TRAF2) and nuclear factor-κB (NF-κB). How these events are integrated determines the eventual cellular response to TNF-α stimulation. In particular, NF-κB regulates transcription of anti-apoptotic factors that can modulate the caspase cascade, and thus NF-κB acts as a checkpoint in a cell's decision to survive or undergo programmed cell death in response to a given stimulus.

When TNF-α is applied to OK cells, markedly reduced viability and induction of apoptosis is observed [47], but this is completely prevented by pretreatment with either insulin or C-peptide. Both insulin and C-peptide activated NF-κB simultaneously, but insulin produced a typical sigmoidal dose response curve with maximal NF-κB activation 100 nM insulin, whereas C-peptide produced a completely different bell shaped curve of NF-κB stimulation, maximal with an applied C-peptide concentration of 5 nM. Pertussis toxin pretreatment had no effect on insulin mediated actions, but was able to substantially block C-peptide effect. These studies also revealed that the ability of C-peptide to prevent TNF-α induced apoptosis was closely associated with its ability to induce the expression, via NF-κB activation, of cell survival genes such as TRAF2 [47].

An overwhelming body of evidence now implicates TGF-β1 as a predominant factor mediating renal injury in diabetic nephropathy manifest predominantly as marked PTC phenotypic changes with tubular atrophy and tubulo-interstitial fibrosis [55, 56]. In diabetes, PTC are stimulated to produce TGF-β1 by a combination of synergistic factors including high glucose and advanced glycation end products [57, 58]. In the proximal tubule, TGF-β1 is a key mediator of epithelial mesenchymal transformation (EMT) whereby epithelial cells lose their healthy differentiated phenotype and assume a myofibroblast-like appearance and functions. This process contributes to tubular atrophy and the development of fibrosis, and results from TGF-β1 mediated modulation of the expression of several epithelial cell recognition and organizational proteins, including the cadherins [59], catenins and the actin cytoskeleton [60]. Therefore, blockade of TGF-β1 actions is a key therapeutic target in diabetic nephropathy.

Application of C-peptide to HK-2 immortalized human proximal tubular cells mitigates the typical TGF-β1-mediated phenotypic and cytoskeletal changes observed at the light microscope level [61]. Phenomena such as TGF-β1-induced loss of the epithelial differentiation marker E-cadherin and up-regulation of the stress protein vimentin in PTC are both blocked by C-peptide (Fig. 4.2). Furthermore, C-peptide also abrogates the up-regulation of expression of both type I and type II TGF-β1 receptors characteristically seen in response to TGF-β1, and in addition abolishes TGF-β1-mediated phosphorylation and transcriptional activity of Smads-2 and -3 [61]. As in previous studies pertussis toxin pretreatment inhibited the actions of C-peptide.

In order to identify PTC genes regulated by C-peptide we performed microarray gene expression profiling in the human proximal cell line, HK-2 [62]. After 48 h exposure to 5 nM C-peptide 1,458 genes showed ≥2 fold change in expression (712 up and 746 down). Following exposure to TGF-β1 for 48 h, there were changes in expression of 1,207 genes ≥2 fold (588 up and 619 down) compared to control conditions. Compared to TGF-β1 alone, cells treated with TGF-β1 and C-peptide together displayed ≥2 fold change in expression of 1,026 genes ($p<0.05$, 506 up and 520 down).

From the list of genes demonstrating >2 fold up- or down-regulation a search was performed for candidates potentially associated with propagation of, or protection from TGF-β1-mediated tubular injury and fibrosis in diabetic nephropathy. Seven genes related to retinoid and hepatocyte growth factor (HGF) signaling were identified (Table 4.2). These genes were of particular interest because recent evidence proposes retinoids as anti-fibrotic agents that may anatagonize the deleterious effects of TGF-β1 on kidney cells acting via HGF [63]. These genes demonstrated either potentially favorable regulation by C-peptide, or deleterious regulation by TGF-β1, or deleterious regulation by TGF-β1 that was antagonized by C-peptide, or a mixture of these effects. These results therefore led us to address the possibility that 9-*cis* RA and HGF may mediate the C-peptide-induced inhibition of TGF-β1-dependent changes of EMT in PTC. Our studies [62] subsequently demonstrated that C-peptide prevented TGF-β1-induced up-regulation of Snail, the transcriptional repressor of E-cadherin, and consequently downregulation of E-cadherin itself (Fig. 4.3). Taken together these results revealed that: (1) C-peptide stimulates

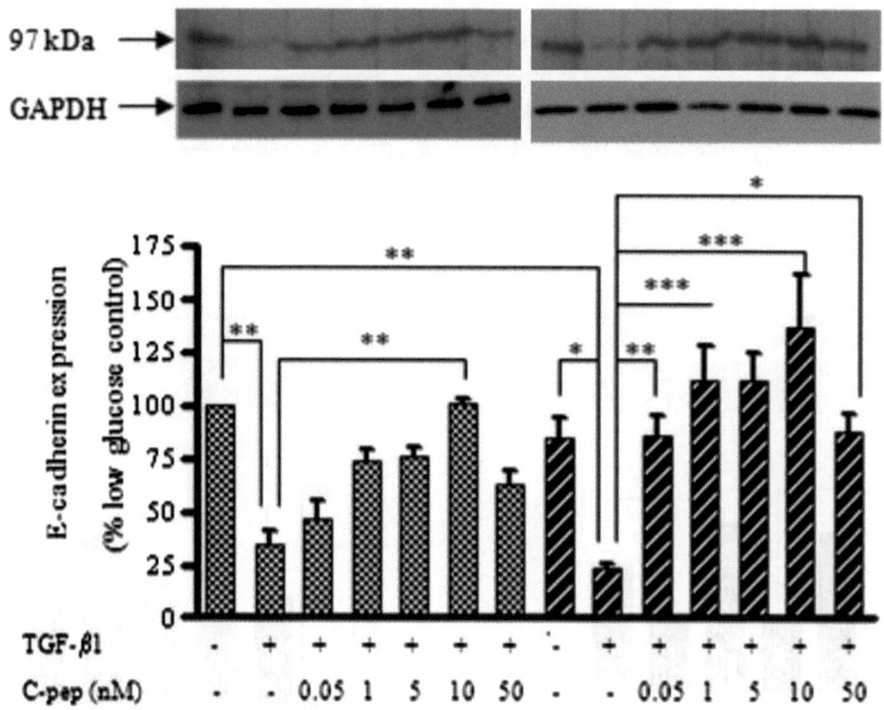

Fig. 4.2 C-peptide reverses TGF-β1 induced changes in E-cadherin expression in HK-2 cells (adapted from Hills et al. [61]). HK-2 cells were grown in low or high glucose alone, or together either with 2 ng/mL TGFβ-1 alone or 2 ng/mL TGFβ-1 and the indicated concentrations of C-peptide, and cell levels of E-cadherin determined by immunoblotting. *Upper panels* are representative immunoblots (low glucose – *left pair*, high glucose – *right pair*) showing E-cadherin expression (*upper blots*) or the same blots stripped and re-probed for GAPDH as a loading control (*lower blots*). Blots were quantified by densitometry and the nonstimulated low glucose control condition normalized to 100% and all other conditions compared to this. *Lower panel* shows the results of densitometry of ≥3 blots. Each *bar* in the histogram represents the same condition in the blots above, chequered pattern is low glucose and cross hatched pattern is high glucose. Key significances are shown, $*p<0.05$, $**p<0.01$, $***p<0.001$

Table 4.2 Changes in expression of retinoic acid and hepatocyte growth factor signaling components in response to C-peptide and/or TGFβ-1

Gene (Homo Sapiens)	Experimental condition			
	C-peptide[a] vs. control (18 h)	C-peptide[a] vs. control (48 h)	TGFβ-1[a] vs. control (48 h)	C-peptide + TGFβ-1[a] vs. TGFβ-1 (48 h)
Cellular retinoic acid binding protein 1 (CRABPI), mRNA	−3.15	−3.0	<±2	−3.1
Cellular retinoic acid binding protein 2 (CRABPII), mRNA	<±2	<±2	<±2	2.9
Retinoic acid receptor, beta (RARβ), transcript variant 1, mRNA	<±2	76	4.8	6.1
Predicted: similar to retinoic acid receptor γ-A (RAR-γ-A) (LOC654040), mRNA	2.2	<±2	−14	7.6
Retinoic acid induced 2	<±2	<±2	−2.3	2.9
Hepatocyte growth factor (hepapoietin A; scatter factor) (HGF), transcript variant 3, mRNA	<±2	32	−9	<±2
Retinoid X receptor, γ (RXRγ), transcript variant 1, mRNA	<±2	<±2	<±2	4.8

Adapted from Hills et al. [62]

[a]*Numbers* represent fold change under condition noted with a *superscript letter* compared to second condition. *Negative numbers* indicate down-regulation by condition noted with *superscript letter a*. Where there was no change in gene expression, either up or down, between conditions or a fold change less than 2, this is indicated as less than ±2

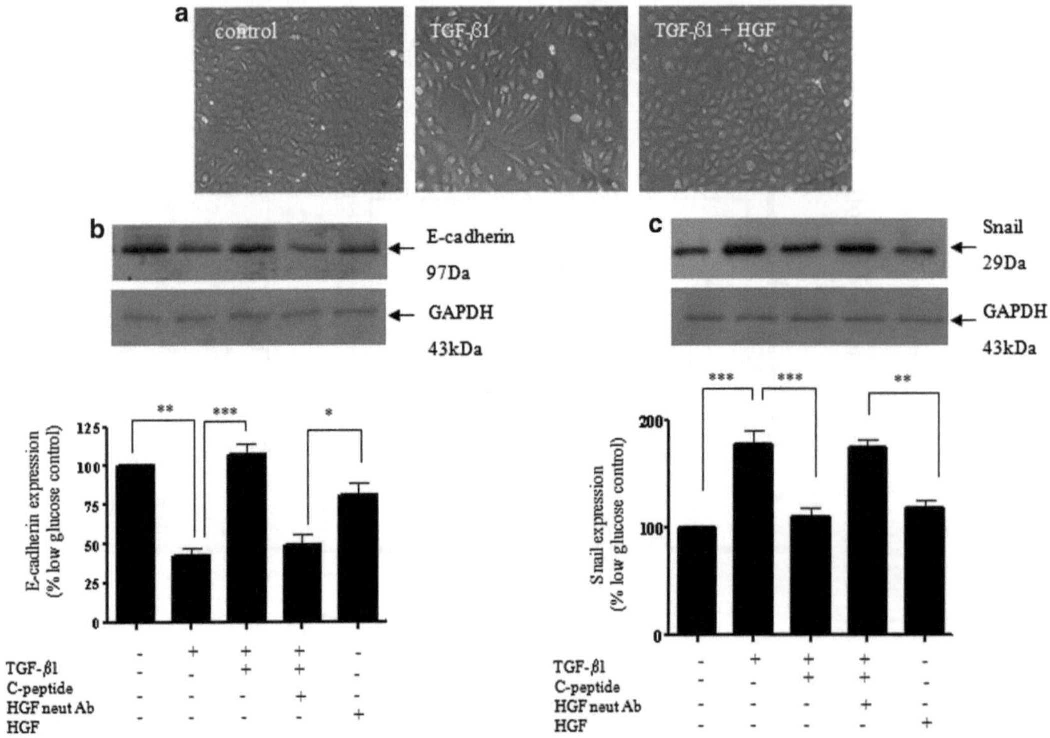

Fig. 4.3 Neutralization of HGF abolishes the C-peptide-mediated reversal of TGF-β1-induced reductions in E-cadherin and Snail expression in HK-2 PTC (adapted from Hills et al. [62]). Assessment of HK-2 morphology was used to determine the anti-fibrotic effects of HGF. Cells were examined by phase contrast microscopy. HK-2 cells were cultured for 48 h under low glucose conditions in control media, in the presence of TGFβ-1 (2 ng/mL) alone, or in combination with HGF (40 ng/mL). (**a**) Representative images are shown (magnification 40×). HK-2 cells were cultured for 48 h in the absence or presence of either TGF-β1 (2 ng/mL), C-peptide (5 nM), HGF (40 ng/mL) or HGF neutralizing antibody (1 μg/mL). The expression levels of E-cadherin (**b**) and Snail (**c**) were then determined by immunoblotting. The upper parts of panels (**b**) and (**c**) are representative immunoblots showing E-cadherin and Snail expression (*upper blots*) or the same blots stripped and re-probed for GAPDH as a loading control (*lower blots*). Band intensities were quantified by densitometry and the nonstimulated, low (glucose) control condition normalized to 100% and all other conditions compared to this. The *lower part* of the panel shows the mean + SEM derived from densitometry of three blots. Each *bar* in the histogram represents the same condition in the blots above. Key significances are shown, $*p<0.05$, $**p<0.01$, $***p<0.001$, $n=3$

expression of HGF and several components of the RA signaling pathway; (2) 9-*cis* RA inhibits TGF-β1-induced changes in expression of the epithelial marker E-cadherin and its transcriptional repressor Snail in a manner similar to C-peptide; (3) 9-*cis* RA blocks TGF-β1-induced up-regulation of vimentin expression whilst preventing the release of β-catenin from the cell periphery in a manner similar to C-peptide; (4) 9-*cis* RA stimulates HGF expression as does C-peptide, and finally (5) the ability of C-peptide to reverse both TGF-β1-induced PTC morphology and changes in expression of both E-cadherin and Snail is dependent on HGF signaling. Therefore, these results indicate a key role for 9-*cis*-RA and HGF in the antagonism of the fibrogenic action of TGF-β1 in HK-2 cells. Further, they support the hypothesis that the anti-fibrotic effects of C-peptide in EMT are driven by downstream enhancement of expression and activity of several elements of RA signaling pathways, which in turn promote increased HGF activity thus negating the pathological effects of TGF-β1.

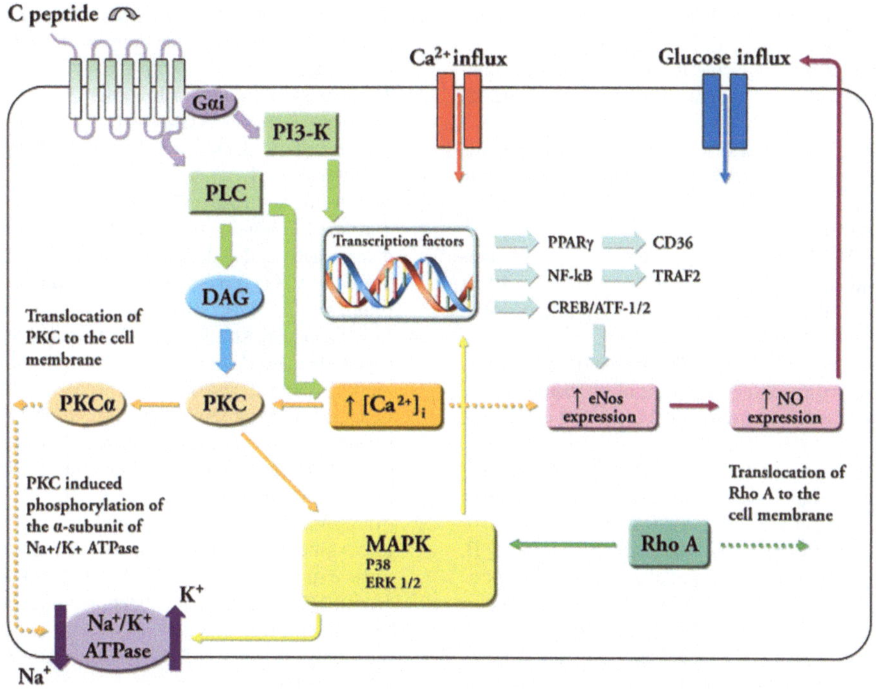

Fig. 4.4 Schematic representation of cellular signaling effects of C-peptide (adapted from Hills and Brunskill [65]). Available evidence suggests that C-peptide binds to a cell membrane receptor which is coupled to a pertussis toxin sensitive G-protein. Activation of this G-protein coupled receptor stimulates both PLC and PI3-K. PLC activation evokes an increase in $[Ca^{2+}]_i$, resulting in the concomitant activation of both endothelial nitric oxide synthase (eNOS) and PKC, the latter of which, together with increased de novo synthesis of DAG stimulates activation of the Na^+,K^+-ATPase via PKCα translocation to the cell membrane. Stimulation of the MAPK pathway also results in both, increased Na^+,K^+-ATPase activity and activation of various transcription factors. Together with the elevated PI3-K levels, MAPK induced transcription factor expression is increased and effects including reduced apoptosis, increased eNOS and CD36 levels are observed (for abbreviations see text)

Summary and Conclusions

Overall the current evidence confirms without doubt that C-peptide is a bioactive peptide with multiple signaling effects (see Fig. 4.4 for a summary of signaling pathways affected). As a consequence C-peptide has a profound influence on gene expression and hence cell phenotype and function. Most importantly however the integration of these effects results in changes in the cellular environment likely to counter the pathophysiological stimuli relevant to the development and pathology of diabetic nephropathy. As such development of C-peptide towards the clinical arena is an important goal in the prevention of diabetic complications.

References

1. Johansson B-L, Borg K, Fernqvist-Forbes E, et al. Beneficial effects of C-peptide on incipient nephropathy and neuropathy in patients with type I diabetes. Diabet Med. 2000;17:181–9.
2. Samnegård B, Jacobson S, Jaremko G, et al. C-peptide prevents glomerular hypertrophy and mesangial matrix expansion in diabetic rats. Nephrol Dial Transplant. 2005;20:532–8.
3. Ekberg K, Brismar T, Johansson B-L, et al. Amelioration of sensory nerve dysfunction by C-peptide in patients with type 1 diabetes. Diabetes. 2003;52:536–41.
4. Ekberg K, Brismar T, Johansson B-L, et al. C-peptide replacement therapy and sensory nerve function in type 1 diabetes neuropathy. Diabetes Care. 2007;30: 71–6.

5. Johansson B-L, Linde B, Wahren J. Effects of C-peptide on blood flow, capillary diffusion capacity and glucose utilization in the exercising forearm of type I (insulin-dependent) diabetic patients. Diabetologia. 1992;35: 1151–8.
6. Johansson B-L, Sundell J, Ekberg K, et al. C-peptide improves adenosine-induced myocardial vasodilation in type 1 diabetes patients. Am J Physiol Endocrinol Metab. 2004;286:E14–9.
7. Stevens M, Zhang W, Li F, Sima A. C-peptide corrects endoneurial blood flow but not oxidative stress in type 1 BB/Wor rats. Am J Physiol Endocrinol Metab. 2004;287:E497–505.
8. Flatt PR, Swanston-Flatt SK, Hampton SM, et al. Specific binding of the C-peptide of proinsulin to cultured B-cells from a transplantable rat islet cell tumor. Biosci Rep. 1986;6:193–9.
9. Rigler R, Pramanik A, Jonasson P, et al. Specific binding of proinsulin C-peptide to human cell membranes. Proc Natl Acad Sci U S A. 1999;96:13318–23.
10. Ohtomo Y, Bergman T, Johansson BL, Jörnvall H, Wahren J. Differential effects of proinsulin C-peptide fragments on Na+, K+-ATPase activity of renal tubule segments. Diabetologia. 1998;41:287–91.
11. Wahren J, Ekberg K, Johansson J, et al. Role of C-peptide in human physiology. Am J Physiol. 2000;278:E759–68.
12. Henriksson M, Nordling E, Melles E, et al. Separate functional features of proinsulin C-peptide. Cell Mol Life Sci. 2005;62:1772–8.
13. Luzi L, Zerbini G, Caumo A. C-peptide: a redundant relative of insulin? Diabetologia. 2007;50:500–2.
14. Wald HP, Scherzer P, Rasch R, Popovtzer MM. Renal tubular Na+, K+-ATPase in diabetes mellitus: relationship to metabolic abnormality. Am J Physiol. 1993;265:E96–101.
15. Raccah D, Lamotte-Jannot MF, Issautier T, Vague P. Effect of experimental diabetes on Na/K-ATPase activity in red blood cells, peripheral nerve and kidney. Diabetes Metab. 1994;20:271–4.
16. Raccah D, Lamotte-Jannot MF, Issautier T, Vague P. Erythrocyte Na(+)-K(+)-ATPase activity, metabolic control, and neuropathy in IDDM patients. Diabetes Care. 1996;19:564–8.
17. Gerbi A, Barbey O, Raccah D, et al. Alteration of Na, K-ATPase isoenzymes in diabetic cardiomyopathy: effect of dietary supplementation with fish oil (n-3 fatty acids) in rats. Diabetologia. 1997;40:496–505.
18. Ohtomo Y, Aperia A, Sahlgren B, Johansson BL, Wahren J. C-peptide stimulates rat renal tubular Na+, K+-ATPase activity in synergism with neuropeptide Y. Diabetologia. 1996;39:199–205.
19. Dufayet De La Tour D, Raccah D, et al. Erythrocyte Na/K ATPase activity and diabetes: relationship with C-peptide level. Diabetologia. 1998;41:1080–4.
20. Forst T, Dufayet De La Tour D, Kunt T, et al. Effects of proinsulin C-peptide on nitric oxide, microvascular blood flow and erythrocyte Na+, K+-ATPase activity in diabetes mellitus type. Clin Sci. 2000;98:283–90.
21. Ido Y, Vindigni A, Chang K, et al. Prevention of vascular and neural dysfunction in diabetic rats by C-peptide. Science. 1997;277:563–6.
22. Tsimaratos M, Roger F, Chabardès D, et al. C-peptide stimulates Na+, K+-ATPase activity via PKC alpha in rat medullary thick ascending limb. Diabetologia. 2003;46:124–31.
23. Maestroni A, Ruggieri D, Dell'Antonio G, Luzi L, Zerbini G. C-peptide increases the expression of vasopressin-activated calcium-mobilizing receptor gene through a G protein-dependent pathway. Eur J Endocrinol. 2005;152:135–41.
24. Li L, Oshida Y, Kusunoki M, Yamanouchi K, et al. Rat C peptide I and II stimulate glucose utilization in STZ-induced diabetic rats. Diabetologia. 1999;42:958–64.
25. Etgen GJ, Fryburg DA, Gibbs EM. Nitric oxide stimulates skeletal muscle glucose transport through a calcium/contraction- and phosphatidylininositol-3 kinase-independent pathway. Diabetes. 1997;46:1915–9.
26. Young ME, Radda GK, Leighton B. Nitric oxide stimulates glucose transport and metabolism in rat skeletal muscle in vitro. Biochem J. 1997;322:223–8.
27. Jensen ME, Messina EJ. C-peptide induces a concentration-dependent dilation of skeletal muscle arterioles only in presence of insulin. Am J Physiol. 1999;276:H1223–8.
28. Joshua IG, Zhang Q, Falcone JC, et al. Mechanisms of endothelial dysfunction with development of type 1 diabetes mellitus: role of insulin and C-peptide. J Cell Biochem. 2005;96:1149–56.
29. Wallerath T, Kunt T, Forst T, et al. Stimulation of endothelial nitric oxide synthase by proinsulin C-peptide. Nitric Oxide. 2003;9:95–102.
30. Kitamura T, Kimura K, Makondo K, et al. Proinsulin C peptide increases nitric oxide production by enhancing mitogen-activated protein-kinase dependent transcription of endothelial nitric oxide synthase in aortic endothelial cells of Wistar rats. Diabetologia. 2003;46:1698–705.
31. Scalia R, Coyle K, Levine B, Booth G, Lefer A. C peptide inhibits leukocyte-endothelium interaction in the microcirculation during endothelial dysfunction. FASEB J. 2000;14:2357–64.
32. Lee SK, Lee JO, Kim JH, et al. C-peptide stimulates nitrites generation via the calcium-JAK2/STAT1 pathway in murine macrophage Raw264.7 cells. Life Sci. 2010;86:863–8.
33. Chang L, Karin M. Mammalian MAP kinase signaling cascades. Nature. 2001;410:37–40.
34. Chen Z, Gibson TB, Robinson F, et al. MAP kinases. Chem Rev. 2001;101:2449–76.
35. Turjanski AG, Vaqué JP, Gutkin JS. MAP kinases and the control of nuclear events. Oncogene. 2007;26: 3240–53.
36. Kitamura T, Kimura K, Jung BD, et al. Proinsulin C peptide rapidly stimulates mitogen activated protein kinases in Swiss 3T3 fibroblasts: requirement of protein phosphoinositide 3-kinase and pertussi toxin-sensitive G protein. Biochem J. 2001;355:123–9.

37. Kitamura T, Kimura K, Jung BD, et al. Proinsulin C peptide activates cAMP response element binding proteins through the p38 mitogen-activated protein kinase pathway in mouse lung capillary endothelial cells. Biochem J. 2002;366:737–44.
38. Al-Rasheed NM, Meakin F, Royal EL, Lewington AJ, Brown J, Willars GB, et al. Potent activation of multiple signaling pathways by C peptide in opossum kidney proximal tubular cells. Diabetologia. 2004;47:987–97.
39. Zhong Z, Davidescu A, Ehren I, et al. C peptide stimulates ERK 1/2 and JNK MAP kinases via activation of protein kinase C in human renal tubular cells. Diabetologia. 2005;48:187–97.
40. Vanhaesebroeck B, Leevers SJ, Ahmadi K, et al. Synthesis and function of 3-phosphorylated inositol lipids. Annu Rev Biochem. 2001;70:535–602.
41. Li Z-G, Zhang W, Sima AAF. C-peptide enhances insulin-mediated cell growth and protection against high glucose-induced apoptosis in SH-SY5Y cells. Diabetes Metab Res Rev. 2003;19:375–85.
42. Walcher D, Aleksic M, Jerg V, et al. C-peptide induces chemotaxis of human CD4-positive cells. Involvement of pertussis toxin–sensitive G-proteins and phosphoinositide 3-kinase. Diabetes. 2004;53:1664–70.
43. Grunberger G, Qiang X, Li Z, Mathews S, et al. Molecular basis for the insulinometric effects of C peptide. Diabetologia. 2001;44:1247–57.
44. Aleksic M, Walcher D, Giehl K, Bach H, Grub M, Durst R, et al. Signaling processes involved in C-peptide induced chemotaxis of CD4-positive lymphocytes. Cell Mol Life Sci. 2009;66:1974–84.
45. Al-Rasheed NM, Chana RS, Baines RJ, Willars GB, Brunskill NJ. Ligand-independent activation of peroxisome proliferator-activated receptor-gamma by insulin and C-peptide in kidney proximal tubular cells: dependent on phosphatidylinositol 3-kinase activity. J Biol Chem. 2004;279:49747–54.
46. Kitazawa M, Shibata Y, Hashimoto S, Ohizumi Y, Yamakuni T. Proinsulin C-peptide stimulates a PKC/IκB/NFκB signaling pathway to activate COX-1 gene transcription in Swiss 3T3 fibroblasts. J Biochem. 2006;139:1083–8.
47. Al Rasheed NM, Willars GB, Brunskill NJ. C-peptide signals via $G\alpha_i$ to protect against TNF-alpha-mediated apoptosis of opossum kidney proximal tubular cells. J Am Soc Nephrol. 2006;17:986–95.
48. Willson TM, Lambert MH, Kliewer SA. Peroxisome proliferator-activated receptor-γ and metabolic disease. Annu Rev Biochem. 2001;70:341–67.
49. Rieusset J, Andreelli F, Auboeuf D, et al. Insulin acutely regulates the expression of the peroxisome proliferator-activated receptor-gamma in human adipocytes. Diabetes. 1999;48:699–705.
50. Kalantarinia K, Awad AS, Siragy HM. Urinary and renal interstitial concentrations of TNF-alpha increase prior to the rise in albuminuria in diabetic rats. Kidney Int. 2003;64:1208–13.
51. Moriwaki Y, Yamamoto T, Shibutani Y, et al. Elevated level of interleukin-18 and tumor necrosis factor-alpha in serum of patients with type 2 diabetes mellitus: relationship with diabetic nephropathy. Metabolism. 2003;52:605–8.
52. Wajant H, Pfizenmaier K, Scheurich P. Tumor necrosis factor signaling. Cell Death Differ. 2003;10:45–65.
53. Baud L, Oudinet JP, Bens M, et al. Production of tumor necrosis factor by rat mesangial cells in response to bacterial lipopolysaccharide. Kidney Int. 1989;35:1111–8.
54. Hruby ZW, Lowry RP. Spontaneous release of tumor necrosis factor alpha by isolated renal glomeruli and cultured glomerular mesangial cells. Clin Immunol Immunopathol. 1991;59:156–64.
55. Kanwar YS, Wada J, Sun L, et al. Diabetic nephropathy: mechanisms of renal disease progression. Exp Biol Med. 2008;233:4–11.
56. Sharma K, Ziyadeh FN. Hyperglycaemia and diabetic kidney disease. The case for transforming growth factor-beta as a key mediator. Diabetes. 1995;44:1139–46.
57. Oldfield MD, Bach LA, Forbes JM, et al. Advanced glycation end products cause epithelial-myofibroblast transdifferentiation via the receptor for advanced glycation end products (RAGE). J Clin Invest. 2001;108:1853–63.
58. Qi W, Chen X, Zhang Y, et al. High glucose induces macrophage inflammatory protein-3 alpha in renal proximal tubule cells via a transforming growth factor-beta 1 dependent mechanism. Nephrol Dial Transplant. 2007;11:3147–53.
59. Tian YC, Fraser D, Attisano L, Philips AO. TGF-beta 1 mediated alterations of renal proximal tubular epithelial cell phenotype. Am J Physiol. 2003;285:F130–42.
60. Humes HD, Nakamura T, Cieslinski DA, et al. Role of proteoglycans and cytoskeleton in the effects of TGF-beta 1 on renal proximal tubule cells. Kidney Int. 1993;43:575–84.
61. Hills CE, Al-Rasheed N, Al-Rasheed N, Willars GB, Brunskill NJ. C-peptide reverses TGF-beta1-induced changes in renal proximal tubular cells: implications for treatment of diabetic nephropathy. Am J Physiol. 2009;296:F614–21.
62. Hills CE, Willars GB, Brunskill NJ. Proinsulin C-peptide antagonizes the pro-fibrotic effects of TGF-β1 via up-regulation of retinoic acid and HGF-related signaling pathways. Mol Endocrinol. 2010;24:822–31.
63. Wen X, Li Y, Hu K, Dai C, Liu Y. Hepatocyte growth factor receptor signaling mediates the anti-fibrotic action of 9-cis-retinoic acid in glomerular mesangial cells. Am J Pathol. 2005;167:947–57.
64. Hills CE, Brunskill NJ. Intracellular signaling by C-peptide. Exp Diabetes Res. 2008, Article ID 635158. doi:10.1155/2008/635158.
65. Hills CE, Brunskill NJ. Cellular and physiological effects of C-peptide. Clin Sci. 2009;116:565–74.

Role of C-Peptide in the Regulation of Microvascular Blood Flow

5

Thomas Forst, Matthias M. Weber, Thomas Kunt, and Andreas Pfützner

Keywords
C-peptide • Microcirculation • Endothelial function • Blood flow

Introduction

Patients with type 1 diabetes mellitus present with an excessive risk for microvascular complications such as retinopathy, nephropathy, and peripheral neuropathy. Endothelial dysfunction is an early feature of vascular disease in patients with type 1 diabetes mellitus. Although elevated blood glucose levels were shown to predict the risk of microvascular complications in type 1 diabetic patients [1], even in patients with good metabolic control, microvascular complications cannot be prevented. Therefore, additional factors beyond glucose control are thought to contribute to the pathogenesis of microvascular complications. Endothelial dysfunction and low-grade inflammation are early features of vascular disease in patients with type 1 diabetes mellitus [2, 3] and precede the development of microvascular complications like retinopathy, nephropathy, and neuropathy. Endothelial dysfunction is characterized by an impaired flow mediated dilatation (FMD) [2], low grade inflammation [4], increased expression of endothelial cell adhesion molecules [4, 5], and the generation of reactive oxygen species (ROS) [6]. ROS attack endothelial cells directly through an inflammatory process and by deactivation of nitric oxide (NO) [7, 8]. An increase in leucocyte-endothelial interactions, increased blood viscosity, and a deterioration in the rheologic properties of blood further add to microcirculatory breakdown and development of tissue damage.

In recent years, C-peptide has been found to have effects on vascular biological activities, including an improvement in endothelial function and microvascular blood flow [9–12]. C-peptide circulates in nanomolar concentrations in healthy individuals, but is almost lacking in type 1 diabetic patients. In the DCCT trial, type 1 diabetic patients with sustained C-peptide secretion showed a significant lower risk for retinopathy or

T. Forst (✉)
Medical Department, Institute for Clinical Research and Development, Parcusstrasse 8, 55116, Mainz, Germany

Department of Endocrinology and Metabolism, Johannes Gutenberg University, Mainz, Germany
e-mail: thomasf@ikfe.de

M.M. Weber
Department of Endocrinology and Metabolism, Johannes Gutenberg University, Mainz, Germany

T. Kunt
Diabetes Center, Berlin, Germany

A. Pfützner
Medical Department, Institute for Clinical Research and Development, Parcusstrasse 8, 55116, Mainz, Germany

A.A.F. Sima (ed.), *Diabetes & C-Peptide: Scientific and Clinical Aspects*, Contemporary Diabetes, DOI 10.1007/978-1-61779-391-2_5, © Springer Science+Business Media, LLC 2012

microalbuminuria compared with those without any residual C-peptide secretion [13, 14]. Even modest beta cell activity was associated with a lower rate of microvascular complications. In a recent cross sectional study, 471 type 1 diabetic patients were followed from 1994 to 2004 [15]. Those patients with the lowest fasting C-peptide levels were found to have the highest rates of microvascular complications. In recent years, numerous efforts have been undertaken to clarify the molecular basis for C-peptides vascular effects.

Effects of C-Peptide on Nitric Oxide (NO)

NO, which is synthesized within the endothelial cell through conversion of the amino acid, l-arginine to l-citrulline by the enzyme endothelial nitric oxide synthase (eNOS), was identified as a powerful vasodilator in the micro- and macrovasculature [16]. The activity of eNOS is regulated by Ca^{2+}-calmodulin. NO triggers the relaxation of vascular smooth muscle cells by increasing generation of cyclic guanosine monophosphate (cGMP) through the induction of guanyl cyclase [17–20]. In patients with diabetes mellitus, the cGMP levels are decreased, suggesting that either the NO release or its action on guanylate cyclase is impaired [21]. In addition to vasorelaxation, NO exerts several effects on blood cells and modulates the interaction between blood cells and the vessel wall. In the blood compartment, NO evokes vasoprotective effects by reducing platelet-vascular wall interactions, reducing the adhesion of circulating monocytes to the endothelial cell and by improving rheological properties of the blood [22, 23].

As shown in Fig. 5.1, eNOS is regulated by several different substrates, all known to be altered in patients with diabetes mellitus. While insulin and C-peptide activate eNOS, hyperglycemia and oxidative stress are strong inhibitors of the NO-release from the endothelial cell. Early in the course of diabetes mellitus, NO secretion from the endothelial cell is decreased, reflecting early endothelial dysfunction and failure of the microcirculation to respond to changing perfusion demands in several tissues [24–26].

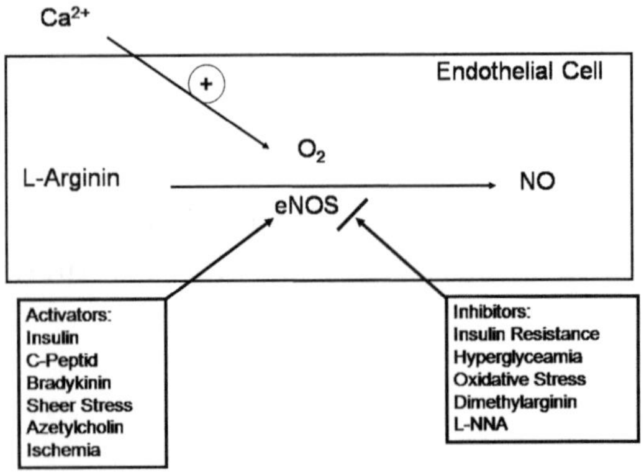

Fig. 5.1 Activators and inhibitors of endothelial NO synthase (eNOS) on the endothelial cell. l-NNA = N^G-nitro-l-arginine. Insulin, C-peptide, acetylcholine, ischemia and an increased shear stress activate the endothelial nitric oxide synthase (eNOS), while dimethylarginine, l-NNA, hyperglycemia, insulin resistance and oxidative stress production leads to an inhibition of the enzyme

In a model of type 1 diabetes mellitus, C-peptide in a range of 1–6 nM increased the release of NO from bovine aortic endothelial cells (BAEC) [27, 28]. In these investigations, C-peptide increased intracellular Ca^{2+} concentration in endothelial cells, which in turn is likely to stimulate NOS III activity. As shown in Fig. 5.2, the release of NO from the endothelial cells was completely abolished by blocking NO synthesis with l-NNA, or by binding Ca^{2+} in the cell culture medium using EDTA. These results strengthen the hypotheses that C-peptide is likely to stimulate eNOS activity by facilitating an influx of Ca^{2+} into the endothelial cell. In a study by Kitamura et al. [12] (see Chap. 6), C-peptide was shown to stimulate NO production by enhancing the mitogen-activated protein-kinase dependent transcription of eNOS in aortic endothelial cells of Wistar rats. In this study, it was shown that C-peptide increases NO release from aortic endothelial cells by enhancing eNOS expression through an ERK-dependent transcriptional pathway.

Jensen and Messina [29] demonstrated a vasodilatory effect of C-peptide in isolated rat cremaster muscle arterioles, which was abolished by the inhibition of NO synthesis using l-NNA. The vasodilatory effect of C-peptide was only obtained in the presence of insulin.

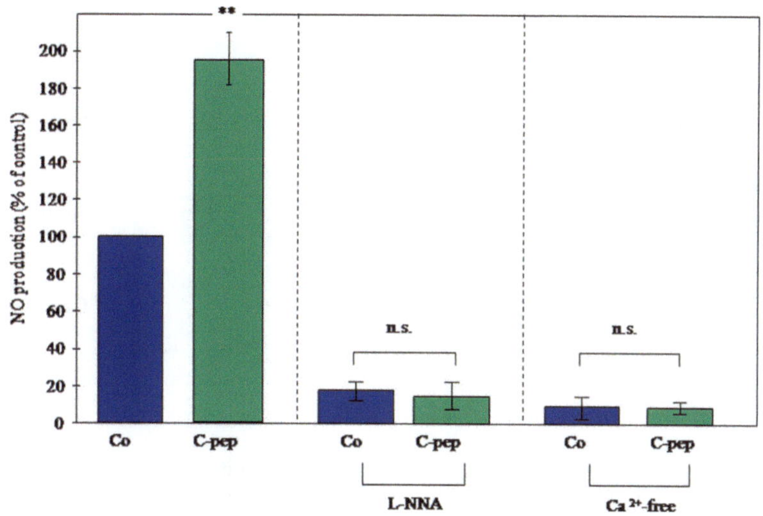

Fig. 5.2 Effect of N^G-nitro-l-arginine (l-NNA) and Ca^{2+}-free Locke's solution on NO release from nonstimulated and C-peptide-stimulated BAEC. Each column represents the mean ± SEM of four experiments, $^{**}p<0.01$ vs. control, $^{***}p<0.001$ vs. control

Many agonists such as acetylcholine are able to initiate the release of NO by increasing the calcium concentration in the endothelial cell [30]. This can be mediated by receptor activation of phospholipase C with subsequent formation of inositol triphosphate and the release of intracellular calcium stores and by enhancing the influx of extracellular calcium into the endothelial cell. Acetylcholine is a strong activator of eNOS and leads to an increased release of NO from the endothelial cell [17–19]. In C-peptide deficient type 1 diabetic patients, the microvascular response to acetylcholine in the skin was investigated during continuous intravenous C-peptide infusion. C-peptide was given at a concentration of 3 $pmol^{-1}\ kg^{-1}\ min^{-1}$ for 1 h and at a concentration of 10 $pmol\ kg^{-1}\ min^{-1}$ for a second hour. Intravenous supplementation of C-peptide in type 1 diabetic patients was found to augment the vascular response to acetylcholine as shown by an increased production of cGMP and an increase in the hyperemic response following acetylcholine. Microvascular skin blood flow as measured by laser Doppler fluxmetry increased by 133% during the low infusion rate but did not increase further during the high infusion rate of C-peptide.

Flow mediated vasodilatation (FMD) depends on an intact endothelial cell function and is considered to be mediated by NO [16]. In type 1 diabetes, FMD is known to be decreased in conduit arteries, such as the brachial or femoral arteries [22, 31, 32]. Fernqvist-Forbes et al. [33] studied the effect of C-peptide administration on FMD in response to reactive hyperemia in type 1 diabetic patients. In addition, the arterial dilatation to glyceryl trinitrate, which is an endothelium independent marker of vascular smooth muscle function, was investigated. When compared with the healthy control group, the type 1 diabetic patients revealed a lower FMD. Following C-peptide administration, blood flow in the brachial artery increased by approximately 35%, and FMD was significantly improved. No effect of C-peptide could be observed on the microvascular response to glyceryltrinitrate.

Effects of C-Peptide on Microvascular Blood Flow

In several studies, C-peptide was shown to affect microvascular blood flow and to improve nerve and renal function in animal models of type 1 diabetes and in humans with type 1 diabetes mellitus [34–37]. In a study by Lindstrom et al. [38], C-peptide supplementation was shown to increase microvascular blood flow in isolated kidneys of

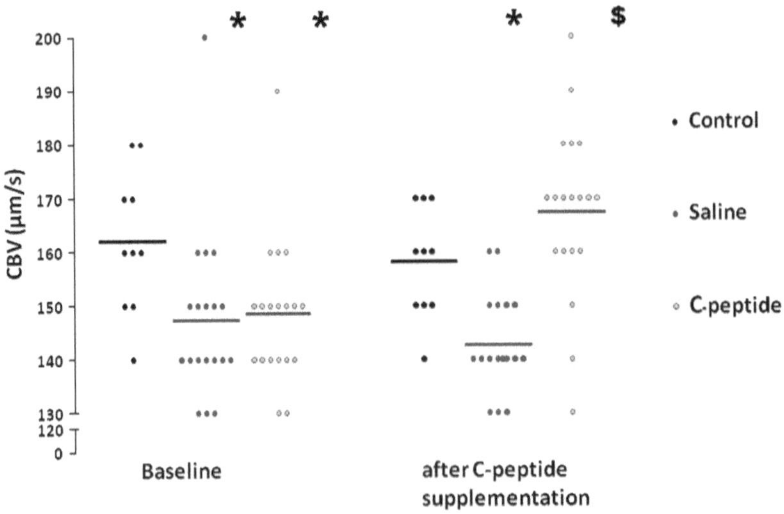

Fig. 5.3 Effect on skin microvascular blood flow at baseline and after intravenous C-peptide supplementation in healthy and in type 1 diabetic subjects. $* = p < 0.05$ vs. healthy subjects; $\$ = p < 0.05$ vs. baseline

the rat due to an increased recruitment of capillaries. In diabetic rats, biosynthetic human C-peptide, given twice daily for 5 weeks normalized blood flow in the anterior uvea, retina, and sciatic nerve [39]. In addition, C-peptide reduced ^{125}I-labeled albumin permeation in retinal and nerve tissue. The effects on microvascular neural blood flow were accompanied by an increase in caudal motor nerve conduction velocity. No effect of C-peptide, neither on microvascular blood flow nor on motor nerve conduction velocity, could be observed in healthy control rats. In accordance with these findings, Cotter et al. [34] observed an increase in sciatic endoneurial blood flow in streptozotocin diabetic rats following the supplementation of physiological C-peptide concentrations. Again, the improvement in nerve microvascular blood flow was accompanied by an improvement in nerve fiber function. Blocking eNOS using l-NNA in these experiments abolished the effects of C-peptide on microvascular blood flow and nerve function (see Chap. 8). In another study, the effect of C-peptides was investigated in skeletal muscle arterioles isolated from rat cremaster muscles [29]. In this study, C-peptide evoked a concentration dependent arteriolar dilatation in a range between 0.3 and 1,000 ng/mL. Addition of insulin at low concentrations, which had no vascular effect by its own, enhanced the vascular effect of C-peptide, indicating a permissive role of both pancreatic peptides in the regulation of microvascular blood flow.

In a study by Johansson et al. [40], C-peptide increased forearm blood flow and capillary diffusion capacity to levels similar to those observed in healthy controls. In accordance with the increase in muscle blood flow, forearm oxygen and glucose uptake increased after C-peptide administration.

In skin microvascular blood flow, the capillary circulation is functionally situated in parallel to the arteriovenous shunts and is thought to have the primary function of skin nutrition. It has been estimated that 80–90% of total skin blood flow passes through thermoregulatory arteriovenous shunts and do not enter the capillary bed [41–43]. While total skin perfusion is increased in diabetes mellitus, nutritional capillary skin blood flow was shown to be reduced in diabetic patients [41, 42, 44]. This discrepancy between nutritional and total skin microcirculation has been explained by diversion of blood through arteriovenous shunts [43, 45].

As shown in Fig. 5.3, short term infusion of C-peptide in type 1 diabetic patients was found to redistribute microvascular blood flow from the subpapillary thermoregulatory blood flow into the nutritive capillary bed [46]. At baseline, nutritive capillary blood flow was significantly lower in type 1 diabetic patients compared to the nondiabetic control group. C-peptide supplementation increased capillary blood flow to a level comparable to that observed in the healthy control group. Thirty minutes after the termination of the C-peptide infusion, capillary blood flow had declined to a level not different from baseline levels. No such effect of C-peptide administration on microvascular skin blood flow could be observed in nondiabetic subjects. A linear relationship was found between plasma C-peptide levels and the capillary blood flow velocity ($r=0.401$; $p<0.0001$).

In contrast, in a study by Polska et al. [47], no effect of C-peptide supplementation in type 1 diabetic patients could be observed on retinal blood flow. Therefore, it may be postulated that C-peptide affects microvascular blood flow in a tissue specific manner.

Effects of C-Peptide on Different Blood Cells and the Interaction between Corpuscular Blood Components and the Vascular Wall

In numerous patients, functional alterations in blood flow can be observed even at the time of diagnosis of type 1 diabetes mellitus [48, 49]. Endothelial dysfunction, increased leukocyte-endothelial adhesion [50], increased blood viscosity [51, 52], and changes in the hemodynamic properties of blood [53, 54] are found during the timecourse of type 1 diabetes mellitus. Blood flow in larger vessels is determined by vessel diameter, blood viscosity, and vessel length according to the law of Hagen-Pouiseuille. In the capillary circulation, especially, if the diameter of the vessel is below the diameter of the erythrocytes, blood flow is dominated by the viscosity and deformability of the erythrocytes. It has been shown, that factors such as decreased erythrocyte deformability and increased erythrocyte aggregation alter microvascular blood flow in patients with diabetes mellitus [51, 53–59].

In a recent study, the effect of C-peptide on erythrocytes obtained from diabetic and nondiabetic subjects was investigated under physiological (0.3–10 Pa) and supraphysiological (>10 Pa) shear stress rates by means of laser diffractoscopy [28]. The erythrocyte deformability in type 1 diabetic patients was significantly reduced compared to erythrocytes from the nondiabetic control group. Incubation of the erythrocytes with different concentrations of C-peptide completely restored erythrocyte deformability in type 1 diabetic patients, but was without any effect on erythrocytes from nondiabetic controls.

Besides the entire C-peptide molecule, the C-terminal fragments of the peptide were also shown to exert physiological effects in several tissues and cell types [39, 60]. Therefore, the physiological effects of C-peptide and the C-terminal fragments of C-peptide on erythrocyte deformability were studied. Incubation of the red blood cells from type 1 diabetes patients with C-peptide completely restored the erythrocyte deformability at all shear stress ranges [23]. Incubation with the C-terminal penta- and hexapeptide also improved erythrocyte deformability, which was not significantly different from that obtained with the entire peptide. In contrast, the middle fragment and the scrambled C-peptide failed to exert any effect on erythrocyte deformability.

Additional efforts were undertaken to elucidate the signal transduction pathway of C-peptide and its fragments in the erythrocytes. Erythrocytes were preincubated with ouabain to inhibit the Na^+-K^+ ATPase and with EDTA to eliminate the Ca^{2+} influx into the erythrocytes. Preincubation with either oubain or EDTA completely abrogated the effect of C-peptide or its fragments on erythrocyte deformability. These data indicate a Ca^{2+}-dependent stimulation of erythrocyte Na^+K^+ATPase, in analogy with the previously established signal transduction pathway for C-peptide in renal tubular cells or peripheral nerve cells [61, 62].

In a recent investigation, C-peptide was shown to increase the release of ATP from erythrocytes due to an activation of GLUT 1 [63] (see Chap. 3). ATP is a recognized stimulus of NO production in the endothelium and the ability of C-peptide to release increased levels of ATP from erythrocytes might be an important mechanism to facilitate the path of erythrocytes to the nutritive capillaries.

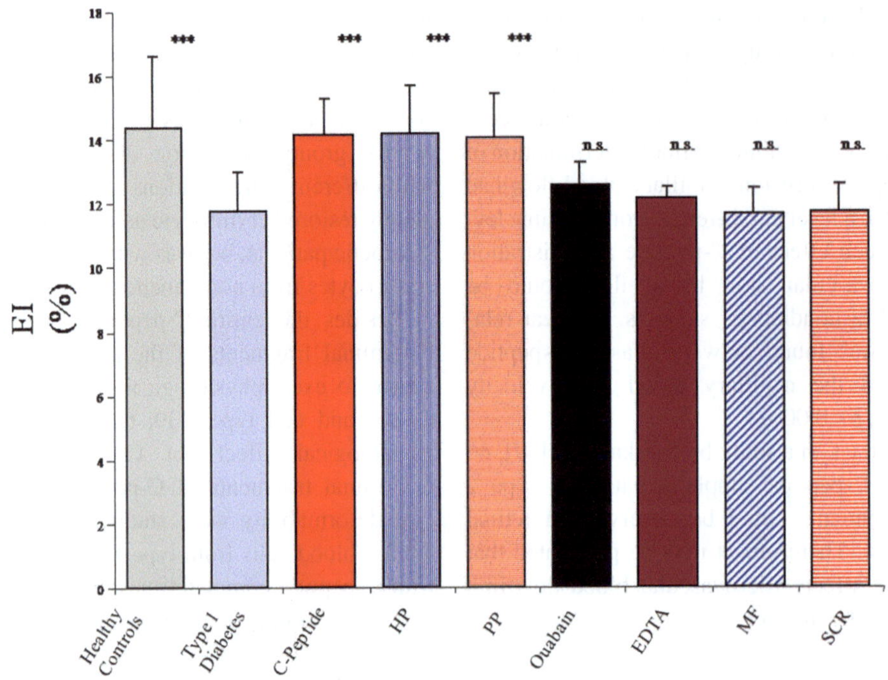

Fig. 5.4 Erythrocyte deformability at a representative physiological shear stress of 1.2 Pa (EI (%)±SD) (HP=C-terminal hexapeptide; PP=C-terminal pentapeptide; MF=middle fragment of C-peptide; SCR=scrambled peptide; ***$p<0.001$ vs. erythrocytes of type 1 diabetic patients)

Figure 5.4 presents the effect of the different C-peptide fragments on erythrocyte deformability and the inhibition with oubain or EDTA at a shear stress rate of 1.2 Pa.

Concerning the possible mechanism of reduced erythrocyte deformability, it is noteworthy that Na^+-K^+-ATPase activity has been shown to be attenuated in several cell types, including erythrocytes in diabetic patients [53, 64, 65] and that it may be restored not only by insulin but C-peptide as well [64]. In order to hypothesize the potential mechanism of the effect of C-peptide, previous studies concerning Na^+K^+ATPase activity in renal tubular cells and erythrocytes of diabetic subjects are of considerable interest [64–67]. Ohtomo et al. were able to show that the attenuated activity of Na^+-K^+-ATPase activity in renal tubular segments of diabetic rats was restored by C-peptide. On the other hand, attenuation of Na^+-K^+-ATPase activity has been demonstrated to correlate with decreased deformability in erythrocytes of type 1 diabetes patients [53]. Impaired Na^+K^+ATPase activity may contribute to the decrease in erythrocyte deformability by increasing the intracellular sodium concentration with subsequent intracellular accumulation of free calcium ions due to competition in the transmembranous exchange [66]. These abnormalities in calcium homeostasis are known to enhance spectrin dimer–dimer interaction and spectrin-protein 4.1-actin interaction [67, 68]. The latter being promoted by adducin, a membrane-skeleton-associated calmodulin-binding protein [69].

The adhesion and migration of circulating monocytes is one of the key events in the early stages of vascular damage. Recently, it could be demonstrated that C-peptide was able to inhibit leukocyte-endothelial interaction in the microcirculation during acute endothelial dysfunction [70]. It emerged that the expression of the endothelial cell adhesion molecule ICAM-1 and P-selectin on microvascular endothelium was attenuated. In another model of vascular injury, C-peptide was able to decrease leucocyte infiltration in isolated rat hearts following ischemia [71]. In hyperglycemic conditions,

C-peptide in physiological concentrations was shown to decrease NF-κB dependent vascular smooth muscle proliferation and neointima formation [72–74].

Nevertheless, the effects of C-peptide in type 2 diabetes mellitus and the development of atherogenesis still appear contradictory. Progression of insulin resistance is temporarily linked to an increased release of insulin and C-peptide from the beta cell. In patients with type 2 diabetes mellitus, an increased deposition of C-peptide was found in early arteriosclerotic lesions located directly adjacent to monocytes and CD4 positive lymphocytes [75, 76]. In a recent study, an improvement in insulin sensitivity using a PPARγ agonist and the complementary reduction in plasma C-peptide levels were associated with a reduction in intima media thickness of the common carotid artery. However, this study could not prove a causal relationship between plasma C-peptide levels and intima media thickness. The results further strengthen the hypothesis that unphysiologically elevated C-peptide levels might harm the vascular wall.

Therefore it seems conceivable, that C-peptide in excessive concentrations, for example in insulin resistant type 2 diabetic patients, might have pro-atherogenic effects, while physiological concentrations fulfill important functions, especially in the regulation of the microcirculation.

Conclusions

As shown in Fig. 5.5, C-peptide affects microvascular blood flow by interfering with several signaling pathways in the endothelial cell. Recent data suggest that C-peptide binds to a G-protein coupled receptor and increases Ca^{2+} influx with subsequent activation of Ca^{2+}-calmodulin. C-peptide supplementation in type 1 diabetic subjects stimulates Na^+/K^+-ATPase and eNOS in erythrocytes and endothelial cells. Increasing activity of eNOS and the release of NO from the endothelial cell interacts with vascular smooth muscle cells on one side, and by interacting with cellular components in the blood on the other side. In the vessel wall, NO increases cGMP levels leading to vasodilatation. Many studies suggest a link between endothelial NO release and erythrocyte deformability [77–79]. At physiological

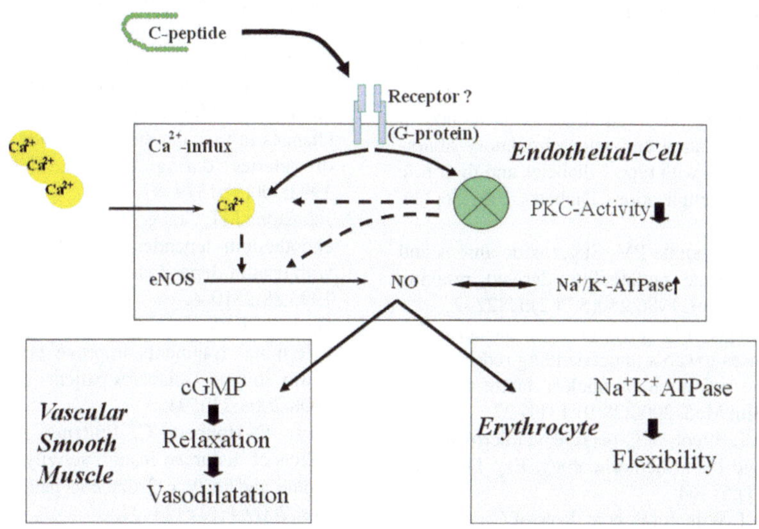

Fig. 5.5 Recent understanding of the molecular effects of C-peptide on endothelial cells, vascular smooth muscle cells, and blood rheology. It is postulated that C-peptide binds to a specific receptor in the cell membrane with subsequent intracellular activation of a G-protein coupled signaling pathway. Increasing intracellular Ca^{2+} concentrations together with a modulation of protein kinase C activity (PKC) activate the eNOS increasing the release of nitric oxide (NO) from the endothelial cell. NO causes vasorelaxation by increasing cGMP levels in the vascular smooth muscle and interacts with several cellular components in the blood. In red blood cells, NO was found to improve their cell membrane fluidity, most likely by an activation of Na-K-ATPase activity

concentrations, NO was found to increase erythrocyte deformability and to improve the hemorheological properties especially in the nutritive capillary bed [79]. Thereby, C-peptide promotes several potent mechanisms in the regulation of nutritive microvascular blood flow and the failure of C-peptide secretion might have important consequences with regard to the development of microvascular complications in patients with type 1 diabetes mellitus.

References

1. Tripathi K. EUCLID study. Lancet. 1997;350(9084):1102–3.
2. Jarvisalo MJ, Raitakari M, Toikka JO, et al. Endothelial dysfunction and increased arterial intima-media thickness in children with type 1 diabetes. Circulation. 2004;109(14):1750–5.
3. Hu H, Li N, Yngen M, et al. Enhanced leukocyte-platelet cross-talk in Type 1 diabetes mellitus: relationship to microangiopathy. J Thromb Haemost. 2004;2(1):58–64.
4. Yngen M, Ostenson CG, Hu H, et al. Enhanced P-selectin expression and increased soluble CD40 ligand in patients with type 1 diabetes mellitus and microangiopathy: evidence for platelet hyperactivity and chronic inflammation. Int J Obes Relat Metab Disord. 2004;47(3):537–40.
5. Clausen P, Jacobsen P, Rossing K, et al. Plasma concentrations of VCAM-1 and ICAM-1 are elevated in patients with type 1 diabetes mellitus with microalbuminuria and overt nephropathy. Diabet Med. 2000;17(9):644–9.
6. Devaraj S, Cheung AT, Jialal I, et al. Evidence of increased inflammation and microcirculatory abnormalities in patients with type 1 diabetes and their role in microvascular complications. Diabetes. 2007;56(11):2790–6.
7. Rubanyi GM, Vanhoutte PM. Superoxide anions and hyperoxia inactivate endothelium-derived relaxing factor. Am J Physiol. 1986;250(5 Pt 2):H822–7.
8. Janssen-Heininger YM, Poynter ME, Baeuerle PA. Recent advances towards understanding redox mechanisms in the activation of nuclear factor kappaB. Free Radic Biol Med. 2000;28(9):1317–27.
9. Forst T, Kunt T. Effects of C-peptide on microvascular blood flow and blood hemorheology. Exp Diabesity Res. 2004;5(1):51–64.
10. Forst T, Kunt T, Wilhelm B, et al. Role of C-peptide in the regulation of microvascular blood flow. Exp Diabetes Res. 2008;2008:176245.
11. Delaney C, Shaw J, Day T. Acute, local effects of iontophoresed insulin and C-peptide on cutaneous microvascular function in type 1 diabetes mellitus. Diabet Med. 2004;21(5):428–33.
12. Kitamura T, Kimura K, Jung BD, et al. Proinsulin C-peptide activates cAMP response element-binding proteins through the p38 mitogen-activated protein kinase pathway in mouse lung capillary endothelial cells. Biochem J. 2002;366(Pt 3):737–44.
13. The Diabetes Control and Complications Trial Research Group. The effect of intensive treatment of diabetes on the development and progression of long-term complications in insulin-dependent diabetes mellitus. N Engl J Med. 1993;329(14):977–86.
14. Steffes MW, Sibley S, Jackson M, et al. Beta-cell function and the development of diabetes-related complications in the diabetes control and complications trial. Diabetes Care. 2003;26(3):832–6.
15. Panero F, Novelli G, Zucco C, et al. Fasting plasma C-peptide and micro- and macrovascular complications in a large clinic-based cohort of type 1 diabetic patients. Diabetes Care. 2009;32(2):301–5.
16. Palmer RM, Ferrige AG, Moncada S. Nitric oxide release accounts for the biological activity of endothelium-derived relaxing factor. Nature. 1987;327(6122):524–6.
17. Calles-Escandon J, Cipolla M. Diabetes and endothelial dysfunction: a clinical perspective. Endocr Rev. 2001;22(1):36–52.
18. Morris SJ, Shore AC, Tooke JE. Responses of the skin microcirculation to acetylcholine and sodium nitroprusside in patients with NIDDM. Diabetologia. 1995;38(11):1337–44.
19. Pieper GM, Siebeneich W, Moore-Hilton G, et al. Reversal by L-arginine of a dysfunctional arginine/nitric oxide pathway in the endothelium of the genetic diabetic BB rat. Diabetologia. 1997;40:910–5.
20. McNally PG, Watt PAC, Rimmer T, et al. Impaired contraction and endothelium-dependent relaxation in isolated resistance vessels from patients with insulin-dependent diabetes mellitus. Clin Sci. 1994;87:31–6.
21. Kamata K, Miyata N, Abiru T, et al. Functional changes in vascular smooth muscle and endothelium of arteries during diabetes mellitus. Life Sci. 1992;50(19):1379–87.
22. Johnstone MT, Craeger SJ, Scales KM, et al. Impaired endothelium-dependent vasodilatation in patients with insulin-dependent diabetes mellitus. Circulation. 1993;88:2510–6.
23. Hach T, Forst T, Kunt T, et al. C-peptide and its C-terminal fragments improve erythrocyte deformability in type 1 diabetes patients. Exp Diabetes Res. 2008;2008:730594.
24. Forst T, Hohberg C, Pfutzner A. Cardiovascular effects of disturbed insulin activity in metabolic syndrome and in type 2 diabetic patients. Horm Metab Res. 2009;41(2):123–31.
25. Forstermann U, Closs EI, Pollock JS, et al. Nitric oxide synthase isozymes. Characterization, purification, molecular cloning, and functions. Hypertension. 1994;23(6 Pt 2):1121–31.
26. Moncada S, Higgs A. The L-arginine-nitric oxide pathway. N Engl J Med. 1993;329(27):2002–12.

27. Wallerath T, Kunt T, Forst T, et al. Stimulation of endothelial nitric oxide synthase by proinsulin C-peptide. Nitric Oxide. 2003;9(2):95–102.
28. Kunt T, Schneider S, Pfutzner A, et al. The effect of human proinsulin C-peptide on erythrocyte deformability in patients with type 1 diabetes mellitus. Diabetologia. 1999;42:465–71.
29. Jensen ME, Messina EJ. C-peptide induces a concentration-dependent dilation of skeletal muscle arterioles only in presence of insulin. Am J Physiol. 1999;276(4 Pt 2):H1223–8.
30. Danthuluri NR, Cybulsky MI, Brock TA. ACh-induced calcium transients in primary cultures of rabbit aortic endothelial cells. Am J Physiol. 1988;255(6 Pt 2):H1549–53.
31. Elliott TG, Cockcroft JR, Groop PH, et al. Inhibition of nitric oxide synthesis in forearm vasculature of insulin-dependent diabetic patients: blunted vasoconstriction in patients with microalbuminuria. Clin Sci (Lond). 1993;85(6):687–93.
32. Clarkson P, Celermajer DS, Donald AE, et al. Impaired vascular reactivity in insulin-dependent diabetes mellitus is related to disease duration and low density lipoprotein cholesterol levels. J Am Coll Cardiol. 1996;28(3):573–9.
33. Fernqvist-Forbes E, Johansson BL, Eriksson MJ. Effects of C-peptide on forearm blood flow and brachial artery dilatation in patients with type 1 diabetes mellitus. Acta Physiol Scand. 2001;172(3):159–65.
34. Cotter MA, Ekberg K, Wahren J, et al. Effects of proinsulin C-peptide in experimental diabetic neuropathy: vascular actions and modulation by nitric oxide synthase inhibition. Diabetes. 2003;52(7):1812–7.
35. Kamiya H, Zhang W, Ekberg K, et al. C-Peptide reverses nociceptive neuropathy in type 1 diabetes. Diabetes. 2006;55(12):3581–7.
36. Johansson BL, Borg K, Fernqvist-Forbes E, et al. Beneficial effects of C-peptide on incipient nephropathy and neuropathy in patients with type 1 diabetes mellitus. Diabet Med. 2000;17(3):181–9.
37. Ekberg K, Juntti-Berggren L, Norrby A, et al. C-peptide improves sensory nerve function in type 1 diabetes and neuropathy. Int J Obes Relat Metab Disord. 2005;48 Suppl 1:A81.
38. Lindstrom K, Johansson C, Johnsson E, et al. Acute effects of C-peptide on the microvasculature of isolated perfused skeletal muscles and kidneys in rat. Acta Physiol Scand. 1996;156(1):19–25.
39. Ido Y, Vindigni A, Chang K, et al. Prevention of vascular and neural dysfunction in diabetic rats by C-peptide. Science. 1997;277(5325):563–6.
40. Johansson BL, Sjoberg S, Wahren J. The influence of human C-peptide on renal function and glucose utilization in type 1 (insulin-dependent) diabetic patients. Diabetologia. 1992;35(2):121–8.
41. Jorneskog G, Brismar K, Fagrell B. Skin capillary circulation is more impaired in the toes of diabetic than non-diabetic patients with peripheral vascular disease. Diabet Med. 1995;12(1):36–41.
42. Jorneskog G, Brismar K, Fagrell B. Skin capillary circulation severely impaired in toes of patients with IDDM, with and without late diabetic complications. Diabetologia. 1995;38:474–80.
43. Boulton AJ, Scarpello JHB, Ward JD. Venous oxygenation in the diabetic neuropathic foot: evidence of arteriovenous shunting. Diabetologia. 1982;22:6–8.
44. Jorneskog G, Ostergren J, Tyden G, et al. Does combined kidney and pancreas transplantation reverse functional diabetic microangiopathy? Transpl Int. 1990;3(3):167–70.
45. Flynn MD, Tooke JE. Aetilogy of diabetic foot ulceration. Diabet Med. 1992;8:320–9.
46. Forst T, Kunt T, Pohlmann T, et al. Biological activity of C-peptide on the skin microcirculation in patients with insulin-dependent diabetes mellitus. J Clin Invest. 1998;101(10):2036–41.
47. Polska E, Kolodjaschna J, Berisha F, et al. C-peptide does not affect ocular blood flow in patients with type 1 diabetes. Diabetes Care. 2006;29(9):2034–8.
48. Tibirica E, Rodrigues E, Cobas RA, et al. Endothelial function in patients with type 1 diabetes evaluated by skin capillary recruitment. Microvasc Res. 2007;73(2):107–12.
49. Forst T, Pfutzner A, Kunt T, et al. Skin microcirculation in patients with type I diabetes with and without neuropathy after neurovascular stimulation. Clin Sci. 1998;94(3):255–61.
50. Kunt T, Forst T, Harzer O, et al. The influence of advanced glycation endproducts (AGE) on the expression of human endothelial adhesion molecules. Exp Clin Endocrinol Diabetes. 1998;106(3):183–8.
51. Ernst E, Matrai A. Altered red and white blood cell rheology in type II diabetes. Diabetes. 1986;35(12):1412–5.
52. Barnes AJ, Locke O, Scudder PR, et al. Is hyperviscosity a treatable component of diabetic microcirculatory disease. Lancet. 1977;2.2:789–91.
53. Finotti P, Palatini P. Reduction of erythrocyte (Na+K+) ATPase activity in type 1 (insulin-dependent) diabetic subjects. Diabetologia. 1986;29:623–8.
54. McMillan DE, Utterback NG, LaPuma J. Reduced erythrocyte deformability in diabetes. Diabetes. 1998;27:895–901.
55. Bareford D, Jennings PE, Stone PC, et al. Effects of hyperglycaemia and sorbitol accumulation on erythrocyte deformability in diabetes mellitus. J Clin Pathol. 1986;39(7):722–7.
56. Chimori K, Miyazaki S, Kosaka J, et al. Increased sodium influx into erythrocytes in diabetes mellitus and hypertension. Clin Exp Hypertens A. 1986;8(2):185–99.
57. Cohen NS, Ekholm JE, Luthra MG, et al. Biochemical characterization of density-separated human erythrocytes. Biochim Biophys Acta. 1976;419(2):229–42.
58. Baba Y, Kai M, Kamada T, et al. Higher levels of erythrocyte membrane microviscosity in diabetes. Diabetes. 1979;28(12):1138–40.

59. Schmid-Schonbein H, Volger E. Red-cell aggregation and red-cell deformability in diabetes. Diabetes. 1976;25(2 Suppl):897–902.
60. Rigler R, Pramanik A, Jonasson P, et al. Specific binding of proinsulin C-peptide to human cell membranes. Proc Natl Acad Sci U S A. 1999;96(23):13318–23.
61. Zhong Z, Davidescu A, Ehren I, et al. C-peptide stimulates ERK1/2 and JNK MAP kinases via activation of protein kinase C in human renal tubular cells. Int J Obes Relat Metab Disord. 2005;48(1):187–97.
62. Zhang W, Yorek M, Pierson CR, et al. Human C-peptide dose dependently prevents early neuropathy in the BB/Wor-rat. Int J Exp Diabetes Res. 2001;2(3):187–93.
63. Meyer JA, Froelich JM, Reid GE, et al. Metal-activated C-peptide facilitates glucose clearance and the release of a nitric oxide stimulus via the GLUT1 transporter. Int J Obes Relat Metab Disord. 2008;51(1):175–82.
64. Ohtomo Y, Aperia A, Sahlgren B, et al. C-peptide stimulates rat renal tubular Na+, K(+)-ATPase activity in synergism with neuropeptide Y. Diabetologia. 1996;39(2):199–205.
65. Ohtomo Y, Bergman T, Johansson BL, et al. Differential effects of proinsulin C-peptide fragments on Na+, K+-ATPase activity of renal tubule segments. Diabetologia. 1998;41(3):287–91.
66. Mazzanti L, Rabini RA, Faloia E, et al. Altered cellular Ca2+ and Na+ transport in diabetes mellitus. Diabetes. 1990;39:850–4.
67. Takakuwa Y, Mohandes N. Modulation of erythrocyte membrane material properties by Ca2+ and calmodulin. J Clin Invest. 1988;82:394–400.
68. Schischmanoff PO, Winardi R, Discher DE, et al. Defining of the minimal domain of protein 4.1 involved in spectrin-actin binding. J Biol Chem. 1995;270(36):21243–50.
69. Gardner K, Bennett V. A new erythrocyte membrane-associated protein with calmodulin binding activity. Identification and purification. J Biol Chem. 1986;261(3): 1339–48.
70. Scalia R, Coyle KM, Levine BJ, et al. A novel role for C-peptide in the regulation of leukocyte endothelium interaction during acute inflammatory events of the microcirculation. FASEB J. 2000;14:A10.
71. Young LH, Ikeda Y, Scalia R, et al. C-peptide exerts cardioprotective effects in myocardial ischemia-reperfusion. Am J Physiol Heart Circ Physiol. 2000;279(4):H1453–9.
72. Mughal RS, Scragg JL, Lister P, et al. Cellular mechanisms by which proinsulin C-peptide prevents insulin-induced neointima formation in human saphenous vein. Int J Obes Relat Metab Disord. 2010;53(8):1761–71.
73. Cifarelli V, Luppi P, Tse HM, et al. Human proinsulin C-peptide reduces high glucose-induced proliferation and NF-kappaB activation in vascular smooth muscle cells. Atherosclerosis. 2008;201(2):248–57.
74. Luppi P, Geng X, Cifarelli V, et al. C-peptide is internalised in human endothelial and vascular smooth muscle cells via early endosomes. Int J Obes Relat Metab Disord. 2009;52(10):2218–28.
75. Marx N, Walcher D, Raichle C, et al. C-peptide colocalizes with macrophages in early arteriosclerotic lesions of diabetic subjects and induces monocyte chemotaxis in vitro. Arterioscler Thromb Vasc Biol. 2004;24(3):540–5.
76. Walcher D, Aleksic M, Jerg V, et al. C-peptide induces chemotaxis of human CD4-positive cells: involvement of pertussis toxin-sensitive G-proteins and phosphoinositide 3-kinase. Diabetes. 2004;53(7):1664–70.
77. Forst T, De La Tour DD, Kunt T, et al. Effects of proinsulin C-peptide on nitric oxide, microvascular blood flow and erythrocyte Na+, K+-ATPase activity in diabetes mellitus type I. Clin Sci. 2000;98(3):283–90.
78. Mesquita R, Picarra B, Saldanha C, et al. Nitric oxide effects on human erythrocytes structural and functional properties – an in vitro study. Clin Hemorheol Microcirc. 2002;27(2):137–47.
79. Bateman RM, Jagger JE, Sharpe MD, et al. Erythrocyte deformability is a nitric oxide-mediated factor in decreased capillary density during sepsis. Am J Physiol Heart Circ Physiol. 2001;280(6):H2848–56.

Is NO-eNOS a Target for C-Peptide Action and Its Protective Effects on Diabetic Nephropathy?

6

Kazuhiro Kimura and Akihiro Kamikawa

Keywords
eNOS • Na^+, K^+-ATPase • NO • PKC and reactive oxygen species.

Introduction

Numerous studies show protective effects of C-peptide on the development of the diabetic complications in type 1 diabetic patients and in its animal models. Recently, we have demonstrated that streptozotocin-induced diabetic rats with almost complete reduction of endogenous insulin and C-peptide increase expression of renal endothelial nitric oxide synthase (eNOS), and that replacement with C-peptide abrogates the increase of eNOS without affecting hyperglycemic state. Here, we first summarize current topics on nitric oxide (NO)-eNOS system in diabetic nephropathy and then we discuss the mechanisms underlying the ameliorating effects of C-peptide on diabetic nephropathy with focus on the NO-eNOS system.

K. Kimura (✉)
Department of Biomedical Sciences, Graduate School of Veterinary Medicine, Hokkaido University, Kita-ku, Kita 18, Nishi 9, Sapporo, 060-0818, Japan
e-mail: k-kimura@vetmed.hokudai.ac.jp

A. Kamikawa
Department of Biomedical Sciences, Graduate School of Veterinary Medicine, Hokkaido University, Kita-ku, Kita 18, Nishi 9, Sapporo, 060-0818, Japan

Department of Basic Veterinary Medicine, Obihiro University of Agriculture and Veterinary Medicine, Obihiro, Hokkaido, Japan

eNOS Expression in Diabetic Nephropathy

Diabetes mellitus is currently considered to be an epidemic disease [1]. More than 30% of individuals with type 1 and type 2 diabetes develop persistent albuminuria, lose renal function, and are at high risk for end-stage renal disease [2]. The natural course of diabetic renal disease can be characterized by a number of phases. As an early pathogenic event, glomerular hyperfiltration can be observed soon after diabetes onset. The hyperfiltration is associated with glomerular hyperperfusion and increased intraglomerular pressure, which may be due to a reduction in the intrarenal vascular resistance with inappropriate dilatation of arterioles. Persistent increase in the glomerular filtration rate (GFR) may develop capillary leakage leading to microalbuminuria and cause structural abnormalities of glomerular capillaries such as thickness of glomerular basement membrane and mesangial expansion. As the disease progresses, characteristic morphologic and histologic changes

A.A.F. Sima (ed.), *Diabetes & C-Peptide: Scientific and Clinical Aspects*, Contemporary Diabetes,
DOI 10.1007/978-1-61779-391-2_6,

occur in the kidney, where protein excretion increases (macroalbuminuria) and GFR falls. As a consequence of the disease progression, end-stage renal disease may occur [2–6].

Endothelial dysfunction and damage are a hallmark of diabetic vascular complications, and are, at least in part, attributed to exceeding and deficient NO production [7–10]. In the early stage of diabetic kidney disease local overproduction of NO may be a cause of hyperperfusion and is critical in the pathogenesis of diabetic nephropathy [7, 11, 12]. Among the three isoforms of NO synthase, eNOS increases in glomerulus and afferent arterioles in response to the hyperglycemic state and this abnormal increase of eNOS is abrogated by daily administration of long-acting insulin [10, 13]. On the other hand, expression of neuronal NOS (nNOS) is irrational, increased, normal, or decreased [10], and expression of inducible NOS (iNOS) protein and mRNA expression are found to be unchanged or barely detectable in the early hyperfiltration stage, and is detectable in the renal cortex of rats with long-term diabetes [10]. Thus, eNOS is suggested to contribute to the changes in glomerular hemodynamics.

In the later stage, NO bioavailability will progressively decrease with advancing nephropathy [7–9]. Deficiency of eNOS in diabetic mice developing advanced diabetic nephropathy is similar to that observed in human diabetic renal disease [14–16], while renal failure due to diabetes is lacking in ordinary animal models of diabetic nephropathy [17]. In humans, two of four eNOS gene polymorphisms (a T to C substitution in the promoter at position −786 and the a-deletion/b-insertion in intron 4) are associated with the risk of advanced nephropathy in type 1 diabetes [18], and the latter polymorphism is linked with increased risk for progression to diabetic nephropathy in type 2 diabetes [19]. Moreover, the other polymorphism (Glu298Asp) causing lowered eNOS activity is closely associated with nondiabetic causes of end-stage renal disease [20, 21]. These findings suggest that decreased expression and activity of eNOS, leading to a decrease in the vascular production of NO, may be a potential culprit in advanced nephropathy in diabetes. However, expression of cortical and glomerular eNOS immunoreactivity is increased in patients with type 2 diabetic nephropathy, and the increase of the expression correlates with more severe vascular complications, whereas iNOS is unchanged but spatially differentially expressed [22].

Regulation of eNOS Activity in Diabetic Kidney

Formation of NO from L-arginine by three isoforms of NOS requires redox-active cofactors, including nicotinamide adenine dinucleotide phosphate (NADPH), flavinmononucleotide (FMN), flavin adenine dinucleotide (FAD), and tetrahydrobiopterin (BH_4), and is activated by an agonist-induced increase in intracellular Ca^{2+}, followed by a complex formation of Ca^{2+}-calmodulin and NOS [23–25]. In rats with experimental diabetic nephropathy, plasma BH_4 levels are decreased with a decrease in glomerular NO levels, although eNOS protein levels were increased [26]. Interestingly, restoration of physiological levels of BH_4 recovered NO production without affecting the increased amounts of eNOS protein. Moreover, asymmetric dimethylarginine (ADMA), an endogenous NOS inhibitor, accumulates in individuals with chronic renal failure and type 1 diabetes [27, 28]. Thus, restriction of cofactors availability and increase in ADMA concentration may be more important factors to control NO production and its availability than expression of the NOS proteins.

ADMA is degraded by dimethylarginine dimethylaminohydrolases (DDAHs), which cleave ADMA into citrulline and dimethylamine. Renal DDAH expression and activity are reduced in diabetic rats with increased and decreased urinary levels of ADMA and NOx, a metabolite of NO [29]. Artificial overexpresssion of DDAH prevents the increase of ADMA and the decrease of NOx, and subsequently decreases urinary albumin excretion [29]. In human endothelial cell culture, high glucose condition decreases DDAH activity and cGMP formation, an indicator of NO formation, and inclusion of antioxidant prevents the decreases of both [30]. Therefore, oxidative stress by hyperglycemia may reduce renal DDAH expression and activity, and as a consequence increased circulating ADMA levels may prevent eNOS activity. Similarly, oxidative stress induces BH_4 oxidation to form BH_2 and other oxidized biopterin species [25, 31, 32], which can cause BH_4 insufficiency. It should be noted that the cofactor insufficiency leads to "uncoupling of eNOS," manifested by a switch from NO to superoxide production [25, 26, 31]. In addition, recent study suggests that diminished intracellular ratio of BH_4 to BH_2, rather than BH_4 depletion per se is the molecular trigger for NO insufficiency, since BH_2 binds to eNOS with equal affinity as BH_4 and can efficiently replace eNOS-bound BH_4, resulting in eNOS uncoupling [32, 33]. Furthermore, BH_4 recycling enzyme, dihydrofolate reductase, may also play a role in eNOS coupling-uncoupling states [34, 35].

Oxidative Stress in Diabetic Kidney

Oxidative stress represents excess production of oxidants or reactive oxygen species (ROS) over antioxidant capacity. ROS form as a natural byproduct of the normal metabolism of oxygen, and antioxidant system such as superoxide dismutase and glutathione peroxidase normally detoxify the reactive intermediates [9]. In the diabetic kidney, a number of pathways enhance generation of ROS. That is, autooxidation of glucose, glycolysis, mitochondrial respiratory chain, polyol pathway, uncoupled eNOS, xanthine oxidase, NAD(P)H oxidase, and advanced glycation [8, 9]. On the other hand, it is reported that cells from type 1 diabetic patients with nephropathy are defective in hyperglycemia-induced expression of glutathione peroxidase and catalase [36]. Thus, excess ROS in diabetic kidney through increased ROS production and/or decreased antioxidant capacity may cause toxic effects on cells by affecting all cellular components including proteins, lipids, and DNA.

Among the ROS producing pathways, mitochondrial production of ROS in response to chronic hyperglycemia may be the key initiator for the other four major biochemical pathways, including increased advanced glycation end-product (AGE) formation, activation of protein kinase C (PKC), and increased flux through the polyol and hexosamine pathways [8, 9, 37]. It is interesting to note that endothelial cells are lacking autoregulation of glucose-transport activity (i.e., glucose-transport activity is suppressed by decreasing expression of GLUT1 protein when exposed to hyperglycemia) [38]. In addition, *in vitro* studies show that ROS further up-regulate GLUT1 expression and subsequent glucose uptake [39], while reduced oxidative stress down-regulates GLUT1 and glucose uptake [40]. Moreover, overexpression of GLUT1 in rat mesangial cells cultured even under normal glucose condition mimic the diabetic phenotype in extracellular matrix synthesis [41]. It is, therefore, likely that endothelial cells exposed to hyperglycemic condition increase the rates of glucose transport, subsequent glucose metabolism and ROS production, which activates the four biochemical pathways and induces GLUT1 expression, resulting in further glucose uptake and ROS production. Such an aggressive feedback loop of glucose uptake, ROS production, and GLUT1 expression may lead to dysfunction of the cells.

It is recently reported that treatment of endothelial cells with nonlethal heat shock (hyperthermia) induces heat shock protein 90 (Hsp90) expression, resulting in prevention of the hyperglycemia-induced increase in ROS formation [40]. The reduction of ROS formation can be explained by the heat shock-dependent down regulation of GLUT1 and glucose uptake and lowering of glucose metabolism even under hyperglycemic condition. Thus, regulation of the glucose transporter activity in endothelial cells is important for controlling ROS production under hyperglycemic conditions. In the same report [40], induction of HSP90 prevents the decreased NO production. This "eNOS coupling" is possibly due to increased association of HSP90 and eNOS, as well as reduced ROS formation.

The Other Regulation of eNOS Activity in Diabetes

As mentioned above, insufficient NO production by eNOS can be caused by reduced eNOS gene expression, inhibition of NOS by ADMA, uncoupling of eNOS due to BH_4 deficiency and dissociation from HSP90. In addition to these mechanisms, deficiency of arginine, a substrate of the enzyme, may be a cause of reduced NO availability in diabetic kidney [42]. Furthermore, the phosphorylation status of eNOS plays a role in the regulation of its activity, since it is well documented that the enzyme activity is controlled through site(s)-specific phosphorylation by various protein kinases, e.g., phosphorylation at Ser-1177 of human eNOS by Akt or AMP-activated protein kinase increases the enzyme activity, while phosphorylation at Thr-497 by PKC decreases the activity [23, 24, 43–45]. Indeed, in hyperglycemia and/or diabetic state, suppression of phosphorylation at Ser-1177 by masking the site with O-linked glycosylation (*O*-GlcNAc) modification through activation of the hexosamine pathway causes a decrease in eNOS activity [46–48].

Ameliorating Effect of C-Peptide on Diabetic Nephropathy

Blood levels of C-peptide are inversely related to the development of diabetic complications including microvascular disturbances and neuropathy [49, 50] (see Chap. 8). Numerous studies show that C-peptide has reno-protective effects in type-1 diabetic patients and in animal models of insulinopenic diabetes [51–60]. Short-term C-peptide administration to type 1 diabetic patients results in decreased GFR by 7% and increased effective renal plasma flow by 3% [51]. Long-term (1–3 months) C-peptide administration to type 1 diabetic patients results in a decrease in the urinary excretion of albumin by 40–55%, reduction of the GFR by 6% and fluorescein leakage across the blood-retinal barrier by 30% [52, 53]. Streptozotocin-induced diabetic rats display increased GFR and increased total protein leakage compared with normal rats [54–59]. Short-term C-peptide administration to these animals reduces GFR and total protein leakage [54, 56, 57], and restores renal functional reserve (RFR: the ability to increase GFR in response to glycine infusion) [54]. In studies of C-peptide administration for 2 and 4 weeks to streptozotocin diabetic rats, physiological doses of C-peptide prevented the development of glomerular hypertrophy and albuminuria with decreased GFR and restoration of RFR [55, 59]. In addition, C-peptide administration prevents the mesangial matrix expansion seen in the posthyperfiltration phase of early diabetic nephropathy [58]. Furthermore, it should be noted that C-peptide administration induces body weight gain regardless of hyperglycemia and glycosuria [59, 60] and reduces urinary sodium waste [59].

C-Peptide Controls NO Availability Through the Regulation of eNOS Expression and Activity

Short-term C-peptide administration to type 1 diabetic patients results in an increase of forearm blood flow [61–63] and brachial artery dilatation [62], which is blocked by NOS inhibitor [63]. Similarly, C-peptide infusion to patients increases skin microcirculation [64], accompanied by increased plasma cyclic GMP, an indicator of NO production [65]. Actually, short-term treatment with C-peptide increases NO release in perfused heart from diabetic rats [66] and bovine aortic endothelial cells [67]. It is of interest to note that NO production from the cells depends on the extracellular Ca^{2+}, but not an eNOS phosphorylation at Ser-1179 (corresponding to Ser-1177 of human eNOS) [67].

Some ameliorative effects of C-peptide on nerve and vascular function are also mediated by NO [68–71], and these beneficial effects are also observed *ex vivo* [68, 69]. For instance, single injection of C-peptide to normal rats inhibits leukocytes-endothelium interactions, increases mRNA expression of eNOS in the lung, and enhances NO production in aortic tissue [68]. In primary cultured aortic endothelial cells, C-peptide increases NO production through mitogen-activated protein kinase (MAPK)-dependent transcriptional enhancement of the eNOS gene [72], although such a transcriptional enhancement of the gene is not seen in bovine aortic endothelial cells [67]. Thus, C-peptide controls NO production through two independent pathways; that is, Ca^{2+}-dependent Ser-1177/1179 phosphorylation-independent activation of eNOS activity and MAPK-mediated eNOS gene expression.

C-Peptide Modifies eNOS Expression in Diabetic Kidney and Circulating NOx Levels

In the kidney, eNOS protein is localized to glomeruli and endothelial cells of arterioles or arcuate arteries, but not to arcuate veins. There is no obvious difference in its localization among nondiabetic and diabetic rats with or without the replacement of insulin and C-peptide [60]. On the other hand, the amounts of eNOS protein are clearly increased in the diabetic kidney when compared with those of nondiabetic control [10, 13, 22, 60], and the diabetes-induced increase of eNOS protein is abrogated by continuous infusion of C-peptide [60]. This abrogation of eNOS expression in the diabetic kidney by C-peptide seems to contradict the previous finding that physiological concentration of C-peptide increases eNOS protein through transcriptional activation of the gene in rat aortic endothelial cells *in vitro* [72], suggesting that there might be other mechanism(s) by which C-peptide regulates eNOS expression.

Contrary to the regulation of eNOS protein levels, replacement of C-peptide increased circulating levels of NOx, oxidative products of NO such as nitrite and nitrate, in the same animal used in [60] (Fig. 6.1). This may be explained by C-peptide's ability to activate eNOS. However, it is most likely that if eNOS is in the uncoupled state as ordinarily found in diabetic animals, eNOS would generate superoxide rather than NO as discussed above. Therefore, increased plasma NOx levels by C-peptide could not be achieved by eNOS activation alone unless C-peptide restores NO-producing eNOS activity as in the coupled state.

Is it possible that C-peptide recovers NO-producing activity? As C-peptide prevents the diabetes-induced activation of renal PKCα, a downstream effector of oxidative stress [60], we speculate that C-peptide reduces oxidative stress as well as PKC activation, which results in maintaining eNOS activity in the coupled state followed by enhanced NO production in the whole body, presumably in the kidney of diabetic animals. There is no evidence showing C-peptide reduces oxidative stress in hyperglycemic condition [71], but this is an interesting hypothesis that should be addressed.

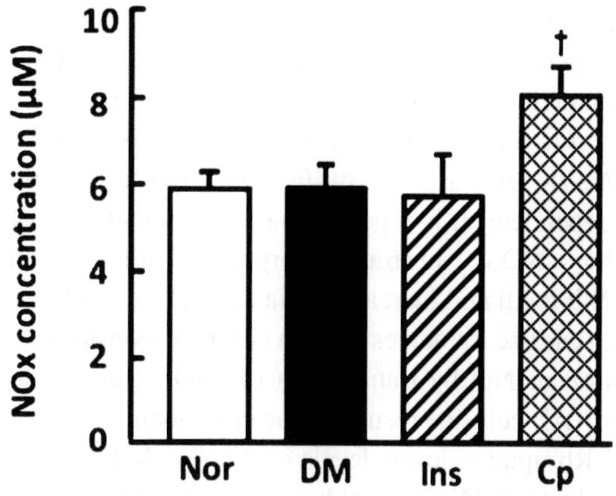

Fig. 6.1 Circulating NOx levels in normal rats (Nor), streptozotocin-induced diabetic rats (DM), DM rats with insulin treatment (Ins) and DM rats with C-peptide treatment (Cp). Detailed experimental conditions are given in ref. [60]

In addition, recent findings show that NOx are not only oxidative products of NO, but also stored forms of NO that regulate vascular tone and blood pressure [73–75]; that is, NO can also be generated from the reduction of nitrite and nitrate in mammals. Accordingly, an increase in NOx levels itself by C-peptide may facilitate and increase NO availability.

C-Peptide Regulates Renal Tubule Na^+/K^+-ATPase Expression and Activity: Possible Link with NO

Several studies report pronounced acute effects of C-peptide on Na^+/K^+-ATPase activity in the renal tubule segment and isolated tubular cells from nondiabetic human and animals [76–79]. In human renal tubular cells, C-peptide stimulates Na^+/K^+-ATPase activity and its translocation to the basolateral membrane through ERK, a well characterized MAPK [76]. In rat renal medullary thick ascending limb tubules (mTAL), C-peptide stimulates Na^+/K^+-ATPase activity in a Ca^{2+}-dependent PKCα-mediated pathway without changing the amounts of the enzyme [77].

On the other hand, acute effects of NO on the Na^+/K^+-ATPase activity *in vitro* seem to be dose dependent. It is reported that supplementation of the NOS substrate L-arginine induces an NO-mediated increase in Na^+/K^+-ATPase activity in cardiac myocytes [80]. In contrast, overproduction of NO by transfection of iNOS gene in an mTAL cell line results in lower ouabain-sensitive ^{86}Rb uptake, lower levels of Na^+/K^+-ATPase α1-subunit mRNA, and reduced rates of de novo Na^+/K^+-ATPase α1-subunit transcription [81]. In addition, if NOS is uncoupled, it can generate superoxide and peroxynitrite, reactive nitrogen species derived from NO and superoxide, which induce inhibition of Na^+/K^+-ATPase activity [80, 82].

In animals or humans with diabetes, decreased Na^+/K^+-ATPase activity has been observed in various tissues including kidney [65, 83–86]. However, the mechanism by which the enzyme activity decreases remains unclear. Overproduction of NO by iNOS may be involved [81], but noticeable changes in the expression of iNOS are not observed in either the kidneys of nondiabetic or diabetic rats [10, 60]. It is important to note, that renomedullary hypoxia doses develop in diabetic kidney [42]. As hypoxia induces and accelerates degradation of Na^+/K^+-ATPase via mitochondrial ROS and the ubiquitin-conjugating system [87], local hypoxia, together with enhanced ROS production in hyperglycemia, may be a mechanism underlying the decrease in Na^+/K^+-ATPase activity.

In the kidney, Na^+/K^+-ATPase α1-subunit is abundantly expressed in the medullary collecting ducts of control animals, but the expression is markedly decreased in the diabetic state with a concomitant decrease in its mRNA expression [88] (see Chap. 7). Replacement of C-peptide for 1 week prevents this decrease [88]. Because C-peptide-induced MAPK activation leads to transcriptional activation and subsequent gene expression [72, 89, 90], one plausible mechanism of C-peptide's action in the renal medulla is that C-peptide simply increases the mRNA expression of the α1-subunit. However, since reduced NO availability in the kidney might be involved in the development of renomedullary hypoxia [42], the other likely mechanism is that C-peptide restores the NO availability which obviates renomedullary hypoxia, thereby preventing Na^+/K^+-ATPase degradation and maintaining its expression.

Prospective

NO-eNOS system is essential for the regulations of vascular responses such as vasorelaxation, inflammation including endothelial interaction with platelets and leukocytes, and vascular smooth muscle cell proliferation [91]. In hyperglycemic condition, due to the lack of autoregulation of glucose-transport activity in endothelial cells, aggressive mitochondrial ROS production exceeds antioxidant capacity and activates several biochemical pathways, leading to dysfunction of the cells such as "eNOS uncoupling" and degradation and inhibition of Na^+/K^+-ATPase (Fig. 6.2).

C-peptide has the ability to activate a variety of signaling and effector molecules including PKC, ERK, eNOS, and Na^+/K^+-ATPase. However, it is unlikely that the beneficial effects of C-peptide replacement in diabetic patients and animal models are fully explained by the activation of these molecules. The fact that C-peptide increases circulating NOx levels suggests that C-peptide could restore eNOS enzyme to the coupling state. The finding that C-peptide prevents hyperglycemia-induced PKC activation, together with restoration of eNOS coupling, implies that C-peptide reduces oxidative stress being upstream signaling of PKC and eNOS.

There is no direct evidence showing that C-peptide reduces oxidative stress. However, it is recently reported that C-peptide reduces high glucose-induced proliferation and NF-κB activation in vascular smooth muscle cells and the brain [92–94] (see Chaps. 9 and 10). As high glucose is known to activate NF-κB via PKC and ROS, these reports support our hypothesis.

Although further studies are necessary to elucidate all mechanisms behind the beneficial roles of C-peptide in diabetic complications, we assume that maintaining a NO-eNOS system by

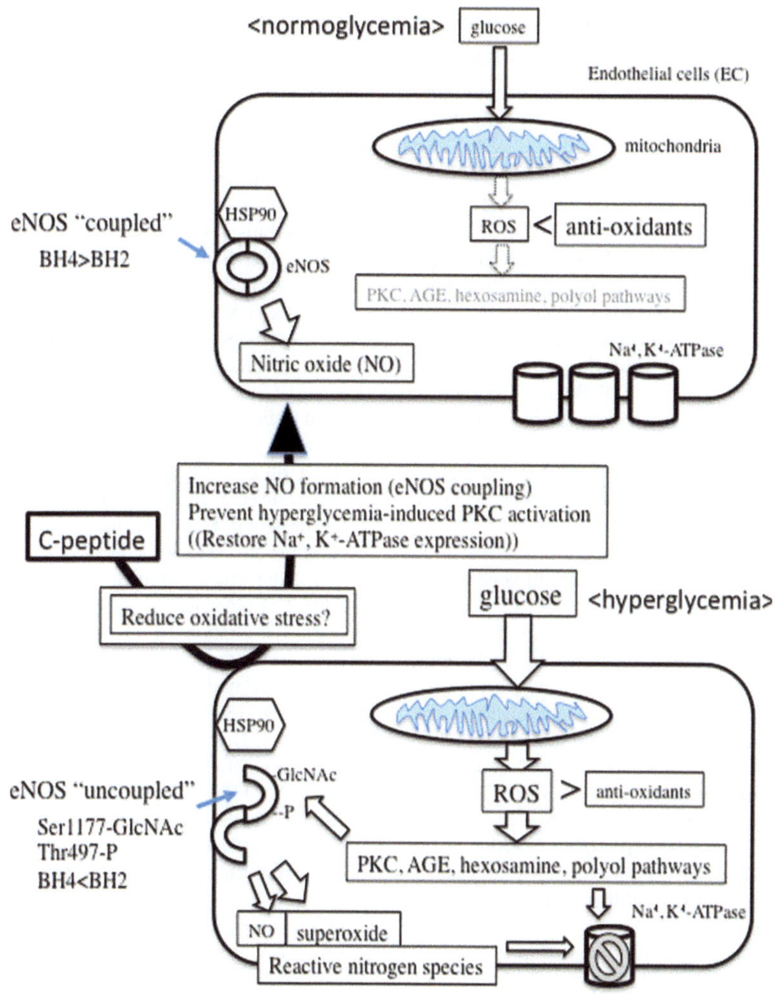

Fig. 6.2 Schematic overview of this chapter. Under normal glucose concentration, endothelial cells are supposed to take up and metabolize glucose in accordance with the energy requirement of the cell. During glucose metabolism reactive oxygen species (ROS) are produced in the mitochondria, but scavenged by antioxidant systems such as glutathione and superoxide dismutase. Thus, there is no oxidative stress. Endothelial nitric oxide synthase (eNOS) forms homodimer, binds to heat shock protein 90 (HSP90) and produces nitric oxide (NO), referred to as eNOS "coupled" state. Na^+, K^+-ATPase is stably expressed. In hyperglycemia, due to the lack of autoregulation of glucose-transport activity in endothelial cells, the cells are supposed to take up and metabolize glucose depending on the glucose gradient. Enhanced glucose flux causes an increase in ROS generation by a number of pathways including autooxidation of glucose, glycolysis, mitochondrial respiratory chain and NAD(P)H oxidase. Thus, the production of ROS exceeds the antioxidant capacity, resulting in an increase in advanced glycation end-product (AGE) formation, activation of protein kinase C (PKC), and increased flux through the polyol and hexosamine pathways. ROS oxidize tetrahydrobiopterin (BH_4), a cofactor of eNOS, to form BH_2, resulting in "eNOS uncoupling" to generate superoxide rather than NO. Modification of eNOS by PKC phosphorylation and hexosamine pathway-mediated *O*-linked glycosylation (*O*-GlcNAc) decrease eNOS activity. Dissociation of HSP90 prevents NO formation. Superoxide and reactive nitrogen species derived from NO and superoxide inhibit Na^+, K^+-ATPase activity, and probably decrease its expression. We have demonstrated that replacement of C-peptide in DM increases circulating NOx levels and prevents hyperglycemia-induced PKC activation, both of which are downstream events of ROS production. We speculate that C-peptide restores eNOS enzyme to the coupling state, through reducing oxidative stress

C-peptide is one of the central mechanisms of C-peptide's actions, possibly through controlling oxidative stress.

References

1. Yach D, Stuckler D, Brownell KD. Epidemiologic and economic consequences of the global epidemics of obesity and diabetes. Nat Med. 2006;12:62–6.
2. Nelson RG, Knowler WC, Pettitt DJ, Bennett PH. Kidney diseases in diabetes. In: Harris MI, Cowie CC, Stern MP, Boyko EJ, Reiber GE, Bennett PH, editors. Diabetes in America. 2nd ed. Washington: NIDDK; 1995. p. 349–400.
3. Mauer SM, Steffes MW, Ellis EN, et al. Structural-functional relationship in diabetic nephropathy. J Clin Invest. 1984;74:1143–55.
4. Krolewski A, Warram J, Christlieb A, Busick E, Kahn C. The changing natural history of nephropathy in type I diabetes. Am J Med. 1985;78:785–94.
5. Brenner BM, Lawler EV, Mackenzie HS. The hyperfiltration theory: a paradigm shift in nephrology. Kidney Int. 1996;49:1774–7.
6. Wolf G, Ziyadeh FN. Molecular mechanisms of diabetic renal hypertrophy. Kidney Int. 1999;56:393–405.
7. Goligorsky MS. Endothelial cell dysfunction and nitric oxide synthase. Kidney Int. 2000;58:1360–76.
8. Giacco F, Brownlee M. Oxidative stress and diabetic complications. Circ Res. 2010;107:1058–70.
9. Forbes JM, Coughlan MT, Cooper ME. Oxidative stress as a major culprit in kidney disease in diabetes. Diabetes. 2008;57:1446–54.
10. Komers R, Anderson S. Paradoxes of nitric oxide in the diabetic kidney. Am J Physiol Renal Physiol. 2003;284:F1121–37.
11. Bank N, Aynedjian HS. Role of EDRF (nitric oxide) in diabetic renal hyperfiltration. Kidney Int. 1993;43:1306–12.
12. Komers R, Allen TJ, Cooper ME. Role of endothelium-derived nitric oxide in the pathogenesis of the renal hemodynamic changes of experimental diabetes. Diabetes. 1994;43:1190–7.
13. Sugimoto H, Shikata K, Matsuda M, et al. Increased expression of endothelial cell nitric oxide synthase (ecNOS) in afferent and glomerular endothelial cells is involved in glomerular hyperfiltration of diabetic nephropathy. Diabetologia. 1998;41:1426–34.
14. Zhao HJ, Wang S, Cheng H, et al. Endothelial nitric oxide synthase deficiency produces accelerated nephropathy in diabetic mice. J Am Soc Nephrol. 2006;17:2664–9.
15. Nakagawa T, Sato W, Glushakova O, et al. Diabetic endothelial nitric oxide synthase knockout mice develop advanced diabetic nephropathy. J Am Soc Nephrol. 2007;18:539–50.
16. Kanetsuna Y, Takahashi K, Nagata M, et al. Deficiency of endothelial nitric-oxide synthase confers susceptibility to diabetic nephropathy in nephropathy resistant inbred mice. Am J Pathol. 2007;170:1473–84.
17. Breyer MD, Böttinger E, Brosius III FC, AMDCC, et al. Mouse models of diabetic nephropathy. J Am Soc Nephrol. 2005;16:27–45.
18. Zanchi A, Moczulski DK, Hanna LS, et al. Risk of advanced diabetic nephropathy in type 1 diabetes is associated with endothelial nitric oxide synthase gene polymorphism. Kidney Int. 2000;57:405–13.
19. Neugebauer S, Baba T, Watanabe T. Association of the nitric oxide synthase gene polymorphism with an increased risk for progression to diabetic nephropathy in type 2 diabetes. Diabetes. 2000;49:500–3.
20. Noiri E, Satoh H, Taguchi J, et al. Association of eNOS Glu298Asp polymorphism with end-stage renal disease. Hypertension. 2002;40:535–40.
21. Persu A, Stoenoiu MS, Messiaen T, et al. Modifier effect of ENOS in autosomal dominant polycystic kidney disease. Hum Mol Genet. 2002;11:229–41.
22. Hohenstein B, Hugo CP, Hausknecht B, et al. Analysis of NO-synthase expression and clinical risk factors in human diabetic nephropathy. Nephrol Dial Transplant. 2008;23:1346–54.
23. Fulton D, Gratton J-P, Sessa WC. Post-translational control of endothelial nitric oxide synthase: why isn't calcium/calmodulin enough? J Pharmacol Exp Ther. 2001;299:818–24.
24. Fleming I, Busse R. Molecular mechanisms involved in the regulation of the endothelial nitric oxide synthase. Am J Physiol. 2003;284:R1–12.
25. Alp NJ, Channon KM. Regulation of endothelial nitric oxide synthase by tetrahydrobiopterin in vascular disease. Arterioscler Thromb Vasc Biol. 2004;24:413–20.
26. Satoh M, Fujimoto S, Haruna Y, et al. NAD(P)H oxidase and uncoupled nitric oxide synthase are major sources of glomerular superoxide in rats with experimental diabetic nephropathy. Am J Physiol Renal Physiol. 2005;288:F1144–52.
27. Vallance P, Leone A, Calver A, Collier J, Moncada S. Accumulation of an endogenous inhibitor of nitric oxide synthesis in chronic renal failure. Lancet. 1992;339:572–5.
28. Tarnow L, Hovind P, Teerlink T, Stehouwer CD, Parving HH. Elevated plasma asymmetric dimethylarginine as a marker of cardiovascular morbidity in early diabetic nephropathy in type 1 diabetes. Diabetes Care. 2004;27:765–9.
29. Shibata R, Ueda S, Yamagishi S, et al. Involvement of asymmetric dimethylarginine (ADMA) in tubulointerstitial ischaemia in the early phase of diabetic nephropathy. Nephrol Dial Transplant. 2009;24:1162–9.
30. Lin KY, Ito A, Asagami T, et al. Impaired nitric oxide synthase pathway in diabetes mellitus: role of asymmetric dimethylarginine and dimethylarginine dimethylaminohydrolase. Circulation. 2002;106:987–92.
31. Shinozaki K, Kashiwagi A, Nishio Y, et al. Abnormal biopterin metabolism is a major cause of impaired endothelium-dependent relaxation through nitric oxide/O_2-imbalance in insulin-resistant rat aorta. Diabetes. 1999;48:2437–45.

32. Crabtree MJ, Smith CL, Lam G, Goligorsky MS, Gross SS. Ratio of 5,6,7,8-tetrahydrobiopterin to 7,8-dihydrobiopterin in endothelial cells determines glucose-elicited changes in NO vs. superoxide production by eNOS. Am J Physiol Heart Circ Physiol. 2008;294:H1530–40.
33. Crabtree MJ, Tatham AL, Al-Wakeel Y, et al. Quantitative regulation of intracellular endothelial nitric-oxide synthase (eNOS) coupling by both tetrahydrobiopterin-eNOS stoichiometry and biopterin redox status. J Biol Chem. 2009;284:1136–44.
34. Crabtree MJ, Tatham AL, Hale AB, Alp NJ, Channon KM. Critical role for tetrahydrobiopterin recycling by dihydrofolate reductase in regulation of endothelial nitric-oxide synthase coupling: relative importance of the de novo biopterin synthesis versus salvage pathways. J Biol Chem. 2009;284: 28128–36.
35. Sugiyama T, Levy BD, Michel T. Tetrahydrobiopterin recycling, a key determinant of endothelial nitric-oxide synthase-dependent signaling pathways in cultured vascular endothelial cells. J Biol Chem. 2009;284:12691–700.
36. Ceriello A, Morocutti A, Mercuri F, et al. Defective intracellular antioxidant enzyme production in type 1 diabetic patients with nephropathy. Diabetes. 2000;49:2170–7.
37. Nishikawa T, Edelstein D, Du XL, et al. Normalizing mitochondrial superoxide production blocks three pathways of hyperglycaemic damage. Nature. 2000;404:787–90.
38. Kaiser N, Sasson S, Feener EP, et al. Differential regulation of glucose transport and transporters by glucose in vascular endothelial and smooth muscle cells. Diabetes. 1993;42:80–9.
39. Cohem G, Riahi Y, Alpert E, Gruzman A, Sasson S. The roles of hyperglycaemia and oxidative stress in the rise and collapse of the natural protective mechanism against vascular endothelial cell dysfunction in diabetes. Arch Physiol Biochem. 2007;113:259–67.
40. Presley T, Vedam K, Druhan LJ, Ilangovan G. Hyperthermia-induced Hsp90/eNOS preserves mitochondrial respiration in hyperglycemic endothelial cells by down-regulating Glut-1 and up-regulating G6PD activity. J Biol Chem. 2010;285:38194–203.
41. Heilig CW, Concepcion LA, Riser BL, et al. Overexpression of glucose transporters in rat mesangial cells cultured in a normal glucose milieu mimics the diabetic phenotype. J Clin Invest. 1995;96: 1802–14.
42. Palm F, Friederich M, Carlsson P-O, et al. Reduced nitric oxide in diabetic kidneys due to increased hepatic arginine metabolism: implications for renomedullary oxygen availability. Am J Physiol Renal Physiol. 2008;294:F30–7.
43. Govers R, Rabelink TJ. Cellular regulation of endothelial nitric oxide synthase. Am J Physiol. 2001;280: F193–206.
44. Makondo K, Kimura K, Kitamura T, et al. Hepatocyte growth factor activates endothelial nitric oxide synthase by Ca^{2+}- and phosphoinositide 3-kinase/Akt-dependent phosphorylation in aortic endothelial cells. Biochem J. 2003;374:63–9.
45. Kolluru GK, Siamwala JH, Chatterjee S. eNOS phosphorylation in health and disease. Biochimie. 2010;92:1186–98.
46. Du XL, Edelstein D, Dimmeler S, et al. Hyperglycemia inhibits endothelial nitric oxide synthase activity by posttranslational modification at the Akt site. J Clin Invest. 2001;108:1341–8.
47. Federici M, Menghini R, Mauriello A, et al. Insulin-dependent activation of endothelial nitric oxide synthase is impaired by *O*-linked glycosylation modification of signaling proteins in human coronary endothelial cells. Circulation. 2002;106:466–72.
48. Musicki B, Kramer MF, Becker RE, Burnett AL. Inactivation of phosphorylated endothelial nitric oxide synthase (Ser-1177) by *O*-GlcNAc in diabetes-associated erectile dysfunction. Proc Natl Acad Sci U S A. 2005;102:11870–5.
49. Wahren J. C-peptide: new findings and therapeutic implications in diabetes. Clin Physiol Funct Imaging. 2004;24:180–9.
50. Sima AAF, Kamiya H, Li ZG. Insulin, C-peptide, hyperglycemia, and central nervous system complications in diabetes. Eur J Pharmacol. 2004;490: 187–97.
51. Johansson BL, Sjoberg S, Wahren J. The influence of human C-peptide on renal function and glucose utilization in type 1 (insulin-dependent) diabetic patients. Diabetologia. 1992;35:121–8.
52. Johansson BL, Kernell A, Sjoberg S, Wahren J. Influence of combined C-peptide and insulin administration on renal function and metabolic control in diabetes type 1. J Clin Endocrinol Metab. 1993;77: 976–81.
53. Johansson BL, Borg K, Fernqvist-Forbes E, et al. Beneficial effects of C-peptide on incipient nephropathy and neuropathy in patients with type 1 diabetes mellitus. Diabet Med. 2000;17:181–9.
54. Sjoquist M, Huang W, Johansson BL. Effects of C-peptide on renal function at the early stage of experimental diabetes. Kidney Int. 1998;54:758–64.
55. Samnegard B, Jacobson SH, Jaremko G, Johansson BL, Sjoquist M. Effects of C-peptide on glomerular and renal size and renal function in diabetic rats. Kidney Int. 2001;60:1258–65.
56. Huang D-Y, Richter K, Breidenbach A, Vallon V. Human C-peptide acutely lowers glomerular hyperfiltration and proteinuria in diabetic rats: a dose-response study. Naunyn Schmiedebergs Arch Pharmacol. 2002;365:67–73.
57. Samnegard B, Jacobson SH, Johansson BL, et al. C-peptide and captopril are equally effective in lowering glomerular hyperfiltration in diabetic rats. Nephrol Dial Transplant. 2004;19:1385–91.
58. Samnegard B, Jacobson SH, Jaremko G, et al. C-peptide prevents glomerular hypertrophy and mesangial matrix expansion in diabetic rats. Nephrol Dial Transplant. 2005;20:532–8.

59. Rebsomen L, Pitel S, Boubred F, et al. C-peptide replacement improves weight gain and renal function in diabetic rats. Diabetes Metab. 2006;32:223–8.
60. Kamikawa A, Ishii T, Shimada K, et al. Proinsulin C-peptide abrogates type-1 diabetes-induced increase of renal endothelial nitric oxide synthase in rats. Diabetes Metab Res Rev. 2008;24:331–8.
61. Johansson BL, Linde B, Wahren J. Effects of C-peptide on blood flow, capillary diffusion capacity and glucose utilization in the exercising forearm of type 1 (insulin-dependent) diabetic patients. Diabetologia. 1992;35:1151–8.
62. Fernqvist-Forbes E, Johansson BL, Erikson MJ. Effects of C-peptide on forearm blood flow and brachial artery dilatation in patients with type 1 diabetes mellitus. Acta Physiol Scand. 2001;172:159–65.
63. Johansson BL, Wahren J, Pernow J. C-peptide increases forearm blood flow in patients with type 1 diabetes via a nitric oxide-dependent mechanism. Am J Physiol Endocrinol Metab. 2003;285:E864–70.
64. Forst T, Kunt T, Pohlmann T, et al. Biological activity of C-peptide on the skin microcirculation in patients with insulin-dependent diabetes mellitus. J Clin Invest. 1998;101:2036–41.
65. Forst T, De La Tour DD, Kunt T, et al. Effects of proinsulin C-peptide on nitric oxide, microvascular blood flow and erythrocyte Na^+, K^+-ATPase activity in diabetes mellitus type I. Clin Sci. 2000;98:283–90.
66. Nakamoto H, Sakane N, Kimura K, et al. Synergistic effects of C-peptide and insulin on coronary flow in early diabetic rats. Metabolism. 2004;53:335–9.
67. Wallerath T, Kunt T, Forst T, et al. Stimulation of endothelial nitric oxide synthase by proinsulin C-peptide. Nitric Oxide. 2003;9:95–102.
68. Scalia R, Coyle KM, Levine BJ, Booth G, Leffer AM. C-peptide inhibits leukocyte-endothelium interaction in the microcirculation during acute endothelial dysfunction. FASEB J. 2000;14:2357–64.
69. Young LH, Ikeda Y, Scalia R, Lefer AM. C-peptide exerts cardioprotective effects in myocardial ischemia-reperfusion. Am J Physiol Heart Circ Physiol. 2000;279:H1453–9.
70. Cotter MA, Ekberg K, Wahren J, Cameron NE. Effects of proinsulin C-peptide in experimental diabetic neuropathy: vascular actions and modulation by nitric oxide synthase inhibition. Diabetes. 2003;52:1812–7.
71. Stevens MJ, Zhang W, Li F, Sima AA. C-peptide corrects endoneurial blood flow but not oxidative stress in type 1 BB/Wor rats. Am J Physiol Endocrinol Metab. 2004;287:E497–505.
72. Kitamura T, Kimura K, Makondo K, et al. Proinsulin C-peptide increases nitric oxide production through mitogen-activated protein kinase-dependent transcriptional enhancement of endothelial nitric oxide synthase in rat aortic endothelial cells. Diabetologia. 2003;46:1698–705.
73. van Faassen EE, Bahrami S, Feelisch M, et al. Nitrite as regulator of hypoxic signaling in mammalian physiology. Med Res Rev. 2009;29:683–741.
74. Bryan NS, Calvert JW, Gundewar S, Lefer DJ. Dietary nitrite restores NO homeostasis and is cardioprotective in eNOS deficient mice. Free Radic Biol Med. 2008;45:468–74.
75. Kapil V, Webb AJ, Ahluwalia A. Inorganic nitrate and the cardiovascular system. Heart. 2010;96:1703–9.
76. Zhong Z, Kotova O, Davidescu A, et al. C-peptide stimulates Na^+/K^+-ATPase via activation of ERK1/2 MAP kinases in human renal tubular cells. Cell Mol Life Sci. 2004;61:2782–90.
77. Tsimaratos M, Roger F, Chabardès D, et al. C-peptide stimulates Na^+/K^+-ATPase activity *via* PKC alpha in rat medullary thick ascending limb. Diabetologia. 2003;46:124–31.
78. Ohtomo Y, Aperia A, Sahlgren B, Johansson BL, Wahren J. C-peptide stimulates rat renal tubular Na^+/K^+-ATPase activity in synergism with neuropeptide Y. Diabetologia. 1996;39:199–205.
79. Ohtomo Y, Bergman T, Johansson BL, Jornvall H, Wahren J. Differential effects of proinsulin C-peptide fragments on Na^+/K^+-ATPase activity of renal tubule segments. Diabetologia. 1998;41:287–91.
80. White CN, Hamilton EJ, Garcia A, et al. Opposing effects of coupled and uncoupled NOS activity on the Na^+-K^+ pump in cardiac myocytes. Am J Physiol Cell Physiol. 2008;294:C572–8.
81. Kone BC, Higham S. Nitric oxide inhibits transcription of the Na^+/K^+-ATPase α1-subunit gene in an MTAL cell line. Am J Physiol. 1999;276:F614–21.
82. Reifenberger MS, Arnett KL, Gatto C, Milanick MA. The reactive nitrogen species peroxynitrite is a potent inhibitor of renal Na-K-ATPase activity. Am J Physiol Renal Physiol. 2008;295:F1191–8.
83. Ido Y, Vindigni A, Chang K, et al. Prevention of vascular and neural dysfunction in diabetic rats by C-peptide. Science. 1997;277:563–6.
84. Sima AA, Zhang W, Sugimoto K, et al. C-peptide prevents and improves chronic type 1 diabetic polyneuropathy in the BB/Wor rat. Diabetologia. 2001;44: 889–97.
85. Raccah D, Lamotte-Jannot MF, Issautier T, Vague P. Effect of experimental diabetes on Na^+/K^+-ATPase activity in red blood cells, peripheral nerve and kidney. Diabete Metab. 1994;20:271–4.
86. Tsimaratos M, Coste TC, Djemli-Shipkolye A, et al. Gamma-linolenic acid restores renal medullary thick ascending limb Na^+, K^+-ATPase activity in diabetic rats. J Nutr. 2001;131:3160–5.
87. Comellas AP, Dada LA, Lecuona E, et al. Hypoxia-mediated degradation of Na, K-ATPase via mitochondrialreactiveoxygenspeciesandtheubiquitin-conjugating system. Circ Res. 2006;98:1314–22.
88. Nordquist L, Shimada K, Ishii T, et al. Proinsulin C-peptide prevents type-1 diabetes-induced decrease of renal Na^+, K^+-ATPase α1-subunit in rats. Diabetes Metab Res Rev. 2010;26:193–9.
89. Kitamura T, Kimura K, Jung BD, et al. Proinsulin C-peptide rapidly stimulates mitogen-activated protein kinases in Swiss 3T3 fibroblasts: requirement of protein

kinase C, phosphoinositide 3-kinase and pertussis toxin-sensitive G protein. Biochem J. 2001;355:123–9.
90. Kitamura T, Kimura K, Jung BD, et al. Proinsulin C-peptide activates CRE binding proteins through the p38 MAP kinase pathway in mouse lung capillary endothelial cells. Biochem J. 2002;366:737–44.
91. Albrecht EW, Stegeman CA, Heeringa P, Henning RH, van Goor H. Protective role of endothelial nitric oxide synthase. J Pathol. 2003;199:8–17.
92. Cifarelli V, Luppi P, Tse HM, He J, Piganelli J, Trucco M. Human proinsulin C-peptide reduces high glucose-induced proliferation and NF-kappaB activation in vascular smooth muscle cells. Atherosclerosis. 2008;201:248–57.
93. Kobayashi Y, Naruse K, Hamada Y, et al. Human proinsulin C-peptide prevents proliferation of rat aortic smooth muscle cells cultured in high-glucose conditions. Diabetologia. 2005;48:2396–401.
94. Sima AAF, Zhang W, Muzik O, et al. Sequential abnormalities in type 1 diabetic encephalopathy and the effects of C-peptide. Rev Diabet Stud. 2009;6: 211–22.

Renoprotective Effects of C-Peptide on Type 1 Diabetes

7

Lina Nordquist, Åsa Kallas, Sara Stridh, Fredrik Palm, and John Wahren

Keywords
Diabetic nephropathy • Oxygen consumption • Glomerular filtration rate • Arteriole

Introduction

Approximately 30% of type 1 diabetes patients develop nephropathy within 10–20 years of the onset of diabetes. Initial glomerular hyperfiltration and early microalbuminuria are commonly followed by progressive deterioration of the glomerular filtration rate (GFR), pronounced albuminuria and eventually the development of end stage renal disease (ESRD), a condition accompanied by 18-fold increased mortality [1]. In addition, retinopathy, hypertension, and cardiovascular disease are frequent co-morbidities attesting to the severity and complexity of the diabetic nephropathy. The first reports of beneficial effects of C-peptide on the diabetic kidney were published by Johansson et al. [2]. In this chapter, we summarize the last 20 years of research on the effects of C-peptide on diabetic nephropathy with regard to both basic science and clinical findings.

L. Nordquist (✉) • S. Stridh
Department of Medical Cell Biology, Division of Integrative Physiology, Biomedical Center, Uppsala University, Box 57175123, Uppsala, Sweden
e-mail: lina.nordquist@mcb.uu.se

Å. Kallas • J. Wahren
Department of Molecular Medicine and Surgery, Karolinska Institutet, Stockholm, Sweden

F. Palm
Department of Medical Cell Biology, Division of Integrative Physiology, Biomedical Center, Uppsala University, Box 57175123, Uppsala, Sweden

Department of Medicine, Division of Nephrology and Hypertension, Georgetown University, Washington, DC, USA

Renal Anatomy and Physiology

Among the essential functions of the kidneys are long-term regulation of blood pressure via direct regulation of the plasma volume, acid-base balance, maintaining water and electrolyte homeostasis to allow survival in a changing environment, production of hormones and excretion of metabolic waste products and water soluble toxins. The human kidney consists of approximately 1,000,000 structural and functional units, nephrons, consisting of the glomerulus, the proximal tubule, the loop of Henle, the distal tubule and the collecting ducts. Blood enters the glomerulus through the afferent arteriole that leads into the glomerular capillaries. In these capillaries, low molecular weight constituents of plasma are filtered across the glomerular membrane into

A.A.F. Sima (ed.), *Diabetes & C-Peptide: Scientific and Clinical Aspects*, Contemporary Diabetes, DOI 10.1007/978-1-61779-391-2_7,

Bowman's space, creating the primary urine. In human kidneys, approximately 180 L of primary urine, equivalent to 1.5 kg of NaCl, are produced daily, but only about 1–2 L and 10–15 g of NaCl are actually excreted [3]. As a consequence, most of the constituents of the primary urine are reabsorbed to the blood by the tubule before the urine exits the kidney and enters the ureters. To achieve this, the different nephron segments contain highly specialized cells that regulate kidney function by altering reabsorption and secretion, as well as directly participating in GFR regulation. Approximately 80% of total renal oxygen consumption is related to electrolyte transport [4]. Na^+ reabsorption is predominately accomplished by the Na^+ gradient created by Na^+/K^+-adenosine triphosphatase (Na^+/K^+-ATPase), located in the basolateral membrane of most tubular cells [5]. Renal proximal tubular cells achieve approximately 2/3 of all tubular electrolyte transport.

Regulators of Glomerular Filtration

To maintain adequate kidney function and facilitate reabsorption, it is essential to regulate the rate by which primary urine is produced by the filtration process across the glomerular capillaries. This rate, commonly referred to as the GFR, is determined by the delta hydraulic pressure in the glomerular capillary (P_{cap}; driving force) and by the opposing pressure of the primary urine in Bowman's space, or the early proximal tubule (P_{tub}). Since the filtration process across the glomerular membrane does not allow proteins to be filtered, difference in oncotic pressure ($\Delta\Pi_{onc}$; i.e., protein concentration in the blood) is also a force opposing filtration of fluids across the glomerular membrane into Bowman's space. Changes in P_{cap} are a result of alterations in the interplay between afferent and efferent glomerular arteriolar resistance, which alters the pressure transmitted into the glomerular capillaries [6, 7]. As defined by the Starling equation, resistances of the afferent and efferent arteriole determine the blood flow, and the relative constriction between the two regulates P_{cap}. Interestingly, $\Delta\Pi_{onc}$ is influenced by GFR per se, since increased GFR will elevate Π_{onc} in the glomerular capillaries, and act as a stabilizing factor opposing large acute changes in GFR [8]. The hydrostatic pressure in the early proximal tubule is determined not only by GFR, but also by the rate of tubular reabsorption, since both these factors influence the hydraulic resistance [9].

In addition to hydraulic and $\Delta\Pi_{onc}$ pressures, GFR is affected by the biophysical characteristics of the glomerular capillary wall. The ultrafiltration coefficient (K_f) is dependent on the hydraulic conductivity, which is determined by the membrane permeability and the size of the glomerular filtration surface area. GFR is also dynamically regulated by tubuloglomerular feedback (TGF); a regulating function described more in detail below.

Development of Diabetic Nephropathy

Approximately 30% of all type 1 diabetic patients will eventually develop diabetic nephropathy, a disease characterized by functional and morphological dysfunction, resulting in progressive renal dysfunction. The first detectable morphological alteration associated with diabetic nephropathy is thickening of the glomerular basement membrane. Later on, mesangial matrix expansion develops, known as diffuse glomerulosclerosis [10]. However, glomerular hyperfiltration and metabolic alterations, such as increased oxygen utilization secondary to increased tubular electrolyte load and oxidative stress, occur before any morphological alterations. Thus, diabetes-induced glomerular hyperfiltration, resulting in glomerular hypertension, is a predictor of later development of diabetic nephropathy, including irreversible morphological damage [11].

Following the initial phase with glomerular hyperfiltration and hypertrophy, diabetic patients commonly enter a quiet, nonsymptomatic phase with development of structural abnormalities. Further on in the progression of diabetic nephropathy follows a phase of incipient nephropathy indicated by the presence of microalbuminuria.

Diabetic nephropathy is considered manifest when patients present with macroalbuminuria, increased blood pressure, and increased serum creatinine levels due to deteriorating GFR [10]. At this stage, glomerulosclerosis and tubulointerstitial fibrosis are common morphological findings. An appreciable number of patients with diabetic nephropathy will eventually develop ESRD, which requires frequent visits to the dialysis unit or kidney transplantation. It should be noted that diabetic patients requiring dialysis have decreased survival rate compared to other patients requiring dialysis [12].

Glomerular Hyperfiltration in Diabetes

Diabetic glomerular hyperfiltration commonly develops in early diabetes mellitus and is closely correlated with the development and progression of diabetic nephropathy. Hyperfiltration has been explained as the result of a reduced vascular resistance of the afferent arteriole [13], likely due to increased proximal electrolyte and glucose reabsorption, leading to a reduced electrolyte load passing the macula densa [14]. This would result in TGF inactivation, i.e., in a reduction of adenosine A_1-receptor stimulation and afferent arteriolar tone, subsequently increasing GFR [15]. Recently, the hypothesis of TGF as cause of diabetic hyperfiltration has been questioned, since adenosine A_1-receptor knockout mice have been reported to develop pronounced hyperfiltration, despite lacking a functional TGF mechanism [16, 17]. Thus, hyperfiltration must develop through other mechanisms. Close to 40 years ago, Leyssac reported that GFR is tightly regulated by the degree of proximal tubular reabsorption [18]. Since it is well established that proximal reabsorption is increased in diabetes [19], this provides an explanation for the glomerular hyperfiltration in this disorder.

There are reports of reduced hydrostatic pressure in the early proximal tubule of diabetic rats, and that this pressure can be increased by inhibiting proximal reabsorption with a carbonic anhydrase inhibitor acetazolamide [20]. Since an increase in net filtration pressure (P_{net}) develops rapidly after inhibition of proximal tubular reabsorption and occurs before activation of TGF, the early P_{tub} is likely a key regulator of GFR during situations of increased tubular reabsorption, including diabetes.

Renal Effects of C-Peptide in Experimental Diabetes

C-peptide exerts beneficial effects in many tissues affected by microvascular diabetes complications. Indirect support is obtained from reports that pancreas or islet transplantation, restoring insulin and C-peptide secretion, results in reduced microalbuminuria and normalized glomerular structural morphology 10 years after restoring normoglycemia and endogenous C-peptide concentrations [21–23].

C-peptide induces a cascade of effects in the diabetic kidney, including reduced glomerular hyperfiltration, reduced albuminuria, and decreased glomerular hypertrophy [24–28]. Interestingly, the intact C-peptide molecule is not required for these beneficial effects since also its carboxy-terminal pentapeptide fragment (EVARQ) reduces the diabetes-induced glomerular hyperfiltration in rats [29]. Possible mechanisms for the beneficial effects of C-peptide on kidney function in diabetes are reviewed below.

Effects on Afferent and Efferent Arteriolar Tone

Reduction of diabetic hyperfiltration can be mediated via effects on either afferent or efferent arteriolar tone, or a combination of the two. Constriction of the afferent arteriole and/or dilation of the efferent arteriole will lower GFR due to reduced P_{cap}, which is a main determinant of P_{net}. The afferent arteriolar diameter is increased in animal models of type 1 diabetes [30], which is an indication that vasodilation could contribute to increasing the P_{cap} and cause an increase in GFR. Dilators of the efferent arteriole (e.g., angiotensin-converting enzyme

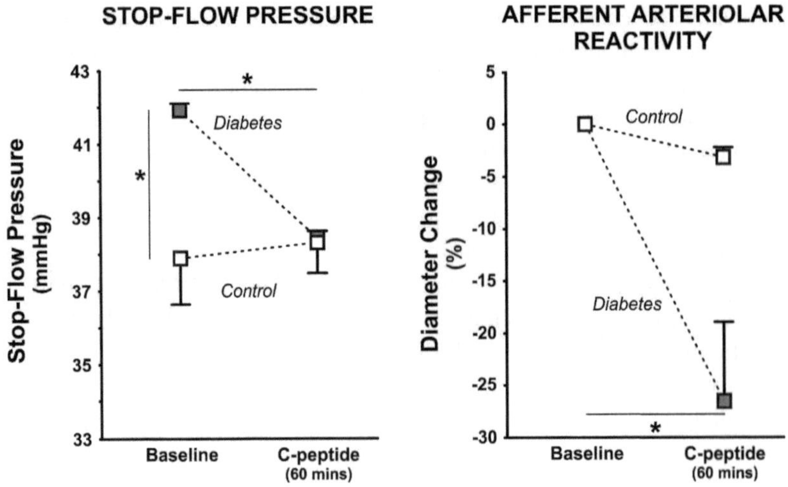

Fig. 7.1 Acute infusion of C-peptide decreases tubular stop-flow pressure in diabetic rats (*left*), and induces constriction of isolated glomerular afferent arterioles isolated from diabetic mice (*right*). Both these mechanisms act to reduce the diabetes-induced glomerular hyperfiltration, which is a known predictor of the progression of diabetic nephropathy. Redrawn from data presented in refs. [26, 37]

inhibitors), as well as afferent constrictors (e.g., low protein diets) are known to reduce GFR and may improve long-term renal function in diabetes [31–34].

C-peptide does not alter total renal blood flow in the diabetic kidney [26, 35, 36]. However, it constricts the afferent arteriole isolated from type 1 diabetic mice (Fig. 7.1) [37]. Interestingly, the constrictory effect of C-peptide on the diabetic afferent arterioles is completely prevented by blockade of the Rho-kinase, indicating that C-peptide causes vasoconstriction by increasing Ca^{2+} sensitivity. In addition, the finding of a vasoconstriction of the afferent arteriole reduced stop-flow pressure (Fig. 7.1) and normalized GFR after C-peptide administration to diabetic rats while maintaining total renal blood flow indicates a pronounced dilation of the efferent arteriole [26]. Similarly, a synchronized effect on renal afferent-efferent arteriole tone has been reported for Ca^{2+} channel blockers and for nitric oxide synthase inhibitors [38, 39]. These observations suggest that C-peptide deficiency in type 1 diabetes may contribute to afferent arteriolar dilation and glomerular hyperfiltration, and that C-peptide may be a useful treatment to reduce the diabetes-induced glomerular hyperfiltration.

Effects on the Renal Tubules and Tubular Cells

It has been widely reported that diabetes-induced hyperfiltration is associated with increased oxygen consumption and renal Na^+/K^+-ATPase activity [40–43]. C-peptide administered to diabetic rats increases fractional urinary Na^+ excretion and lithium clearance in vivo, the latter being inversely related to proximal tubular Na^+ transport (Fig. 7.2) [26]. This is caused by C-peptide-induced inhibition of Na^+/K^+-ATPase activity reducing the driving force for tubular Na^+ transport. These effects have been studied in vitro on freshly isolated tubular cells from diabetic rat kidneys and are manifested as reduced oxygen consumption related to tubular electrolyte transport (Fig. 7.2) [26].

C-peptide may exert state-specific effects related to prevailing glucose concentrations. Under normoglycemic conditions, C-peptide phosphorylates the Na^+/K^+-ATPase α-subunit in tubular cells, thus stimulating Na^+/K^+-ATPase and tubular Na^+ transport [44, 45]. Interestingly, activation of Na^+/K^+-ATPase is also achieved by the C-terminal penta- and hexapeptides of C-peptide [46]. Analogous state-specific effects have been

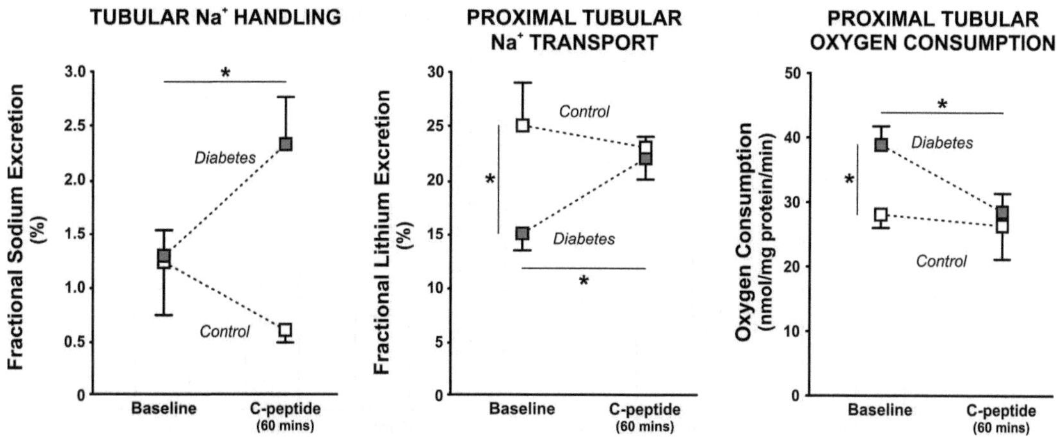

Fig. 7.2 C-peptide acutely reduces tubular Na^+ reabsorption (*left*) and increases Li^+ clearance (*middle*; inversely related of proximal tubular Na^+ reabsorption) in diabetic rats in vivo. Furthermore, C-peptide reduces electrolyte transport-related oxygen consumption in proximal tubular cells isolated from diabetic rats (*right*). Together, these results demonstrate that C-peptide effectively inhibits tubular Na^+ reabsorption, which might affect both blood pressure regulation and renal oxygenation. Redrawn from data presented in ref. [26]

observed for C-peptide on endothelial nitric oxide synthase [47, 48]. The background to the divergent effects of C-peptide on tubular electrolyte handling during normoglycemia and hyperglycemia are currently not fully understood, but may be related to differences in oxidative stress state.

C-Peptide and Kidney Oxygenation

Although the kidneys make up only about 0.5% of total body mass, they account for approximately 10% of whole body oxygen consumption. Oxygen consumption is increased in tubular cells isolated from diabetic kidneys (Fig. 7.2) [26, 49, 50], which translates into increased total oxygen consumption by the diabetic kidney [51]. The increased oxygen utilization results in renal hypoxia [49–51], which has been proposed as a pivotal mechanism for the onset and progression of diabetic nephropathy [52]. Nangaku and coworkers have proposed hypoxia in the tubulointerstitium as a final pathway to fibrosis and ESRD [53–56]. Several reports have emphasized a connection between increased renal Na^+/K^+-ATPase activity and augmented oxygen consumption, and also to glomerular hyperfiltration [40–43]. Interestingly, C-peptide inhibits Na^+/K^+-ATPase and therefore reduces the oxygen consumption in freshly isolated proximal tubular cells from diabetic rat kidneys [26]. In addition, red blood cell deformability is reduced in diabetes and by improving red cell compliance, C-peptide exerts a positive influence on renal blood flow and oxygen availability [57].

C-Peptide and Renal Structural Abnormalities

C-peptide directly influences renal function in diabetes, but has also been shown to increase cell proliferation [58] and to reduce renal structural abnormalities commonly associated with prolonged diabetes duration [28, 59]. Glomerular mesangial matrix expansion and capillary basement membrane thickening are among the first detectable morphological alterations during the early development of diabetic nephropathy, resulting in increased glomerular volume and augmented width of the podocyte interdigital processes [60]. Apoptotic cell loss due to pro-apoptotic cytokines is a feature of diabetic nephropathy. Accumulation of extracellular matrix, a common cause of glomerulosclerosis, eventually results in tubular damage and development of ESRD [61, 62]. Tubular cells can induce tubulointerstitial fibrosis [63], a process known as epithelial-mesenchymal transformation.

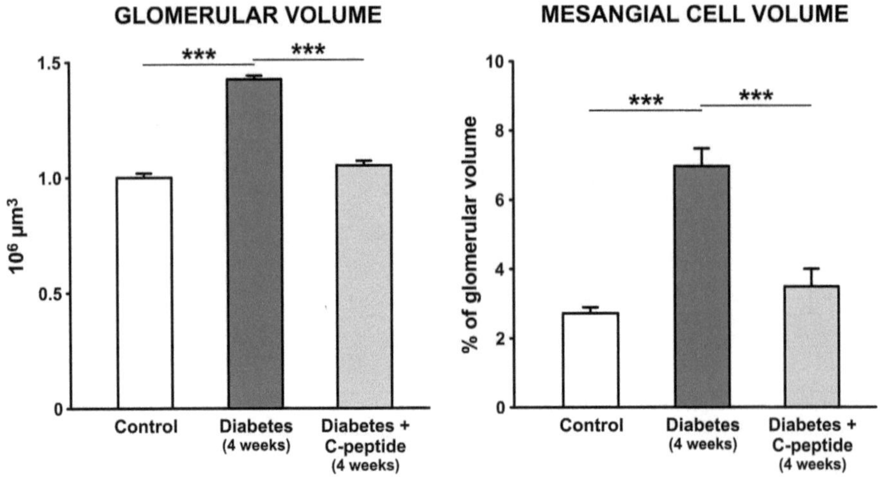

Fig. 7.3 Chronic C-peptide treatment prevents the diabetes-induced increase in glomerular volume and diminishes mesangial matrix expansion. Redrawn from data presented in ref. [59]

Administration of C-peptide in physiological concentrations to diabetic rats and mice prevents glomerular hypertrophy and early intraglomerular morphological alterations [28, 64]. Likely, structural improvements following C-peptide administration are secondary to reduced glomerular mesangial matrix expansion (Fig. 7.3) [59]. Little is known about the mechanisms involved in effects of C-peptide on the renal structural abnormalities in diabetes, but signaling pathways involve effects on transcription factors, as well as inhibition of disease mediators. Transforming growth factor (TGF)-β is a well known pro-fibrotic factor involved in diabetes-induced fibrosis, as well as other morphological dysfunctions [65]. Brunskill and colleagues recently reported that C-peptide will block pathological TGF-β1 signaling pathways, thereby inhibiting epithelial-mesenchymal transformation in human kidney proximal tubular cells [24]. Another well-known culprit in diabetic nephropathy is tumor necrosis factor (TNF)-α, a pro-inflammatory, pro-apoptotic cytokine [66]. In opossum kidney proximal tubular cells, C-peptide protects against TNF-α-induced proximal tubular cell toxicity and apoptosis [67], most likely via activation of transcription factor NF-kappaB [67]. C-peptide-induced pathways and renal intracellular signaling are further described in Chap. 4. Regardless of the precise mechanisms involved, the beneficial effects of C-peptide in preventing diabetes-induced renal structural abnormalities strongly support a role for C-peptide as a potential therapy for nephropathy in type 1 diabetes.

Renal Effects of C-Peptide in Patients with Type 1 Diabetes

The results from the first studies involving effects of C-peptide on renal function in patients with type 1 diabetes without overt signs of renal disease were reported in 1992 [2]. C-peptide was infused intravenously at two rates for 2 h, reaching concentrations in the physiological range (0.7 and 2.1 nmol/L for the low and high infusion rate, respectively). All patients presented with glomerular hyperfiltration in the basal state and the GFR decreased by 7% after C-peptide administration (Fig. 7.4). Furthermore, blood flow increased slightly and the filtration fraction decreased from 19 to 17% in response to C-peptide infusion. These results in diabetic patients are in good agreement with the reports from recent animal studies, and may in part reflect an increased intrarenal vascular tone of the preglomerular afferent arterioles whereas the efferent arterioles dilate in order to maintain total renal blood flow. The higher C-peptide

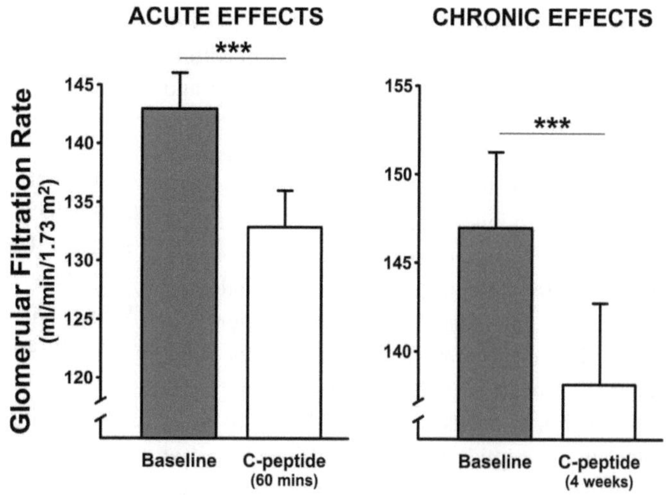

Fig. 7.4 C-peptide administration for 60 min decreases glomerular hyperfiltration in diabetic patients (*left*), an effect that is sustained also after chronic administration for 4 weeks (*right*). Redrawn from data presented in refs. [2, 69]

concentrations in the group receiving the higher infusion rate were not associated with more pronounced effects. In the same study, C-peptide was also infused in healthy subjects, in whom it was found to have no detectable effect on any of the renal parameters. This is consistent with the reports showing that C-peptide binding to cell membranes saturates already at low nanomolar concentrations [68]. Further elevation of the concentration of C-peptide above physiological levels in healthy individuals will thus not elicit any further effects.

In subsequent studies, prolonged periods of C-peptide administration have been employed. In a double-blind randomized study, type 1 patients with incipient nephropathy received replacement doses of C-peptide for 1 month administered by subcutaneous infusion via a pump together with the patients' regular insulin therapy [69]. All patients displayed elevated GFR and mild microalbuminuria at the start of the study. In the C-peptide-treated patients, GFR fell by 6% and the urinary albumin excretion decreased by approximately 50% (Fig. 7.5), whereas no significant change was observed in the controls receiving insulin and placebo. Blood pressure was unchanged but indices of glycemic control improved slightly in the C-peptide group, but not in the controls, which may possibly have contributed to the positive outcome of the C-peptide administration.

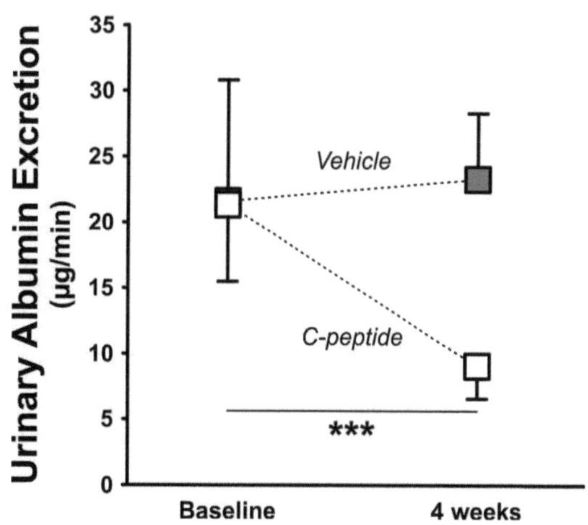

Fig. 7.5 Chronic C-peptide administration for 3 months reduces urinary albumin excretion in diabetic patients. Redrawn from data presented in ref. [70]

In a study involving type 1 patients with longer diabetes duration, microalbuminuria and slightly more advanced renal dysfunction, C-peptide was administered for 3 months in replacement doses via four daily subcutaneous injections [70]. Prestudy urinary albumin excretion was in the range 25–220 µg/min and measurements were done after 1, 2, and 3 months. Albumin excretion decreased gradually throughout the study period and was reduced by approximately 40% at the end of the study in the patients receiving C-peptide. Notably, albumin excretion remained unchanged or was slightly increased in the vehicle-treated controls. Indices of glycemic control were similar in the C-peptide group and the controls and all patients were normotensive throughout the study, demonstrating that the renal effect most likely was directly related to the C-peptide administration. Taken together, the findings in type 1 patients confirm that the beneficial results for C-peptide obtained in animal studies translate into positive effects in patients. It should be noted that the above studies were undertaken in patients free of medications other than insulin. It needs to be established to what extent the C-peptide effects are influenced, if at all, by chronic blockade of the renin angiotensin aldosterone system in diabetic patients, since this is the current standard therapy for patients with diabetic nephropathy. Further studies are warranted involving longer study duration, larger patient groups and type 1 patients with more advanced renal disease.

Concluding Comments: What Next for C-Peptide?

The available experimental and clinical data show that C-peptide exerts a number of beneficial effects on diabetes-induced functional and structural abnormalities of the kidneys in type 1 diabetes, as summarized in Fig. 7.6. In fact, C-peptide treatment emerges as a compelling new therapeutic option for type 1 nephropathy. Improved understanding of the mechanisms by which C-peptide reduces hyperfiltration and albuminuria in vivo is needed. Likewise, additional data characterizing the influence of C-peptide on glomerular and tubular structural abnormalities are required. It is noted that most of the present data have been generated in cell systems or via animal experiments, while only few human studies have been carried out so far. This is a consequence of the costs associated

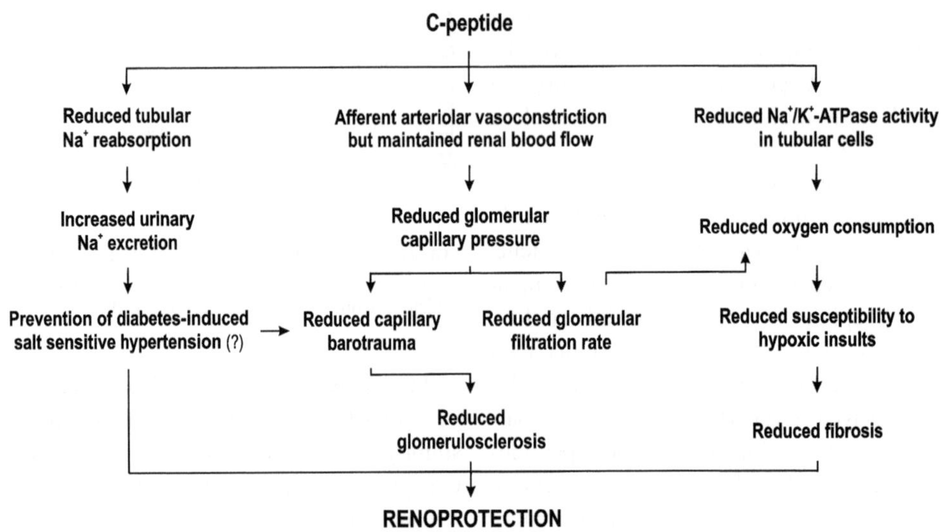

Fig. 7.6 Schematic overview of the reported renoprotective effects of C-peptide. C-peptide constricts the glomerular afferent arteriole which reduces the capillary pressure, resulting in protection against glomerular barotrauma and glomerulosclerosis. The inhibition of the Na^+/K^+-ATPase together with the reduced tubular electrolyte load, due to the reduced glomerular filtration rate, reduce the oxygen utilization and protects against hypoxic insults. The reduced tubular Na^+ reabsorption increases the urinary Na^+ excretion that is proposed to reduce the salt sensitive hypertension commonly associated with prolonged diabetes duration. Together, these effects of C-peptide prevent the development of glomerulosclerosis and interstitial fibrosis and protect against the development of diabetic nephropathy

with conducting clinical trials, which cannot readily be accommodated in an academic setting. Consequently, a commitment from the pharmaceutical industry is warranted at this time. Clinical trials involving C-peptide administration together with regular insulin therapy for prolonged periods of time (12–24 months) in type 1 patients at different stages of nephropathy are urgently needed in order to advance our knowledge of the therapeutic potential of C-peptide. Furthermore, the possible interaction between C-peptide therapy and the present standard care for diabetic nephropathy such as blockade of the renin angiotensin aldosterone system needs to be evaluated.

References

1. Groop PH, Thomas MC, Moran JL, et al. The presence and severity of chronic kidney disease predicts all-cause mortality in type 1 diabetes. Diabetes. 2009;58(7):1651–8.
2. Johansson BL, Sjoberg S, Wahren J. The influence of human C-peptide on renal function and glucose utilization in type 1 (insulin-dependent) diabetic patients. Diabetologia. 1992;35(2):121–8.
3. Yamasue K, Tochikubo O, Kono E, Maeda H. Self-monitoring of home blood pressure with estimation of daily salt intake using a new electrical device. J Hum Hypertens. 2006;20(8):593–8.
4. Lassen NA, Munck O, Thaysen JH. Oxygen consumption and sodium reabsorption in the kidney. Acta Physiol Scand. 1961;51:371–84.
5. Katz AI, Epstein FH. The role of sodium-potassium-activated adenosine triphosphatase in the reabsorption of sodium by the kidney. J Clin Invest. 1967;46(12): 1999–2011.
6. Ren YL, Garvin JL, Ito S, Carretero OA. Role of neuronal nitric oxide synthase in the macula densa. Kidney Int. 2001;60(5):1676–83.
7. Persson AE, Gushwa LC, Blantz RC. Feedback pressure-flow responses in normal and angiotensin-prostaglandin-blocked rats. Am J Physiol. 1984;247(6 Pt 2):F925–31.
8. Brenner BM, Troy JL. Postglomerular vascular protein concentration: evidence for a causal role in governing fluid reabsorption and glomerulotubular balance by the renal proximal tubule. J Clin Invest. 1971;50(2):336–49.
9. Karlsen FM, Holstein-Rathlou NH, Leyssac PP. A re-evaluation of the determinants of glomerular filtration rate. Acta Physiol Scand. 1995;155(4):335–50.
10. Brenner BM, editor. Brenner and rector's: the kidney. 8th ed. Philadelphia: Saunders; 2004.
11. Mogensen CE. Early glomerular hyperfiltration in insulin-dependent diabetics and late nephropathy. Scand J Clin Lab Invest. 1986;46(3):201–6.
12. Koch M, Thomas B, Tschope W, Ritz E. Survival and predictors of death in dialysed diabetic patients. Diabetologia. 1993;36(10):1113–7.
13. Hostetter TH, Troy JL, Brenner BM. Glomerular hemodynamics in experimental diabetes mellitus. Kidney Int. 1981;19(3):410–5.
14. Thomson SC, Vallon V, Blantz RC. Kidney function in early diabetes: the tubular hypothesis of glomerular filtration. Am J Physiol Renal Physiol. 2004;286(1): F8–15.
15. Wright FS, Schnermann J. Interference with feedback control of glomerular filtration rate by furosemide, triflocin, and cyanide. J Clin Invest. 1974;53(6):1695–708.
16. Sallstrom J, Carlsson PO, Fredholm BB, et al. Diabetes-induced hyperfiltration in adenosine A(1)-receptor deficient mice lacking the tubuloglomerular feedback mechanism. Acta Physiol (Oxf). 2007;190: 253–9.
17. Faulhaber-Walter R, Chen L, Oppermann M, et al. Lack of A1 adenosine receptors augments diabetic hyperfiltration and glomerular injury. J Am Soc Nephrol. 2008;19(4):722–30.
18. Leyssac PP. Dependence of glomerular filtration rate on proximal tubular reabsorption of salt. Acta Physiol Scand. 1963;58:236–42.
19. Hryciw DH, Lee EM, Pollock CA, Poronnik P. Molecular changes in proximal tubule function in diabetes mellitus. Clin Exp Pharmacol Physiol. 2004;31(5–6):372–9.
20. Leyssac PP, Karlsen FM, Skott O. Dynamics of intrarenal pressures and glomerular filtration rate after acetazolamide. Am J Physiol. 1991;261(1 Pt 2): F169–78.
21. Fiorina P, Folli F, Zerbini G, et al. Islet transplantation is associated with improvement of renal function among uremic patients with type I diabetes mellitus and kidney transplants. J Am Soc Nephrol. 2003;14(8):2150–8.
22. Fioretto P, Steffes MW, Sutherland DE, Goetz FC, Mauer M. Reversal of lesions of diabetic nephropathy after pancreas transplantation. N Engl J Med. 1998;339(2):69–75.
23. Perkins BA, Ficociello LH, Silva KH, et al. Regression of microalbuminuria in type 1 diabetes. N Engl J Med. 2003;348(23):2285–93.
24. Hills CE, Al-Rasheed N, Al-Rasheed N, Willars GB, Brunskill NJ. C-peptide reverses TGF-beta1-induced changes in renal proximal tubular cells: implications for treatment of diabetic nephropathy. Am J Physiol Renal Physiol. 2009;296(3):F614–21.
25. Sjoquist M, Huang W, Johansson BL. Effects of C-peptide on renal function at the early stage of experimental diabetes. Kidney Int. 1998;54(3):758–64.
26. Nordquist L, Brown RD, Fasching A, Persson P, Palm F. Proinsulin C-peptide reduces diabetes-induced glomerular hyperfiltration via efferent arteriole dilation and

inhibition of tubular sodium reabsorption. Am J Physiol Renal Physiol. 2009;297:F1265–72.
27. Samnegard B. Renal effects of C-peptide in experimental type-1 diabetes mellitus. Stockholm: Danderyd Hospital and Department of Surgical Sciences, Karolinska Institute; 2005.
28. Samnegard B, Jacobson SH, Jaremko G, Johansson BL, Sjoquist M. Effects of C-peptide on glomerular and renal size and renal function in diabetic rats. Kidney Int. 2001;60(4):1258–65.
29. Nordquist L, Moe E, Sjoquist M. The C-peptide fragment EVARQ reduces glomerular hyperfiltration in streptozotocin-induced diabetic rats. Diabetes Metab Res Rev. 2007;23(5):400–5.
30. Ikenaga H, Bast JP, Fallet RW, Carmines PK. Exaggerated impact of ATP-sensitive K(+) channels on afferent arteriolar diameter in diabetes mellitus. J Am Soc Nephrol. 2000;11(7):1199–207.
31. Myers BD, Deen WM, Brenner BM. Effects of norepinephrine and angiotensin II on the determinants of glomerular ultrafiltration and proximal tubule fluid reabsorption in the rat. Circ Res. 1975;37(1):101–10.
32. Aurell M. Aspects of the role of intraglomerular pressure as a cause of progressive renal damage. Drugs. 1988;35 Suppl 5:42–7.
33. Inman SR, Stowe NT, Nally Jr JV, Brouhard BH, Vidt DG. Dietary protein does not alter intrinsic reactivity of renal microcirculation to angiotensin II in rodents. Am J Physiol. 1995;268(2 Pt 2):F302–8.
34. Dullaart RP, Beusekamp BJ, Meijer S, van Doormaal JJ, Sluiter WJ. Long-term effects of protein-restricted diet on albuminuria and renal function in IDDM patients without clinical nephropathy and hypertension. Diabetes Care. 1993;16(2):483–92.
35. Huang DY, Richter K, Breidenbach A, Vallon V. Human C-peptide acutely lowers glomerular hyperfiltration and proteinuria in diabetic rats: a dose-response study. Naunyn Schmiedebergs Arch Pharmacol. 2002;365(1):67–73.
36. Samnegard B, Jacobson SH, Johansson BL, et al. C-peptide and captopril are equally effective in lowering glomerular hyperfiltration in diabetic rats. Nephrol Dial Transplant. 2004;19(6):1385–91.
37. Nordquist L, Lai EY, Sjoquist M, Patzak A, Persson AE. Proinsulin C-peptide constricts glomerular afferent arterioles in diabetic mice. A potential renoprotective mechanism. Am J Physiol Regul Integr Comp Physiol. 2008;294(3):R836–41.
38. Feng MG, Navar LG. Nitric oxide synthase inhibition activates L- and T-type Ca2+ channels in afferent and efferent arterioles. Am J Physiol Renal Physiol. 2006;290(4):F873–9.
39. Hayashi K, Wakino S, Sugano N, et al. Ca2+ channel subtypes and pharmacology in the kidney. Circ Res. 2007;100(3):342–53.
40. Korner A, Eklof AC, Celsi G, Aperia A. Increased renal metabolism in diabetes. Mechanism and functional implications. Diabetes. 1994;43(5):629–33.
41. Wald H, Scherzer P, Rasch R, Popovtzer MM. Renal tubular Na(+)-K(+)-ATPase in diabetes mellitus: relationship to metabolic abnormality. Am J Physiol. 1993;265(1 Pt 1):E96–101.
42. Ku DD, Sellers BM, Meezan E. Development of renal hypertrophy and increased renal Na, K-ATPase in streptozotocin-diabetic rats. Endocrinology. 1986; 119(2):672–9.
43. Scherzer P, Nachliel I, Bar-On H, Popovtzer MM, Ziv E. Renal Na-K-ATPase hyperactivity in diabetic Psammomys obesus is related to glomerular hyperfiltration but is insulin-independent. J Endocrinol. 2000;167(2):347–54.
44. Ohtomo Y, Aperia A, Sahlgren B, Johansson BL, Wahren J. C-peptide stimulates rat renal tubular Na+, K(+)-ATPase activity in synergism with neuropeptide Y. Diabetologia. 1996;39(2):199–205.
45. Zhong Z, Kotova O, Davidescu A, et al. C-peptide stimulates Na+, K+-ATPase via activation of ERK1/2 MAP kinases in human renal tubular cells. Cell Mol Life Sci. 2004;61(21):2782–90.
46. Ohtomo Y, Bergman T, Johansson BL, Jornvall H, Wahren J. Differential effects of proinsulin C-peptide fragments on Na+, K+-ATPase activity of renal tubule segments. Diabetologia. 1998;41(3):287–91.
47. Kamikawa A, Ishii T, Shimada K, et al. Proinsulin C-peptide abrogates type-1 diabetes-induced increase of renal endothelial nitric oxide synthase in rats. Diabetes Metab Res Rev. 2008;24(4):331–8.
48. Kitamura T, Kimura K, Makondo K, et al. Proinsulin C-peptide increases nitric oxide production by enhancing mitogen-activated protein-kinase-dependent transcription of endothelial nitric oxide synthase in aortic endothelial cells of Wistar rats. Diabetologia. 2003;46(12):1698–705.
49. Palm F, Cederberg J, Hansell P, Liss P, Carlsson PO. Reactive oxygen species cause diabetes-induced decrease in renal oxygen tension. Diabetologia. 2003;46(8):1153–60.
50. Palm F, Hansell P, Ronquist G, et al. Polyol-pathway-dependent disturbances in renal medullary metabolism in experimental insulin-deficient diabetes mellitus in rats. Diabetologia. 2004;47(7):1223–31.
51. Palm F, Fasching A, Hansell P, Kallskog O. Nitric oxide originating from NOS1 controls oxygen utilization and electrolyte transport efficiency in the diabetic kidney. Am J Physiol Renal Physiol. 2010;298(2):F416–20.
52. Palm F. Intrarenal oxygen in diabetes and a possible link to diabetic nephropathy. Clin Exp Pharmacol Physiol. 2006;33(10):997–1001.
53. Mackensen-Haen S, Bader R, Grund KE, Bohle A. Correlations between renal cortical interstitial fibrosis, atrophy of the proximal tubules and impairment of the glomerular filtration rate. Clin Nephrol. 1981;15(4):167–71.
54. Nangaku M. Chronic hypoxia and tubulointerstitial injury: a final common pathway to end-stage renal failure. J Am Soc Nephrol. 2006;17(1):17–25.

55. Risdon RA, Sloper JC, De Wardener HE. Relationship between renal function and histological changes found in renal-biopsy specimens from patients with persistent glomerular nephritis. Lancet. 1968;2(7564):363–6.
56. Nangaku M. Hypoxia and tubulointerstitial injury: a final common pathway to end-stage renal failure. Nephron Exp Nephrol. 2004;98(1):e8–12.
57. Kunt T, Schneider S, Pfutzner A, et al. The effect of human proinsulin C-peptide on erythrocyte deformability in patients with type I diabetes mellitus. Diabetologia. 1999;42(4):465–71.
58. Al-Rasheed NM, Meakin F, Royal EL, et al. Potent activation of multiple signalling pathways by C-peptide in opossum kidney proximal tubular cells. Diabetologia. 2004;47(6):987–97.
59. Samnegard B, Jacobson SH, Jaremko G, et al. C-peptide prevents glomerular hypertrophy and mesangial matrix expansion in diabetic rats. Nephrol Dial Transplant. 2005;20(3):532–8.
60. Osterby R. Lessons from kidney biopsies. Diabetes Metab Rev. 1996;12(3):151–74.
61. Steffes MW, Osterby R, Chavers B, Mauer SM. Mesangial expansion as a central mechanism for loss of kidney function in diabetic patients. Diabetes. 1989;38(9):1077–81.
62. Striker LJ, Doi T, Elliot S, Striker GE. The contribution of glomerular mesangial cells to progressive glomerulosclerosis. Semin Nephrol. 1989;9(4):318–28.
63. Manotham K, Tanaka T, Matsumoto M, et al. Transdifferentiation of cultured tubular cells induced by hypoxia. Kidney Int. 2004;65(3):871–80.
64. Maezawa Y, Yokote K, Sonezaki K, et al. Influence of C-peptide on early glomerular changes in diabetic mice. Diabetes Metab Res Rev. 2006;22(4):313–22.
65. August P, Suthanthiran M. Transforming growth factor beta signaling, vascular remodeling, and hypertension. N Engl J Med. 2006;354(25):2721–3.
66. Hasegawa G, Nakano K, Sawada M, et al. Possible role of tumor necrosis factor and interleukin-1 in the development of diabetic nephropathy. Kidney Int. 1991;40(6):1007–12.
67. Al-Rasheed NM, Willars GB, Brunskill NJ. C-peptide signals via Galpha i to protect against TNF-alpha-mediated apoptosis of opossum kidney proximal tubular cells. J Am Soc Nephrol. 2006;17(4):986–95.
68. Rigler R, Pramanik A, Jonasson P, et al. Specific binding of proinsulin C-peptide to human cell membranes. Proc Natl Acad Sci U S A. 1999;96(23):13318–23.
69. Johansson BL, Kernell A, Sjoberg S, Wahren J. Influence of combined C-peptide and insulin administration on renal function and metabolic control in diabetes type 1. J Clin Endocrinol Metab. 1993;77(4):976–81.
70. Johansson BL, Borg K, Fernqvist-Forbes E, et al. Beneficial effects of C-peptide on incipient nephropathy and neuropathy in patients with type 1 diabetes mellitus. Diabet Med. 2000;17(3):181–9.

8 The Mechanisms Underlying the Effects of C-Peptide on Type 1 Diabetic Neuropathy

Hideki Kamiya, Wei-Xian Zhang, and Anders A.F. Sima

Keywords
Neuropathy • C-peptide • Axonal degeneration • Nodal degeneration • Regeneration

Introduction

Diabetic polyneuropathy (DPN) is the most common chronic complication of diabetes occurring in approximately 60% of diabetic patients [1–3]. It affects somato-sensory, nociceptive and autonomic peripheral nerves. These involvements may lead to serious consequences such as sensory loss and foot ulcerations, sometimes necessitating limb amputation. A common bothersome symptom is neuropathic pain. Autonomic neuropathy may impact on cardiac and gastrointestinal functions [2, 3].

Initially, DPN was believed to be primarily a Schwann cell disorder [4, 5] and to be the same disease process in type 1 and type 2 diabetes [6]. Only in the late 1970s, based mainly on experimental studies, was DPN characterized as a primary axonopathy affecting both the peripheral and central sensory axons [7–9]. A decade later, extensive histopathological studies of human sural nerve biopsies confirmed axonopathy as the primary abnormality and revealed differences with respect to DPN in type 1 vs. type 2 diabetic patients and hence firmly established DPN as a primary axonopathy [10–12].

The pathogenesis of DPN is not fully understood. For decades, the view has been held that hyperglycemia, common to both type 1 and type 2 diabetes, is the overriding culprit. Hence, it was argued that if we can control hyperglycemia, we should be able to prevent and cure DPN and other diabetic complications [13–16].

In past decades, several attempts have been made to address the underlying mechanisms

H. Kamiya
Department of Pathology, Wayne State University and Detroit Medical Center, 540 E. Canfield Avenue, Detroit, MI 48201, USA

Department of Endocrinology and Diabetes, Graduate School of Medicine, University of Nagoya, Nagoya 466-8550, Japan

W.-X. Zhang
Department of Pathology, Wayne State University and Detroit Medical Center, 540 E. Canfield Avenue, Detroit, MI 48201, USA

A.A.F. Sima (✉)
Department of Pathology, Wayne State University and Detroit Medical Center, 540 E. Canfield Avenue, Detroit, MI 48201, USA

Department of Neurology, Wayne State University and Detroit Medical Center, Detroit, MI 48201, USA
e-mail: asima@med.wayne.edu

A.A.F. Sima (ed.), *Diabetes & C-Peptide: Scientific and Clinical Aspects*, Contemporary Diabetes, DOI 10.1007/978-1-61779-391-2_8,

emanating from hyperglycemia therapeutically. Hence an array of aldose reductase inhibitors were developed to inhibit an activated polyol pathway. Although some effects could be demonstrated, the clinical benefits from such interventions were limited ([17–21]; review see [22]). Hyperglycemia has been shown to cause oxidative stress in peripheral nerves [2, 16, 23]. Several antioxidants have been subjected to clinical trial in patients with DPN, such as α-lipoic acid, γ-linoleic acid and tocopherol. Although some beneficial effects on somatic and autonomic neuropathies were demonstrated, they have been limited [23–25]. Aminoguanidine, an inhibitor of AGE formation, although promising in animal models, clinical trials in humans were discontinued because of adverse effects. Acetyl-L-carnitine, which promotes fatty acid β-oxidation has proven beneficial in animal models, but again clinical trials have met with limited benefits [26–28]. Lately, it has become evident that common comorbidities of diabetes may also impact on DPN. In a recent study, we showed that hyperlipidemia is a strong predictor of progression of DPN [29].

Now, it should be emphasized that many of the clinical trials in the past were performed in patients with established and at times advanced DPN and were usually of limited duration. One may argue that DPN at an advanced stage is less responsive to interventions. Rather any intervention is more likely to be effective when initiated at an early preferably preclinical stage of DPN. It should be mentioned though that large-scale clinical trials employing tight glycemic control through multiple daily insulin injections have provided positive results [12, 13, 30, 31].

Lately, it has become increasingly evident that insulin deficiency, the characteristic hallmark of type 1 diabetes, may play an important initiating pathogenetic role in type 1 DPN [3, 32–34]. Insulin deficiency underlies hyperglycemia and a myriad of other abnormalities. The beneficial effects from long-term trials designed to control hyperglycemia by intensive insulin therapy, one may argue, could be the effect of improved insulin function rather than that of hyperglycemic control per se.

Insulin and C-Peptide Actions

Insulin Action

One factor that probably underlies the differences of DPN in type 1 vs. type 2 diabetes is the degree of perturbed insulin signaling due to insulin deficiency in the former [35, 36]. Besides its hypoglycemic effects ,insulin signaling exerts a multitude of metabolic and molecular effects not always being recognized. It has prominent effects of Na^+/K^+-ATPase and nitric oxide (NO) activities, whose deficiencies are the key metabolic abnormalities underlying the acute nerve dysfunction in DPN [16, 37–41]. Insulin provides strong neurotrophic effects on its own and possesses gene regulatory functions on other key neurotrophic factors such as IGF-1, NGF, and NT-3 and their receptors, besides having a regulatory effect on the insulin receptor (IR) itself [16, 33, 42, 43]. Downstream from its wide-ranging effects on neurotrophism, it indirectly modifies the synthesis and expression of key neuroskeletal proteins such as neurofilaments and neurotubulins and their postranslational modifications [35, 36, 44]. Similar effects are provided with respect to cell adhesive molecules, their modifications and interactions being important for the integrity of various protective barrier functions in peripheral nerve [3, 45]. Furthermore, insulin exerts anti-inflammatory, anti-oxidative and anti-apoptotic effects, whose perturbations play contributing pathogenetic roles in DPN [32, 46–48]. A further effect is its interaction with caveolin-1 with secondary effects on neuroregulin and Erb B2 signaling in Schwann cells, pertinent in demyelination in peripheral nerve [49]. Interestingly in DPN caveolin-1 is downregulated, whereas in diabetic encephalopathy it is upregulated (see Chap. 9). Thus, considering these effects provided by insulin itself, it is perhaps not totally unexpected that strict hyperglycemic control alone will not provide total protection against DPN.

C-Peptide and Insulin Interaction

Following the discovery of C-peptide by Steiner et al. [50], it was assumed that it would have insulin-like effects. However, no effects on glycolysis or lipid metabolism could be demonstrated. In the 1990s, clinical effects on blood flow and early neuropathy and nephropathy were demonstrated [51, 52], which led to renewed interest in C-peptide physiology. It was demonstrated that C-peptide binds to cell membranes and it was suggested that C-peptide acted via a G-protein coupled receptor mechanism [53]. Detailed studies showed that C-peptide autophosphorylates the IR via interaction with protein tyrosine phosphatase [54, 55]. From this followed stimulation of p38-MAP-kinase and PI-3 kinase activities and diminished activation of JNK phosphorylation with subsequent dose-related effects on Na^+/K^+-ATPase activity and NO [46, 56–58]. Hence, insulin-like or insulinomimetic effects were established, although C-peptide does not bind to the IR, but rather acts via interaction with protein tyrosine phosphatase thereby regulating insulin signaling [55, 59].

Despite longstanding efforts to identify a specific C-peptide receptor, it remains elusive. Instead, recent studies have revealed interesting stoichiometric relationships between insulin and C-peptide with consequences as to insulin signaling activities. It has been shown that at high insulin concentrations, C-peptide has an inhibitory effect on insulin signaling activities, conversely in the presence of low insulin concentrations, C-peptide enhances insulin signaling [34, 54, 60]. Both insulin and C-peptide exist in oligomeric forms, which are in equilibrium with the dominant fractions of monomeric forms. It has been shown that C-peptide may alter the equilibrium between oligomeric and monomeric insulin by binding to metal ions specifically Zn^{2+} and hence, it may regulate available monomeric insulin for binding to its receptor and activation of signaling. This would thus provide a second mechanism for the insulinomimetic effect of C-peptide ([59, 61–63]; see also Chap. 3).

Additional mechanisms of C-peptide that have been recently described and which pertain to DPN, are its internalization into endosomes and regulation of ribosomal RNA [64, 65]. C-peptide is taken up into nuclear nucleoli in which it binds to histones of the promoter region of genes for ribosomal RNA [66]. This may provide an additional mechanism explaining its growth factor effects and regulatory effects on gene expression of neurotrophic factors and their receptors via activation of early gene responses as previously demonstrated [36, 46, 67]. Additional effects elicited by C-peptide are its anti-apoptotic and antiinflammatory effects ([68–71]; see also Chaps. 9 and 11).

The Effect of C-Peptide on the Progressive Changes of DPN

Effects on the Early Dysmetabolism and the Acute Nerve Conduction Defect

The results referred to below, have been mainly obtained from the spontaneously type 1 diabetic BB/Wor-rat. This model develops spontaneously and acutely type 1 diabetes and shows complete insulin and C-peptide deficiencies due to an immune mediated β-cell destruction [38, 72] similar to that occurring in human type 1 diabetes. The BB/Wor-rat requires daily sustenance doses of insulin in order to survive and is maintained at high hyperglycemic levels.

The two key abnormalities in acute DPN are the aberrations in Na^+/K^+-ATPase and NO activities, which underlie the acute nerve conduction defects [37, 73, 74]. Impaired Na^+/K^+-ATPase activity in DPN has consequences as for Na^+ permeation at the node of Ranvier and results in decreased transmembranous potentials and intra-axonal Na^+ accumulation with consequent swelling of the intranodal axon [10, 37, 38, 75]. The nodal defect in Na^+/K^+-ATPase activity is likely the consequence of an insulin-deficiency-mediated defect in protein kinase C activity and phosphorylation of Na^+/K^+-ATPase [76].

Subacutely diabetic BB/Wor-rat given C-peptide replacement show a dose-dependent increase in Na^+/K^+-ATPase activity, diminished nodal swelling (Fig. 8.1), and restoration of nerve conduction velocity [57] (Fig. 8.2). In peripheral nerve the insulin receptor (IR) is located to the nodal axolemma and hence, colocalizes with nodal Na^+-channels, Na^+/K^+-ATPase and glucose transporters. It is also localized to nodal microvilli and terminal Schwann cell loops of the paranodal apparatus [77]. At the latter sites it colocalizes with specialized

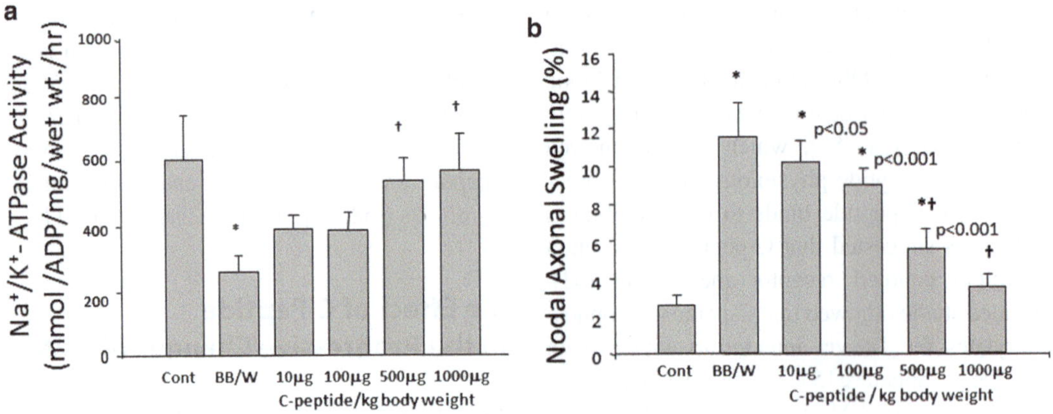

Fig. 8.1 Na^+/K^+-ATPase activity (**a**) in sciatic nerve from control and 2-month diabetic BB/Wor-rats. Note dose-related increases in Na^+/K^+-ATPase activities in sciatic nerves from rats given increasing daily subcutaneous doses of human C-peptide. The increasing activity of Na^+/K^+-ATPase activity corresponded to a decreasing frequency of nodal axonal swelling (**b**) as assessed morphometrically (adapted from ref. [57]). $^*p<0.001$ vs. age-matched controls; $^†p<0.001$ vs. age-matched non-treated diabetic rats

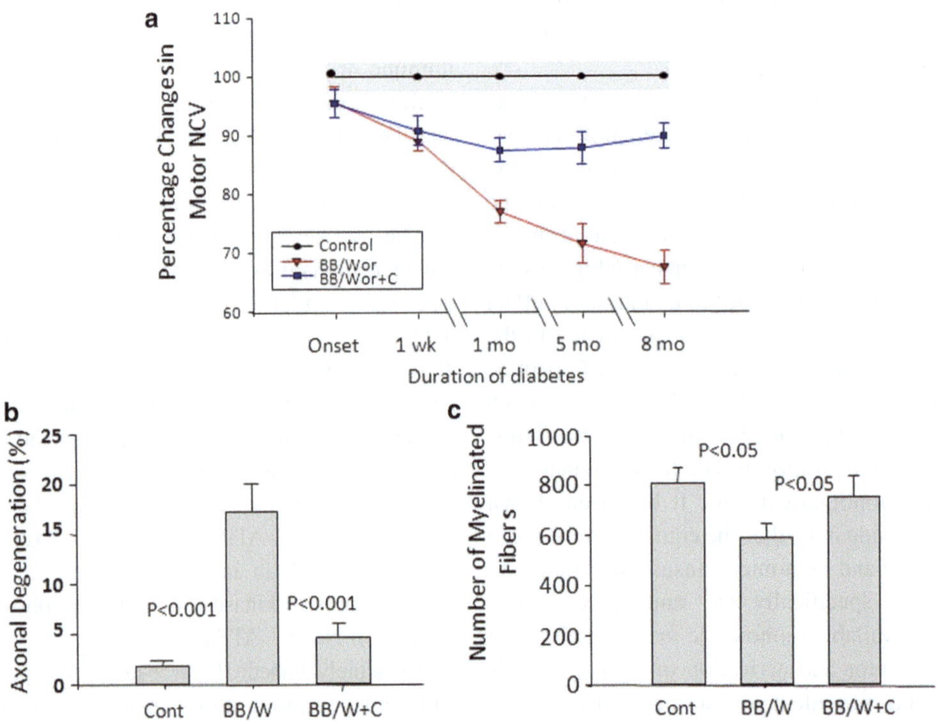

Fig. 8.2 (**a**) Percentage change in motor NCV in diabetic and C-peptide replaced BB/Wor-rats over an 8 month period. Note in untreated diabetic BB/Wor-rats a progressive decline in NCV which reaches 70% of normal NCV at 8 months. Diabetic rats replaced with C-peptide from onset of diabetes show an incomplete but significant attenuation of NCV slowing to approximately 90% of normal at 8 months. The residual 10% defect is presumably the hyperglycemic component of the NCV slowing (see text). (**b**) Percent of fibers demonstrating axonal degenerative changes reached 17% in nontreated diabetic rats after 8 months of diabetes. Axonal degeneration was significantly prevented in rats receiving full C-peptide replacement. (**c**) The loss of myelinated fibers in the sural nerve of 8-month diabetic rats amounted to approximately 27%. This fiber loss was significantly prevented by full C-peptide replacement (adapted from refs. [34, 73])

cell adhesive molecules like caspr, contactin, neurofascin, and $RPTP_{\beta}$, which comprise the axoglial junctions of the ion-channel barrier of the paranodal apparatus (see below).

An additional mechanism implicated in the acute nerve conduction slowing is decreased endoneurial blood flow, secondary to diminished endothelial NO release because of impaired expression of eNOS [40, 78]. This has been linked to both an activation of the polyol-pathway via a NADPH-mediated mechanism and to changes in protein kinase activity in insulin signaling and calcium levels [40, 78]. Full C-peptide replacement of experimental type 1 diabetic rat models normalizes the expression of eNOS, endoneurial blood flow, and vascular conductance in the presence of unaltered hyperglycemic blood levels [41, 58]. Hence, the early effects of C-peptide on Na^+/K^+-ATPase activity and endoneurial vascular NO underlie the corrective effects of the acute nerve conduction defect and appear to be independent of hyperglycemia (Fig. 8.2).

Nodal and Paranodal Degeneration and C-Peptide

A characteristic abnormality occurring in type 1 DPN in humans and animal models is progressive degeneration of the nodal and paranodal apparati [10, 79–81]. The paranodal tight junctions adhering the terminal myelin loops to the paranodal axolemma, and comprise the paranodal ion-channel barrier, important for the normal placement and confinement of α-Na^+-channels to the nodal axolemma. The progressive degeneration and breakdown of this barrier in type 1 DPN allows for lateralization of the α-Na-channels away from the node and correlates with the chronic less reversible nerve conduction defect [75, 81–83].

As mentioned above, this barrier system is made up of a series of interacting adhesive proteins. Not only are these structural proteins, like caspr, contactin, and RPTB-β downregulated in type 1 DPN, but their binding to each other and activation are perturbed. So, for instance, the phosphorylation of RPTB-β and the binding of p85 to the SH_3 domains of caspr are compromised, abnormalities which are caused by impaired insulin signaling [84–87]. Full C-peptide replacement in the BB/Wor-rat prevents and corrects the underlying molecular defects and restores the structural integrity of the ion-channel barrier (Fig. 8.3) [45].

At the node itself the voltage-gated α-Na-channels are anchored to the nodal axolemma by auxiliary β_1- and β_2-Na-channel subunits, which in turn interact with RPTP-β, a ligand for the contactin receptor, and $ankyrin_G$. The signaling induced by RPTP-β is mediated via tyrosine phosphorylation sites regulated by NGF and insulin [87]. In the diabetic BB/Wor-rat, $ankyrin_G$ and β_1-Na-channel expression is markedly downregulated, whereas the expression of α-Na-channel is unaltered. In C-peptide replaced animals these abnormalities are prevented and the anchoring of α-Na-channel is therefore secured [45]. These effects of C-peptide therefore prevent the breach of the paranodal ion-channel barrier and secure the anchoring of the Na-channels to the nodal axolemma with profound effects on the otherwise progressive and structurally related nerve conduction defect [16, 45, 73] (Fig. 8.2).

The Effect of C-Peptide on Altered Neurotrophism

Insulin along with proinsulin C-peptide have extensive neurotrophic and neuroprotective effects on their own, as well as gene regulatory roles on the endogenous and peripheral NGF, NT-3, and IGF systems [43, 68, 88] (Fig. 8.4). In peripheral nerve the IR is localized to the nodal and paranodal apparati as described above. In addition it is found in the Schmidt-Lantermann incisures and in small dorsal root ganglia (DRG) [77, 89]. Furthermore, in endoneurial vessels it colocalizes with endothelial tight junctions and in adjacent ad- and ab-lumen endothelial cells. The latter location may suggest a function similar to that of paranodal apparatus in maintaining the inter-endothelial junctions, which make up the peripheral nerve blood barrier [77].

In acutely type 1 diabetic rats the expression of the IR is unaltered in peripheral nerve, but

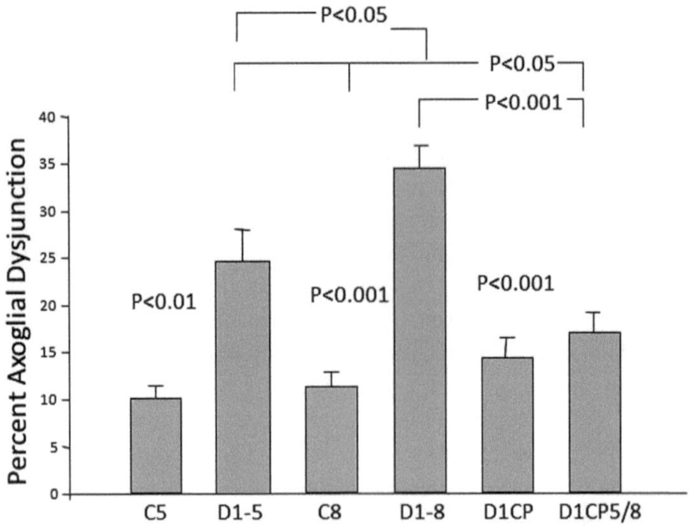

Fig. 8.3 Morphometric assessment of axoglial junction loss. Note in control rats about 10% of axoglial junctions are not closed (C5 and C8). In nontreated diabetic rats there was a progressive loss of paranodal junctions from 5 to 8 months duration of diabetes (D1-5 and D1-8). Rats treated with full C-peptide replacement from onset of diabetes (DICP) showed a significant prevention of axoglial dysjunction. Animals treated with full C-peptide replacement from 5 to 8 months of diabetes (DICP 5/8) showed significant repair of paranodal junctions (adapted from ref. [91])

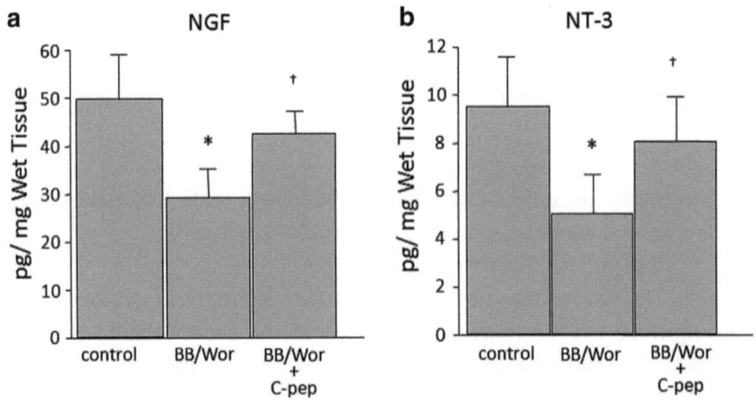

Fig. 8.4 Concentration of NGF (**a**) and NT-3 (**b**) in sciatic nerve at 8 months duration of diabetes. These neurotrophic factors are suppressed to approximately 50% of normal in nontreated diabetic rats. Diabetic rats replaced with C-peptide from onset of diabetes showed significant prevention of neurotrophic factor suppression (adapted from refs. [3, 103])

increases with duration of diabetes [45]. In contrast to peripheral nerve, in DRG the expression of IR decreases progressively with duration of diabetes. By comparison, IR expression is downregulated in sciatic nerve in the hyperinsulinemic type 2 diabetic BBZDR/Wor-rats and unchanged in DRG's in this model [35, 90]. The abnormalities of IR expression in the type 1 diabetic rat model are normalized by full C-peptide replacement [73, 91] (Fig. 8.5).

The gene regulatory effects of insulin/C-peptide are mediated by transcription factors as mentioned above of which NFκB is a prominent one. In addition, early gene responses like c-fos, c-jun, and the first waves of IGF and NGF are elicited by insulin/C-peptide [35, 42]. These factors and early gene responses are compromised in type 1 DPN with consequences as to the gene expression of NGF, IGF-1, and NT-3 and their respective receptors [33, 42, 45] (Fig. 8.5). Full C-peptide

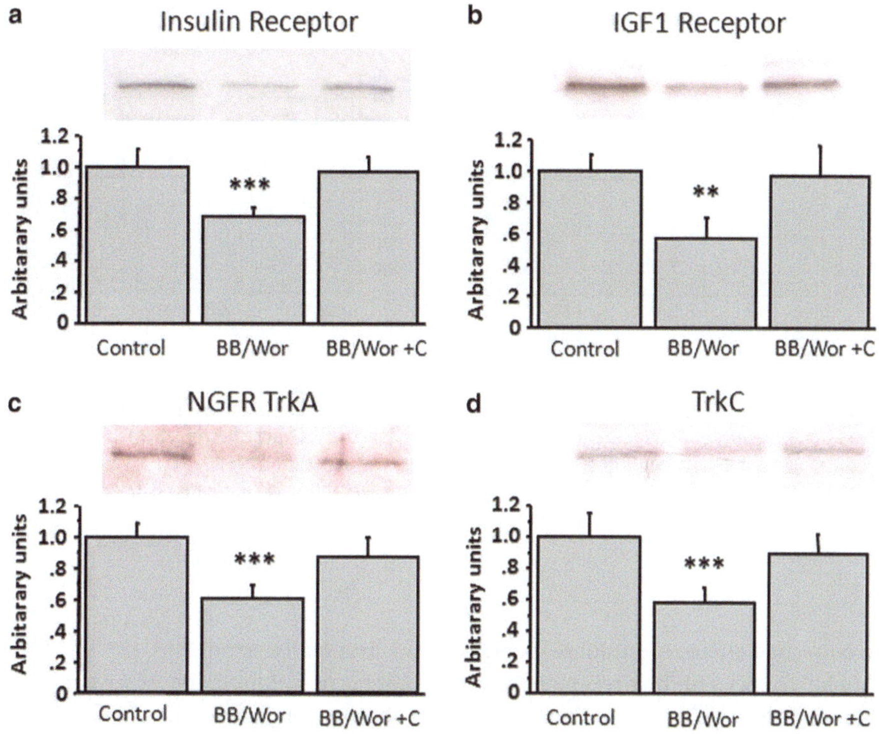

Fig. 8.5 Protein expression of neurotrophic factor receptors in dorsal root ganglia. Note significant decreases in the expression of insulin receptor (**a**), IGF-1 receptor (**b**), NGF-TrkA receptor (**c**) and that of NT-3 TrkC (**d**). Full replacement of C-peptide from onset to 8 months of diabetes prevented the decrease in neurotrophic factor receptors (adapted from refs. [3, 103]). ***$p<0.001$; **$p<0.005$ vs. age-matched control rats

replacement in the BB/Wor-rat has a corrective effect on this cascade of events with downstream effects on the expression of neurotrophic factors and their function (Figs. 8.4 and 8.5). Interestingly, confirming the initiating effects elicited by insulin signaling, similar corrective effects are achieved by intrathecal insulin treatment of the STZ-rat, a treatment that does not affect hyperglycemia [33].

C-Peptide, Neuroskeletal Proteins and Axonal Atrophy

Axonal atrophy and secondary dyingback of peripheral and central axons of DRG cells is the very hallmark of DPN and is more evident and severe in DPN accompanying type 1 diabetes as compared to type 2 DPN. Cytoskeletal neurofilaments and tubulins are the major building blocks of the axon. Their expressions and phosphorylation status impact on their interaction, axonal function, such as axonal transport, axonal size, and the regenerative capacity of axons [88, 92, 93]. Experimental animal models of type 1 diabetes demonstrate reduced mRNA and protein expression of NF's and tubulins in DRG's, aberrant phosphorylation ,and decreased axonal transport. NF's are unique to the nervous system and consist of three NF's; NFL, NFM, and NFH, signifying low, medium, and high molecular weight NF's. In the axon they assemble in staggered fashion and interact with tubulins by phosphorylation and provide the skeleton for axonal transport. Several kinases are involved in phosphorylation of NF's like cyclin-dependent kinase Cdk5, MAP kinases Erk 1/2, SAPK [92] ,and GSKβ [88, 93]. As mentioned

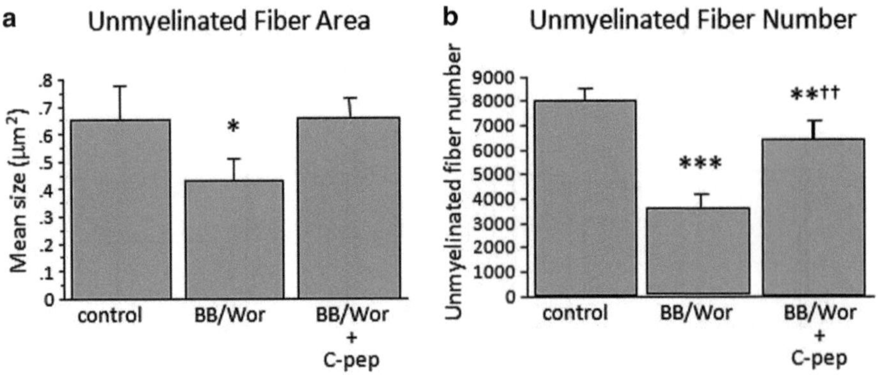

Fig. 8.6 Morphometric analyses of unmyelinated C-fibers in sural nerve after 8 months of diabetes. Diabetes causes a significant atrophy of unmyelinated fibers (**a**), which is fully prevented following full C-peptide replacement. The number of unmyelinated fibers is reduced to less than half in diabetic rats (**b**). This loss of C-fibers is partially prevented by C-peptide replacement (adapted from ref. [103]). *$p<0.05$; **$p<0.005$; ***$p<0.001$ vs. control rats; ††$p<0.001$ vs. untreated BB/Wor-rats

above, the corrective effects of insulin/C-peptide on neurotrophic factors and their receptors result in downstream correction of neurofilament and tubulin mRNA, protein expression, and normalization of the aberrant phosphorylation of NF's [44, 94–97]. This in turn translates into beneficial effects on both myelinated and unmyelinated axonal size and number [44, 73] (Figs. 8.2 and 8.6) with further effects on axonal conductivity and transport functions and the regenerative capacity of damaged axons (see below). However, it should be mentioned that although full C-peptide substitution significantly prevents the progressive nerve conduction defect, it is not completely prevented (see Fig. 8.2). This led us to suggest that the conduction defect consist of an insulin/C-peptide deficiency component and a hyperglycemic component [3, 34, 60]. The latter not being effected by C-peptide substitution. Thus, in the progressive development of type 1 DPN, insulin and C-peptide deficiencies affects insulin signaling activities which result in (1) impaired expression of neurotrophic factors with secondary adverse effects on neuroskeletal proteins and (2) increased expression of so-called stress-kinases. This series of events result in malalignment and disassembly of neurofilaments and tubulins and consequent axonal degeneration and eventually axon loss [8, 9]. The clinical consequence of these progressive changes is loss of sensory modalities, the characteristic clinical hallmark of type 1 DPN.

Nociceptive Neuropathy and C-Peptide

Chronic pain is a common complaint by diabetic patients and can severely compromise quality of life of affected patients [1]. The underlying mechanisms are not fully understood but are the subject of active research. Treatment options are few with limited benefits and are at times associated with severe side effects [27, 28, 98, 99].

Abnormal pain sensation can be either exaggerated responses to painful stimuli, hyperalgesia, or painful responses to normal stimuli or allodynia. Nociceptive sensation originates from damage to unmyelinated and small myelinated Aβ fibers originating from small nociceptive DRG neurons. Such damage induces increased excitability through upregulation of tetrodotoxin-resistant Na^+-channels and β-adrenergic receptors [100, 101]. The resultant high frequency firing pattern enhances nociception with further amplification by sensitizing spinal interneurons. Pain sensation is further modulated in the brainstem in the para-aqueductal gray matter and at thalamic levels [102].

In the BB/Wor-rat model, hyperalgesia and increased firing frequency occur early and progress with diabetes duration [90]. These phenomena are prevented and reversed by C-peptide replacement [73, 103, 104]. The positive effects correlate with normalization of the insulin and NGF-TrkA receptors in small nociceptive DRG neurons (Fig. 8.5) and nociceptive interneurons in the spinal cord [89, 103] and with normalization of substance P and calcitonin gene-related peptide (CGRP) synthesis in nociceptive DRG neurons. Furthermore, C-peptide replacement prevents and improves the atrophy and loss of nociceptive fibers in the sensory nerve trunk [103–105] (Fig. 8.6). These results suggest that C-peptide has a modulating effect on painful diabetic neuropathy. It should be kept in mind though that C-peptide does not influence hyperglycemia. Hyperglycemia associated mechanisms such as spinal cyclooxygenase-2 and release of spinal prostaglandin E_2 are probably co-conspirators to nociceptive neuropathy [99, 102, 106].

Nerve Fiber Regeneration is Promoted by C-Peptide

The progressive degeneration and loss of myelinated and unmyelinated fibers that characterize DPN, can be potentially ameliorated through an increased regenerative capacity of such fibers. However, regenerated myelinated fibers will not fully restore their initial functions such as nerve conduction velocity. The reason for this is the shorter internodal distances in a regenerated myelinated fiber which means a slower nerve conduction, since the time consuming event in conductivity is the depolarization of the nodal potential. Thus, the regenerated nerve fiber conducts at a slower velocity, because of a greater number of nodes per unit length.

As mentioned above, early gene responses and defects in the expression of neurotrophic factors and neuroskeletal proteins are more severely affected in type 1 BB/Wor-rat than in its type 2 diabetic counterpart, the BBZDR/Wor-rat [35, 43]. This observation suggests that insulin deficiency is an important underlying factor not only in nerve degeneration but also in nerve fiber regeneration. Nerve fiber regeneration is a complex event requiring correct timing of molecular events. C-peptide substitution results in an immediate correction of early gene responses as shown by the normalization of mRNA and expression of IGF-1 protein and its receptor. C-peptide replacement also induces sequentially c-fos and lesion-induced upregulation of NGF and the attenuated upregulation of the NGF-TrkA-receptor is restored [42, 44].

The early upregulation of NGF following degeneration of the axon induces macrophage recruitment necessary for phagocytosis of axonal debris and secretion of interleukins and other neurotrophic factors [107, 108]. An orderly regeneration of nerve fibers requires amplification of neurotrophic factors in the neuronal cell somata and the presence of insulin to induce neuroskeletal protein synthesis [95–97, 109, 110]. C-peptide-replaced rats show a timely upregulation of neurotrophic factors in DRG's of axonotomized rats [44]. Insulin and NGF signaling activities upregulate NFM and NFL and indirectly β-tubulin by stabilizing their mRNA's [95, 97].

The normal elongation and growth of the regenerating axon require that the upregulation of β-tubulin precedes the upregulation of NF's. In the type 1 diabetic BB/Wor-rat the necessary downregulation of NF's does not occur nor does it demonstrate the important initial upregulation of β-tubulins (Fig. 8.7). C-peptide replacement not only restores the expression of the neuroskeletal proteins but normalizes the equally important timing and sequence in the synthesis and delivery of the cytoskeletal building blocks to the regenerating axon (Fig. 8.7) [44]. It is therefore evident that C-peptide substitution has profound effects on normalizing the intricate molecular events and their timing enabling a normal regenerative capacity of previously degenerated nerve fibers resulting in increased regenerative capacity (Fig. 8.7).

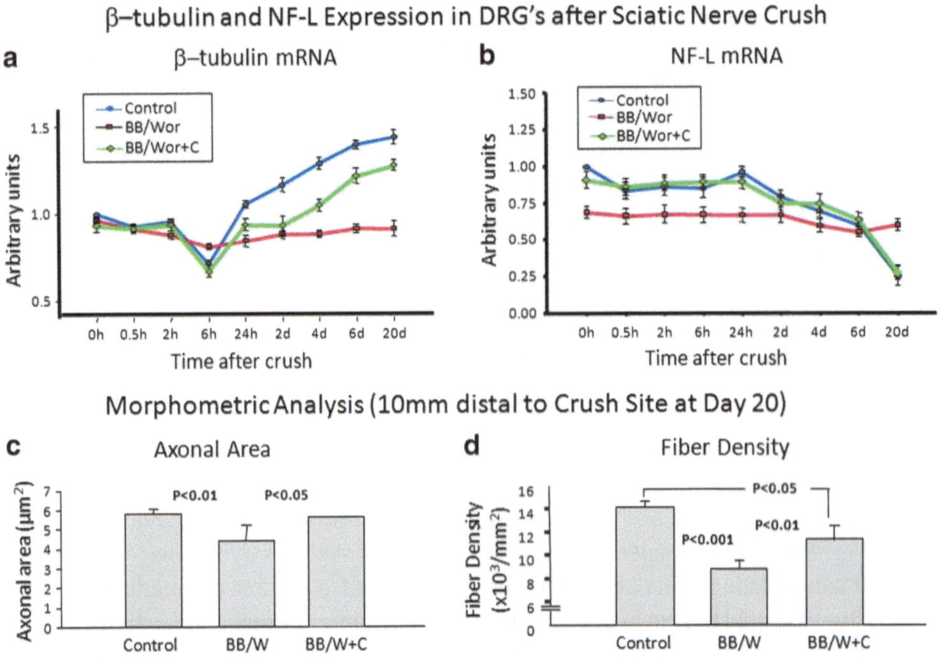

Fig. 8.7 Time sequence of β-tubulin mRNA (**a**) and NF-L mRNA expression after sciatic nerve crush in control, diabetic and C-peptide-replaced diabetic BB/Wor-rat. In (**a**) from 6 h after crush there is a progressive upregulation of β-tubulin mRNA, whereas NF-L mRNA (**b**) becomes increasingly downregulated in normal control rats. In diabetic rats these regulations do not take place, instead the mRNA expression levels remain fairly constant throughout the observation period. In C-peptide replaced animals there is a significant normalization of the post-crush upregulation of β-tubulin and downregulation of NF-L. These corrections in the dynamics of neuroskeletal gene expression resulted in normalization of axonal areas of regenerating fibers (**c**) and a significant increase in the number of regenerating fibers (**d**) (adapted from ref. [44])

Summary and Conclusions

As outlined here and previously [16, 34, 79], it is evident that DPN is a complex and a highly dynamic disease process. Based on current findings and those in other chapters of this volume, it is evident that type 1 diabetes is a disorder of two hormones; insulin and C-peptide, which are lacking due to the destruction of the pancreatic β-cell from which they originate. As demonstrated by large-scale clinical trials intended to control hyperglycemia by frequent insulin injections, complete preventative effects cannot be achieved. Instead they showed that hyperglycemic control is not sufficient to prevent or reverse the progression of type 1 DPN. It is becoming increasingly clear that insulin and C-peptide have a multitude of effects pertaining to the various pathobiological aspects in this dynamic and progressive disorder. They range from early metabolic effects on neuronal NA^{+}/K^{+}-ATPase activity and NO, responsible for the acute functional deficits. They display effects on gene regulatory mechanisms on neurotrophic factors and their receptors and cell-adhesive molecules and their postranslational modifications essential to their function. As outlined in this chapter, such effects lead downstream to perturbed expression of neuroskeletal proteins and their assembly and ultimately axonal degeneration and loss, the very hallmarks of type 1 DPN. Further effects not dealt with in this chapter are those on inflammation and apoptosis (see Chap. 9).

A decade of research focusing on C-peptide and its effects on DPN, has been indeed stimulating.

Full C-peptide restitution has demonstrated step by step beneficial effects on the progressive pathophysiologic web of this most common complication of diabetes. The initial in vivo studies in the BB/Wor-rat were followed by clinical trials in patients with type 1 diabetes (see Chap. 12), which have confirmed the beneficial effects on somatic and autonomic DPN.

When considering the fact that no targeted therapy exists for this disorder and in view of the substantial amount of scientific and clinical information that has accumulated over the last decade regarding C-peptide, its physiology and pathobiological role, it is surprising that the pharmaceutical industry is regarding the therapeutical rational for this naturally occurring hormone with such ignorance. One would believe that while awaiting the ultimate cure for this rapidly increasing disorder, C-peptide substitution in addition to insulin therapy would be a pretty good alternative.

References

1. Greene DA, Sima AAF, Feldman EL, Stevens MJ. Diabetic neuropathy. In: Porte Jr D, Sherwin RS, editors. Ellenberg and rifkin diabetes mellitus. 5th ed. Stanford: Appleton & Lange; 1997. p. 1009–76.
2. Feldman EL, Stevens MJ, Russell JW, et al. Somatosensory neuropathy. In: Porte DS, Sherwin RS, Baron A, editors. The diabetes mellitus manual. New York: McGraw-Hill; 2005. p. 366–84.
3. Sima AAF, Kamiya H. Diabetic neuropathy differs in type 1 and type 2 diabetes. Ann N Y Acad Sci. 2006;1084:235–49.
4. Thomas PK, Lascelles RG. Schwann cell abnormalities in diabetic neuropathy. Lancet. 1965;1:1355–7.
5. Thomas PK, Lascelles RG. The pathology of diabetic neuropathy. Q J Med. 1966;35:489–509.
6. Thomas PK, Eliasson SG. Diabetic neuropathy. In: Dyck PJ, Thomas PK, Lambert EH, editors. Peripheral neuropathy. Philadelphia: WB Saunders Co.; 1975. p. 956–81.
7. Sima AAF, Robertson DM. Peripheral neuropathy in mutant diabetic mouse [C57/B1/KS(db/db)]. Acta Neuropathol (Berl). 1978;41:85–9.
8. Sima AAF, Bouchier M, Christensen H. Axonal atrophy in sensory nerves of the diabetic BB-Wistar rat, a possible early correlate of human diabetic neuropathy. Ann Neurol. 1983;13:264–72.
9. Sima AAF, Yagihashi S. Central-peripheral distal axonopathy in the spontaneously diabetic BB-rat: ultrastructural and morphometric findings. Diabetes Res Clin Pract. 1986;1:289–98.
10. Sima AAF, Nathaniel V, Bril V, McEwen TAJ, Greene DA. Histopathological heterogeneity of neuropathy in insulin-dependent and non-insulin-dependent diabetes, and demonstration of axo-glial dysjunction in human diabetic neuropathy. J Clin Invest. 1988;81:349–64.
11. Greene DA, Sima AAF, Pfeifer MA, Albers JW. Diabetic neuropathy. Annu Rev Med. 1990;41: 303–17.
12. Reichard P, Pihl M, Rosenquist U, Sule J. Complications in IDDM are caused by elevated blood glucose level: the Stockholm Diabetes Intervention Study (SDIS) at 10-year follow-up. Diabetologia. 1996;39:1483–8.
13. The Diabetes Control Complications Trial Research Group. The effect of intensive treatment of diabetes on the development and progression of long-term complications in insulin-dependent diabetes mellitus. N Engl J Med. 1993;329:977–86.
14. Dyck PJ, Zimmerman BR, Vileu TH, et al. Nerve glucose, fructose, sorbitol, myoinositol, and fiber degeneration and regeneration in diabetic neuropathy. N Engl J Med. 1988;319:542–8.
15. Hale PJ, Nattrass M, Silverman SH, et al. Peripheral nerve concentrations of glucose, fructose, sorbitol and myoinositol in diabetic and non-diabetic patients. Diabetologia. 1987;30:464–7.
16. Sima AAF. New insights into the metabolic and molecular basis for diabetic neuropathy. Cell Mol Life Sci. 2003;60:2445–64.
17. Sima AAF, Bril V, Nathaniel V, et al. Regeneration and repair of myelinated fibers in sural nerve biopsies from patients with diabetic neuropathy treated with an aldose reductase inhibitor. N Engl J Med. 1988;319:548–55.
18. O'Hare JP, Morgan MH, Alden P, et al. Clinical and neuropsychological studies of one year's treatment with sorbinil. Diabet Med. 1988;5:537–42.
19. Boulton AJM, Levin S, Comstock J. A multicentre trial of the aldose reductase inhibitor tolrestat, in patients with symptomatic diabetic neuropathy. Diabetologia. 1990;33:431–7.
20. Sima AAF, Greene DA, Brown MB, et al. Effect of hyperglycemia and the aldose reductase inhibitor tolrestat on sural nerve biochemistry and morphometry in advanced diabetic peripheral polyneuropathy. J Diabetes Complications. 1993;7:157–69.
21. Greene DA, Arezzo J, Brown M. Effects of aldose reductase inhibition on nerve conduction and morphometry in diabetic neuropathy. Neurology. 1999; 53:580–91.
22. Veves A. Aldose reductase inhibitors for the treatment of diabetic neuropathy. In: Veves A, Malik RA, editors. Diabetic neuropathy. Clinical management. Totowa: Humana Press; 2007. p. 309–20.
23. Ziegler D, Gries FA. Alpha-lipoic acid in the treatment of diabetic peripheral and cardiac autonomic neuropathy. Diabetes. 1997;46 Suppl 2:562–6.

24. Ziegler D, Schatz H, Conrad F, et al. Effects of treatment with the antioxidant alpha-lipoic acid on cardiac autonomic neuropathy in NIDDM patients. A 4-month randomized controlled multicenter trial (DEKAN Study). Deutsche Kardiale Autonome Neuropathie. Diabetes Care. 1997;20:369–73.
25. Keen H, Payan J, Allawi J, et al. Treatment of diabetic neuropathy with gamma-linolenic acid. The gamma linolenic acid multicenter trial group. Diabetes Care. 1993;16:8–15.
26. Stevens MJ, Lattimer SA, Feldman EL, et al. Acetyl-L-carnitine deficiency as a cause of altered nerve myo-inositol content, Na^+ K^+-ATPase activity and motor conduction velocity in the streptozotocin diabetic rat. Metabolism. 1996;45:865–72.
27. Sima AAF, Calvani M, Mehra M, Amato A. Acetyl-L-carnitine improves pain, vibratory perception and nerve morphology in patients with chronic diabetic peripheral neuropathy: an analysis of two randomized, placebo-controlled trials. Diabetes Care. 2005;28:96–101.
28. Evan JD, Jacobs TF, Evans EV. Role of acetyl-L-carnitine in the treatment of diabetic peripheral neuropathy. Ann Pharmacother. 2008;42:1686–91.
29. Wiggins TD, Sullivan KA, Pop-Busui R, et al. Elevated triglycerides correlate with progression of diabetic neuropathy. Diabetes. 2009;58:1634–40.
30. UK Prospective Diabetes Study (UKPDS) Group. Intensive blood glucose control with sulphonylureas or insulin compared with conventional treatment and risk of complications in patients with type 2 diabetes. Lancet. 1998;352:S37–53.
31. Burger AJ, Weinrauch LA, D'Elia JA, Aronson D. Effect of glycemic control on heart rate variability in type 1 diabetic patients with cardiac autonomic neuropathy. Am J Cardiol. 1999;84:687–91.
32. Cheatham B, Kahn R. Insulin action and the insulin signaling network. Endocr Rev. 1995;16:117–42.
33. Brussee V, Cunningham FA, Zochodne DW. Direct insulin signaling of neurons reverses diabetic neuropathy. Diabetes. 2004;53:1824–30.
34. Sima AAF, Kamiya H. Insulin, C-peptide and diabetic neuropathy. Sci Med. 2004;10:308–19.
35. Pierson CR, Zhang W, Murakawa Y, Sima AAF. Early gene responses of trophic factors differ in nerve regeneration in type 1 and type 2 diabetic neuropathy. J Neuropathol Exp Neurol. 2002;61:857–71.
36. Pant HC, Veeranna, Grant P. Regulation of axonal neurofilament phosphorylation. Curr Top Cell Regul. 2000;36:133–50.
37. Greene DA, Yagihashi S, Lattimer SA, Sima AAF. Nerve Na+-K+-ATPase, conduction and myo-inositol in the insulin deficient BB-rat. Am J Physiol. 1984;247:E534–9.
38. Sima AAF, Brismar T. Reversible diabetic nerve dysfunction. Structural correlates to electrophysiological abnormalities. Ann Neurol. 1985;18:21–9.
39. Vague P, Dufayet D, Coste T, et al. Association of diabetic neuropathy with Na/K ATPase gene polymorphism. Diabetologia. 1997;40:506–11.
40. Stevens MJ, Dananberg J, Feldman EL, et al. The linked roles of nitric oxide, aldose reductase and (Na+, K+)-ATPase in the slowing of nerve conduction in the streptozotocin diabetic rat. Metabolism. 1996;45:865–72.
41. Stevens MJ, Zhang W, Li F, Sima AAF. C-peptide corrects endoneurial blood flow but not oxidative stress in type 1 BB/Wor-rats. Am J Physiol. 2004;287:E497–505.
42. Xu G, Sima AAF. Altered immediate early gene expression is impaired in diabetic nerve: implications in regeneration. J Neuropathol Exp Neurol. 2001;60(10):972–83.
43. Pierson CR, Zhang W, Murakawa Y, Sima AAF. Insulin deficiency rather than hyperglycemia accounts for impaired neurotrophic responses and nerve fiber regeneration in type 1 diabetic neuropathy. J Neuropathol Exp Neurol. 2003;62:260–71.
44. Pierson CR, Zhang W, Sima AAF. Proinsulin C-peptide replacement in type 1 diabetic BB/Wor-rats prevents deficits in nerve fiber regeneration. J Neuropathol Exp Neurol. 2003;62:765–79.
45. Sima AAF, Zhang W, Li Z-G, Murakawa Y, Pierson CR. Molecular alterations underlie nodal and paranodal degeneration in type 1 diabetic neuropathy and are prevented by C-peptide. Diabetes. 2004;53:1556–63.
46. Bierhaus A, Schiekofer S, Schwarninger M, et al. Diabetes associated sustained activation of the transcription factor nuclear factor-kappa B. Diabetes. 2001;50:2792–806.
47. Ramasamy R, Vanucci SJ, Yau SO, et al. Advanced glycation end product and RAGE: a common thread in aging, diabetes, neurodegeneration and inflammation. Glycobiology. 2004;15:16R–28.
48. Cifarelli V, Luppi P, Tse HM, et al. Human proinsulin C-peptide reduces high glucose induced proliferation and NF-kappaB activation in smooth muscle cells. Atherosclerosis. 2008;201:248–57.
49. McGuire JF, Rouen S, Siegfreid E, Wright DE, Dobrowsky RT. Caveolin-1 and altered neuroregulin signaling contribute to the pathophysiological progression of diabetic peripheral neuropathy. Diabetes. 2009;58:2677–86.
50. Steiner DF, Cunningham L, Spigelman L, Aben B. Insulin biosynthesis: evidence for a precursor. Science. 1967;157:697–700.
51. Johansson B-L, Linde B, Wahren J. Effect of C-peptide on blood flow, capillary diffusion capacity and glucose utilization in the exercising forms of type 1 (insulin-dependent) diabetic patients. Diabetologia. 1992;35:1151–8.
52. Johansson B-L, Borg K, Fernquist-Forbes E, et al. Beneficial effects of C-peptide on incipient nephropathy and neuropathy in patients with type 1 diabetes mellitus. Diabet Med. 2000;17:181–9.
53. Rigler R, Pramanik A, Jonasson P, et al. Specific binding of the proinsulin C-peptide to human cell membranes. Proc Natl Acad Sci USA. 1999;46:13318–23.

54. Grunberger G, Qiang X, Li Z-G, et al. Molecular basis for the insulinomimetic effects of C-peptide. Diabetologia. 2001;44:1247–57.
55. Li Z-G, Qiang X, Sima AAF, Grunberger G. C-peptide attenuates protein tyrosine phosphatase activity and enhances glycogen synthesis in L6 myoblasts. Biochem Biophys Res Commun. 2001;26:615–9.
56. Othomo Y, Aperia A, Sahlgren B, Johansson B-L, Wahren J. C-peptide stimulates rat renal tubular Na^+, K^+-ATPase activity in synergism with neuropeptide Y. Diabetologia. 1996;39:199–205.
57. Zhang W, Yorek M, Pierson CR, et al. Human C-peptide dose dependently prevents early neuropathy in the BB/Wor-rat. Int J Exp Diabetes Res. 2001;2(3):187–94.
58. Cotter MA, Ekberg K, Wahren J, Cameron NE. Effects of proinsulin C-peptide in experimental diabetic neuropathy: vascular actions and modulation by nitric oxide synthase inhibition. Diabetes. 2003;52:1812–7.
59. Jägerbrink T, Landahl E, Shafqat J, Jörnvall H. Proinsulin C-peptide interaction with protein tyrosine phosphatase 1B demonstrated with a labeling reaction. Biochem Biophys Res Commun. 2009;387:31–5.
60. Sima AAF. Diabetic neuropathy in type 1 and type 2 diabetes and the effects of C-peptide. Neurol Sci. 2004;220:133–6.
61. Shafqat J, Melles E, Sigmudsson K, et al. Proinsulin C-peptide elicits disaggregation of insulin resulting in enhanced physiological insulin effects. Cell Mol Life Sci. 2006;63:1805–11.
62. Medawala W, McCahill P, Giebink A, et al. A molecular level understanding of zinc activation of C-peptide and its effects on cellular communications in the bloodstream. Rev Diabet Stud. 2009;6:148–58.
63. Jörnvall H, Lindahl E, Astorga-Wells J, et al. Oligomerization and insulin interactions of proinsulin C-peptide: threefold relationships to properties of insulin. Biochem Biophys Res Commun. 2010;391:1561–6.
64. Lindahl E, Nyman U, Melles E, et al. Cellular internalization of proinsulin C-peptide. Cell Mol Life Sci. 2007;64:479–86.
65. Luppi P, Geng X, Cifarelli V, Drain P, Trucco M. C-peptide is internalized in human endothelial and vascular smooth muscle cells via early endosomes. Diabetologia. 2009;52:2218–28.
66. Lindahl E, Nyman U, Zaman F, et al. Proinsulin C-peptide regulates ribosomal RNA expression. J Biol Chem. 2010;285:3462–9.
67. Xu G, Murakawa Y, Pierson CR, Sima AAF. Altered β-tubulin and neurofilament expression and impaired axonal growth in diabetic nerve regeneration. J Neuropathol Exp Neurol. 2002;61:164–75.
68. Li Z-G, Zhang W, Sima AAF. C-peptide enhances insulin-mediated cell growth and protection against high glucose induced apoptosis in SH-SY5Y cells. Diabetes Metab Res Rev. 2003;19:375–85.
69. Sima AAF, Li Z-G. The effect of C-peptide on cognitive dysfunction and hippocampal apoptosis in type 1 diabetes. Diabetes. 2005;54:1497–505.
70. Luppi P, Cifarelli V, Tse H, Piganelli J, Trucco M. Human C-peptide antagonizes high glucose-induced endothelial dysfunction through the nuclear factor-κB pathway. Diabetologia. 2008;51:1534–43.
71. Sima AAF, Zhang W, Kreipke CW, Rafols JA, Hoffman WH. Inflammation in diabetic encephalopathy is prevented by C-peptide. Rev Diabet Stud. 2009;6:37–42.
72. Sima AAF. Can the BB-rat help to unravel diabetic neuropathy? Annotation. Neuropathol Appl Neurobiol. 1985;11:253–64.
73. Sima AAF, Kamiya H. Is C-peptide replacement the missing link for successful treatment of neurological complications in type 1 diabetes? Curr Drug Targets. 2008;9:37–46.
74. Cameron NE, Cotter MA. Metabolic and vascular factors in the pathogenesis of diabetic neuropathy. Diabetes. 1997;46 Suppl 2:S31–7.
75. Brismar T, Sima AAF. Changes in nodal function in nerve fibres of the spontaneously diabetic BB-Wistar rat. Potential clamp analysis. Acta Physiol Scand. 1981;113:499–506.
76. Greene DA, Lattimer SA, Sima AAF. Sorbitol, phosphoinositides and sodium-potassium ATPase in the pathogenesis of diabetic complications. N Engl J Med. 1987;316:599–606.
77. Sugimoto K, Murakawa Y, Zhang W-X, Xu G, Sima AAF. Insulin receptor in rat peripheral nerve: its localization and alternatively spliced isoforms. Diabetes Metab Res Rev. 2000;16(5):354–63.
78. Kutanyra T, Kimura K, Makondo K, et al. Proinsulin C-peptide increases nitric oxide production by enhancing mitogen-activated protein-kinase-dependent transcription of endothelial nitric oxide synthase in aortic enothelial cells of Wistar-rats. Diabetologia. 2003;46:1698–705.
79. Sima AAF. Heterogeneity of diabetic neuropathy. Front Biosci. 2008;13:4809–16.
80. Sima AAF, Zhang W-X, Tai J, Tze WJ, Nathaniel V. Diabetic neuropathy in STZ-induced diabetic rat and effect of allogenic islet cell transplantation. Morphometric analysis. Diabetes. 1988;37:1129–36.
81. Sima AAF, Lattimer SA, Yagihashi S, Greene DA. "Axo-glial dysjunction": a novel structural lesion that accounts for poorly reversible slowing of nerve conduction in the spontaneously diabetic BB-rat. J Clin Invest. 1986;77:474–84.
82. Cherian PV, Kamijo M, Angelides KJ, Sima AAF. Nodal Na+-channel displacement is associated with nerve conduction slowing in the chronically diabetic BB/W-rat. Prevention by an aldose reductase inhibitor. J Diabetes Complications. 1996;10:192–200.
83. Brismar T, Sima AAF, Greene DA. Reversible and irreversible nodal dysfunction in diabetic neuropathy. Ann Neurol. 1987;21:504–7.
84. Peles E, Nativ M, Lustig M, et al. Identification of a novel contactin-associated transmembrane receptor

with multiple domains implicated in protein-protein interactions. EMBO J. 1997;16:978–88.
85. Ratcliffe CF, Qu V, McCormick KA, et al. A sodium channel signaling complex: modulation by associated receptor protein tyrosine phosphatase β. Nat Neurosci. 2000;3:437–44.
86. Peles E, Nativ M, Campbell PL, et al. The carbonic anhydrase domain of receptor tyrosine phosphatase beta is a functional ligand for the axonal recognition molecule contactin. Cell. 1995;82:251–60.
87. Johnson KG, Van Vactor D. Receptor protein tyrosine phosphases in nervous system development. Physiol Rev. 2003;83:1–24.
88. Purves T, Middlemas A, Agthong S, et al. A role for mitogen-activated protein kinases in the etiology of diabetic neuropathy. FASEB J. 2001;15:2508–14.
89. Sugimoto K, Murakawa Y, Sima AAF. Expression and localization of insulin receptor in rat dorsal root ganglion and spinal cord. J Pheripher Nerve Syst. 2002;7:44–53.
90. Kamiya H, Murakawa Y, Zhang W, Sima AAF. Unmyelinated fiber sensory neuropathy differs in type 1 and type 2 diabetes. Diabetes Metab Res Rev. 2005;21:448–58.
91. Sima AAF, Zhang W-X, Sugimoto K, et al. C-peptide prevents and improves chronic type 1 diabetic neuropathy in the BB/Wor-rat. Diabetologia. 2001;44:889–97.
92. Terada M, Yasuda H, Kikkawa R. Delayed Wallerian degeneration and increased neurofilament phosphorylation in sciatic nerves of rats with streptozotocin-induced diabetes. J Neurol Sci. 1998;155:23–30.
93. Brownlees J, Yates A, Bajaj NP, et al. Phosphorylation of neurofilament heavy chain side-arms by stress activated protein kinase – 1b/Jun N-terminal kinase-3. J Cell Sci. 2000;113:401–7.
94. Kamiya H, Zhang W, Sima AAF. Dynamic changes of neuroskeletal proteins underlie impaired axonal maturation and progressive degeneration in type 1 diabetes. Exp Diabetes Res. 2009;2009:793281.
95. Fernyhough P, Mill JF, Roberts JL, Ishii DN. Stabilization of tubulin mRNA's by insulin and insulin-like growth factor-1 during neurite formation. Mol Brain Res. 1989;6:109–20.
96. Verge VNK, Tetzlatt W, Bisby MA, Richardson PM. Influence of nerve growth factor on neurofilament gene expression in mature primary sensory neurons. J Neurosci. 1990;10:2018–25.
97. Fernyhough P, Willars GB, Lindsay RM, Tomlinson DR. Insulin and insulin-like growth factor I enhance regeneration in cultured adult rat sensory neurons. Brain. 1993;607:117–24.
98. Gilron I, Flatters SJ. Gabapentin and pregabalin for the treatment of neuropathic pain: a review of laboratory and clinical evidence. Pain Res Manag. 2006;11(Suppl A):16–29.
99. Ramos KM, Jiang Y, Svensson CI, Calcutt NA. Pathogenesis of spinally mediated hyperalgesia in diabetes. Diabetes. 2007;56:1569–76.
100. Burchiel KJ, Russel LC, Lee RP, Sima AAF. Spontaneous activity of primary afferent neurons in diabetic BB-Wistar rats. A possible mechanism of chronic diabetic pain. Diabetes. 1985;34:1210–3.
101. Hirade M, Yasuda H, Omatsu-Kanbe M, Kikkawa R, Kitasato H. Tetrodotoxin-resistant sodium channels of dorsal root ganglion neurons are readily activated in diabetic rats. Neuroscience. 1999;90:933–7.
102. Bachouja M-M. Pathophysiology of neuropathic pain. In: Veves A, Malik RA, editors. Diabetic neuropathy. Clinical management. Totowa: Humana Press; 2007. p. 339–50.
103. Kamiya H, Zhang W, Sima AAF. C-peptide prevents nociceptive sensory neuropathy in type 1 diabetes. Ann Neurol. 2004;56:827–35.
104. Kamiya H, Zhang W, Ekberg K, Wahren J, Sima AAF. C-peptide reverses nociceptive neuropathy in type 1 diabetic BB/Wor-rat. Diabetes. 2006;55:3581–7.
105. Kamiya H, Zhang W, Sima AAF. Degeneration of Golgi and neuronal loss in DRG's in diabetic BB/Wor-rats. Diabetologia. 2006;49:2763–74.
106. Kapur D. Neuropathic pain and diabetes. Diabetes Metab Res Rev. 2003;19:S9–15.
107. Kamijo M, Merry AC, Akdas G, Cherian PV, Sima AAF. Nerve fiber regeneration following axotomy in the diabetic BB/W-rat. The effect of ARI-treatment. J Diabetes Complications. 1996;10:183–91.
108. Sima AAF, Levitan I, Ristic H, Kamijo M. Nerve fiber regeneration in the spontaneously diabetic BB/W-rat. In: Hotta N, Greene DA, Ward JD, Sima AAF, Boulton AJM, editors. Diabetic neuropathy: new concepts and insights. Amsterdam: Elsevier; 1995. p. 27–36.
109. Ide C. Peripheral nerve regeneration. Neurosci Res. 1996;25:101–21.
110. Ishii DN, Glazner GW, Pu S. Role of insulin-like growth factor in peripheral nerve regeneration. Mol Neurobiol. 1997;14:67–116.

C-Peptide and Type 1 Diabetic Encephalopathy

9

Anders A.F. Sima and Wei-Xian Zhang

Keywords
Diabetic encephalopathy • C-peptide • Gray matter changes • White matter atrophy

Introduction

Diabetic encephalopathies are recently recognized complications affecting both type 1 and type 2 diabetic patients [1, 2]. With the increasing incidences of both types of diabetes, the central nervous system (CNS) complications are likely to increase in frequency. Similar to other so-called microvascular complications, diabetic encephalopathies differ in type 1 and type 2 diabetes, suggesting differences in underlying causative mechanisms [2]. Type 2 diabetes is associated with an increased incidence of Alzheimer's disease and vascular multiinfarct dementia [3–6].

Neuropsychological studies in type 1 diabetic children have demonstrated deficits in attention, processing speed, executive function, and memory [7–11]. Morphometric imaging studies have revealed volumetric deficits in both gray and white matter structures, particularly in so-called limbic areas involved in cognition [12, 13]. Such deficits tend to be more evident in children with early onset of diabetes and progress with duration of diabetes [7, 8, 14, 15]. In contrast to earlier belief, recurrent episodes of hypoglycemia due to strict insulin therapy do not appear to play a role in evolving cognitive deficits, except for cases with extreme and prolonged hypoglycemia [16–19]. Instead, experimental studies in various diabetic animal models seem to suggest that insulin and C-peptide deficiencies seem to play major underlying pathobiological roles in the development of type 1 diabetic encephalopathy [20–24]. The incidence of type 1 diabetic encephalopathy is likely to increase in pace with the global increase in the incidence of type 1 diabetes. A further contributing and probably enhancing factor is that type 1 diabetes occurs at increasingly younger ages, at ages when the brain is still developing and therefore particularly vulnerable to metabolic insults [25–27].

A.A.F. Sima (✉)
Department of Pathology, Wayne State University and Detroit Medical Center, 540 E. Canfield Avenue, Detroit, MI 48201, USA

Department of Neurology, Wayne State University and Detroit Medical Center, Detroit, MI 48201, USA
e-mail: asima@med.wayne.edu

W.-X. Zhang
Department of Pathology, Wayne State University and Detroit Medical Center, 540 E. Canfield Avenue, Detroit, MI 48201, USA

A.A.F. Sima (ed.), *Diabetes & C-Peptide: Scientific and Clinical Aspects*, Contemporary Diabetes,
DOI 10.1007/978-1-61779-391-2_9,

Animal studies of type 1 diabetic encephalopathy have shown sequential abnormalities demonstrating early neurobehavioral deficits, associated with down-regulation of neurotrophic factors, activation of inflammatory responses, apoptotic activities, and neurostructural deficits [20–24]. In this sequence of developing abnormalities, those of the white matter appear to precede those of gray matter structures [2, 24].

In this chapter, we will describe the clinical characteristics of the progressive changes occurring in type 1 diabetic patients. The sequential mechanistic changes occurring in the spontaneously diabetic BB/W-rat will be discussed in detail and the beneficial effects of C-peptide substitution in this model will be reviewed with regard to prevention and modifications in the evolution of type 1 diabetic encephalopathy.

Clinical Studies

Functional and Neuropsychological Findings

Prolonged latencies of evoked potentials, such as visual, auditory, and somatosensory potentials, are common subclinical findings in type 1 diabetic patients reflecting both peripheral and central abnormalities [28]. The visually evoked P100 wave is generated in visual cortex. Auditory-evoked potentials with delayed latencies between waves are reflective of slowed pontine and mesencephalic conductivity and have been documented in type 1 diabetic patients [28–32]. Increased latencies of somatosensory-evoked potentials are more variable and reflect also the peripheral component [33–35]. Evoked potential endogenous to the CNS such as the P300 wave is commonly reported with increased latencies in type 1 diabetic patients and is reflective of cognitive and mnemonic functions [16, 36, 37]. Such changes indicative of CNS dysfunction are usually evident early in the course of diabetes and are present before demonstrable cognitive deficits have developed [32]. They have been reported to be partially reversible with tight blood glucose control [38].

The term diabetic encephalopathy was introduced by Reske-Nielsen et al. [39] in 1965 describing pathological changes in brains of young patients with long-term type 1 diabetes. Patients with type 1 diabetes have since repeatedly been reported as showing modest and progressive defects on neuro-psychological testings. An extensive meta-analyses comprising 33 studies [40] demonstrated defects in major cognitive domains in type 1 diabetic patients. Although some changes were relatively mild, overall cognitive deficiencies were highly significant between diabetic and age-matched control subjects, despite the fact that the number of patients, onset of diabetes, and duration varied greatly between individual studies. Diabetic children are likely to perform more poorly at school than their nondiabetic peers, with lower scores on academic achievement tests and verbal intelligence [10, 15, 41]. Neuropsychological tests have revealed deficits in various cognitive spheres such as crystallized intelligence, psychomotor speed, sustained and visual attention, mental flexibility, visuoperceptual function, learning, and memory skills [8, 9, 40, 42, 43]. Verbal IQ scores appear to decline with duration of diabetes and to be more severe with earlier onset of disease [14, 44]. Besides age of onset, gender seems to have an effect, in that boys perform worse than girls [7, 45]. In contrast to earlier opinions, recent studies have not associated cognitive deficits with repeated episodes of hypoglycemia [16–19].

Imaging Studies

Neuroradiological studies have examined brain volumes in patients with type 1 diabetes. Both gray and white matter abnormalities have been described. A high incidence of mesotemporal lobe sclerosis was demonstrated as being evident already after 7 years of diabetes. This structural deficit was unrelated to previous episodes of severe hypoglycemia [12]. Significant white matter atrophy in parahippocampal, temporal, and frontal white matter measured volumetrically was reported in patients 12 years after onset of diabetes. Such white matter changes were associated with decreased volumes of insular cortex, hippocampus, and thalamic structures [12, 46]. Voxel-based morphometric analyses have reported decreased densities in thalami, superior and middle temporal gyri, and frontal cortex in patients with long-standing type 1 diabetes [13, 46]. Detailed neuropathological reports on brains of type 1 diabetic patients are rare. However, the neuroradiological abnormalities described above are consistent with recent neuropathological reports on patients with early onset of diabetes who succumbed to ketoacidosis. The postmortem exams of these patients showed severe neuronal loss in hippocampus and frontal cortex accompanied by white matter atrophy of frontal and temporal lobes. These neuropathological findings were associated with severe down-regulation of the insulin and IGF-1 receptors, increased expression of receptor for advanced glycation end products (RAGE), and neuroinflammatory factors such as TNF-α and interleukins and correlated with MRS studies of neurometabolites reflective of neuronal viability [47–49]. Therefore, radiological and limited structural studies suggest that limbic temporal and frontal structures are particularly vulnerable and are likely to underlie compromised cognition such as attention, information processing, executive function, and memory as suggested by impaired functional connectivity [50].

Several studies have demonstrated a relationship between encephalopathy and other chronic complications such as retinopathy, neuropathy, and nephropathy, [43, 44] suggesting that similar metabolic perturbations may underlie type 1 diabetic encephalopathy. Of the common complications, a relationship between retinopathy and encephalopathy has been specifically and repeatedly reported [32, 44, 51].

Neuroradiological studies have demonstrated focal white and gray matter lesions, diffuse high-intensity periventricular white matter lesions, and enlarged perivascular spaces as characteristic of type 1 diabetic encephalopathy [40, 44, 51]. Such lesions are not likely to be diabetes-induced per se, but appear to be characteristic lesions seen in hypertensive encephalopathy, such as random focal infarcts, periventricular leukoariosis, and enlarged perivascular spaces, so-called "êtat criblé." Now, it may be argued that hypertension often accompanies diabetes in early middle-aged patients as in some of these studies. However, in order to come to grips with the mechanisms of what we understand as "type 1 diabetic encephalopathy," it will be imperative to separate type 1 diabetes from other comorbid systemic disorders that may in themselves cause CNS pathology [52].

The recent increase in the incidence of type 1 diabetes and its onset at increasingly younger ages are evident not only in developed countries, but alarmingly so in heavily populated countries such as India, China, and also in the Middle East [53–56]. The reason for this very concerning trend is not known. Various factors have been suggested such as formula feeding rather than breast feeding during early infancy, increased incidence of Cesarean section deliveries, and the increasing incidence of infant and childhood obesity triggering inflammation potentially causing autoimmune mechanisms targeting pancreatic β-cells [57–59].

Experimental Studies

Studies in Streptozotocin-Induced Diabetes in Rodents

Early studies in rats with streptozotocin (STZ)-induced diabetes demonstrated white matter deficits and neuronal loss in frontal cortex [60]. Neurobehavioral deficits in STZ-rats were demonstrated by employing the Morris water maze paradigm [61]. Such deficits were prevented with insulin treatment from onset of diabetes [62]. Impaired water maze learning was associated with abnormal long-term potentiation reflective of synaptic plasticity, which was also prevented by insulin treatment [62]. On the other hand, interventional treatment with insulin to normoglycemic levels did not reverse water maze learning deficits, but had a partial effect on long-term potentiation [62]. These data suggest that both pro- and postsynaptic activities are affected in hippocampus [63]. Data obtained from the STZ-induced diabetic Swiss Webster wild-type mouse show progressive cerebral atrophy and cognitive decline [23]. The cerebral atrophy in this model was mainly due to white matter abnormalities as cortical neuronal loss was not demonstrated. White matter atrophy was accompanied by up-regulation of the RAGE [23, 24]. The described abnormalities were associated with down-regulation of insulin-signaling intermediaries, the transcription factor cyclic adenosine monophosphate (cAMP), the response element-binding protein, (CREB) and synaptophysin. Administration of intranasal insulin, which does not effect systemic hyperglycemia, corrected insulin-signaling intermediaries, slowed the development of neurobehavioral deficits and prevented white matter atrophy [24]. These data are consistent with and support our previous data and notion put forward that insulin deficiency per se plays a pivotal role in the development of type 1 diabetic encephalopathy [2, 22, 64].

Insulin-Signaling and C-Peptide

Insulin possesses a variety of functions in the CNS. It is a potent neurotrophic factor in and by itself. It exerts gene regulatory effects on other neurotrophic factors like NGF, IGF-1, NT-3, and their receptors and it has anti-inflammatory and antiapoptotic effects [2, 21, 65–70]. As mentioned earlier, a specific C-peptide receptor has not been identified. Instead, there is accumulating data demonstrating insulin-like effects by C-peptide [71, 72]. C-peptide elicits disaggregation of hexameric insulin, probably via a Zn^{2+}-related mechanism thereby enhancing the effect of insulin [73, 74]. A further insulin-enhancing effect is its inhibition of intracellular protein tyrosine phosphatase (PTP) activity resulting in increased autophosphorylation of the insulin receptor (IR) [69, 75]. These effects are believed to be charge-based interactions ([76], see Chap. 3).

C-peptide binds to cell membranes of a variety of cells [77–79], although there is no evidence that it binds specifically to the IR. Instead, it has been suggested that it binds to a G-protein-coupled receptor [77, 78] or that some C-peptide effects may be mediated by nonchiral interactions [80]. Recent data have demonstrated internalization of C-peptide into cytosolic ribosomes ([81], see Chap. 10), and to nuclear nucleoli, where it binds to histones of the promotor region of genes for ribosomal RNA ([82], see Chap. 3). These findings are highly relevant suggesting a growth factor effect of C-peptide that may explain its cell proliferative effects, antiapoptotic effects, and regulatory effects on the gene expression of several neurotrophic factors and their receptors both in peripheral nerve and CNS [2, 20, 22, 68, 69, 83–85].

An additional effect by C-peptide, pertinent to type 1 diabetic encephalopathy, is its anti-inflammatory effect [68, 86]. Innate inflammation is a common accompaniment to a variety of neurodegenerative disorders. It has been suggested that activation of the inflammatory cascade is initiated by hyperglycemia-induced NFκB [86, 87]. This is probably not the major initiating mechanism, since treatment with C-peptide, which does not effect hyperglycemia, has an ameliorating effect on inflammation. We have suggested that an additional mechanism is the impaired insulin-signaling mechanisms. Impaired signaling activity of the insulin pathway results in phosphorylation of IκB [21, 70, 88–90] with disinhibition of NFκB and hence increased expression. As mentioned earlier, impaired insulin-signaling affects the expression of various neurotrophic factors with secondary downstream adverse effects on the synthesis of neuroskeletal proteins and their phosphorylation both in peripheral nerve and CNS [2, 20, 91, 92]. These downstream effects underlie in part neurodegeneration and inhibit regenerative capacities. Hence, to date a variety of mechanisms have been identified leading to adverse effects on the CNS under conditions of C-peptide deficiency in type 1 diabetes.

Neurobehavioral Deficits in Type 1 Diabetes

Early behavioral testing, using the radial arm paradigm [93], shows significant deficits already in 2-month diabetic BB/Wor-rats. Type I and

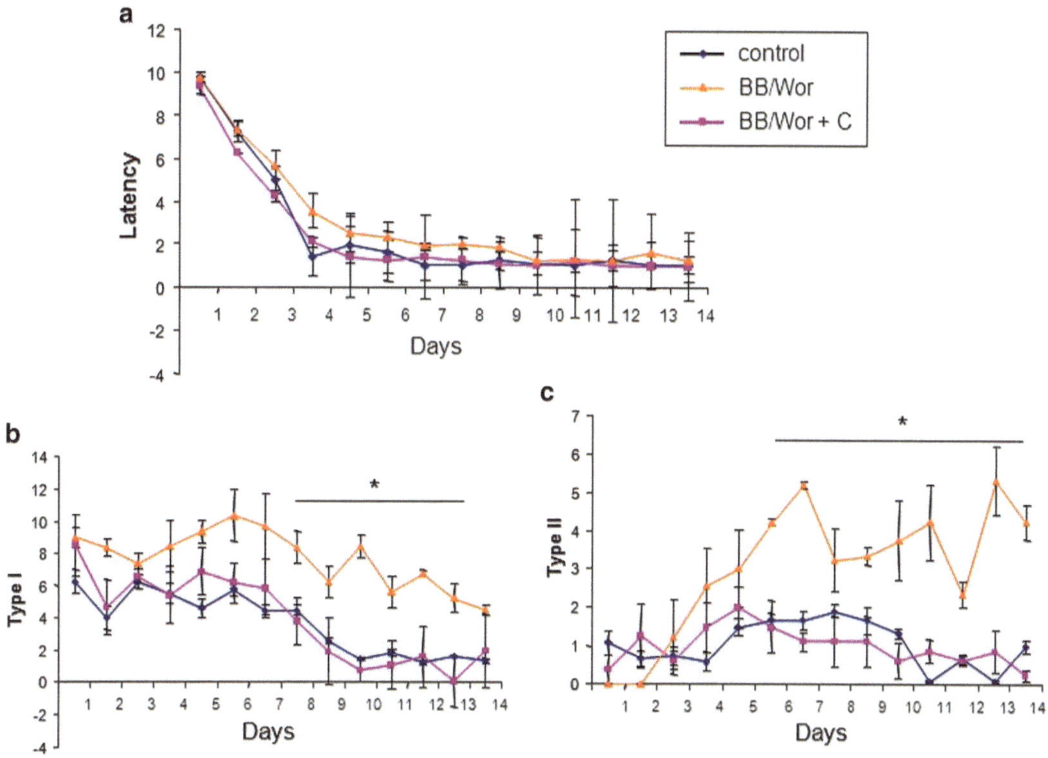

Fig. 9.1 Behavioral testing using the radial arm paradigm [93]. This test records the time (latency) it takes for the animal to retrieve baits placed in three cued arms out of eight radial arms. Type I error signifies entrance into an arm without a bait (reference memory). Type II error is recorded when entering an arm from which the bait has already been retrieved (working memory). At 2 months duration of diabetes, diabetic BB/Wor-rats showed no increase in total latencies (**a**). However, the number of type I and type II errors reflecting impaired reference and working memory, respectively, were significantly increased in diabetic rats (**b**, **c**) after approximately 7 days of previous training. Full replacement of rat-II C-peptide fully prevented these abnormalities. Such errors have been closely related to hippocampal activity, long-term potentiation, and mossy fiber pathology. Data reproduced with permission from ref. [85]

Type II errors signifying impaired reference and working memory, respectively, are significantly more common in diabetic rats [20]. Full C-peptide replacement from onset of diabetes resulted in complete prevention of these deficits (Fig. 9.1). On the other hand, latencies of the radial arm performances were not altered in 2-month diabetic BB/Wor-rats. Studies using the Morris water maze system [94] in which multiple cognitive components are invoked, such as problem solving, formation of internal representation of the environment, and storage and retrieval of relevant information and memory, showed no significant deficits at 2 months (Fig. 9.2a), but only after 6 months of diabetes could significantly prolonged latencies be elicited [2, 20, 22] (Fig. 9.2b). C-peptide replacement from onset of diabetes resulted in significant prevention of the shortcomings in the Morris water maze testing at 8 months duration of diabetes [22] (Fig. 9.2c). These results indicate that progressive learning and memory deficiencies occur in a duration-dependent fashion and that they can be significantly prevented by full C-peptide replacement. The changes are indicative of altered synaptic plasticity and are associated with depression of long-term potentiation and enhanced long-term depression [22, 62, 63].

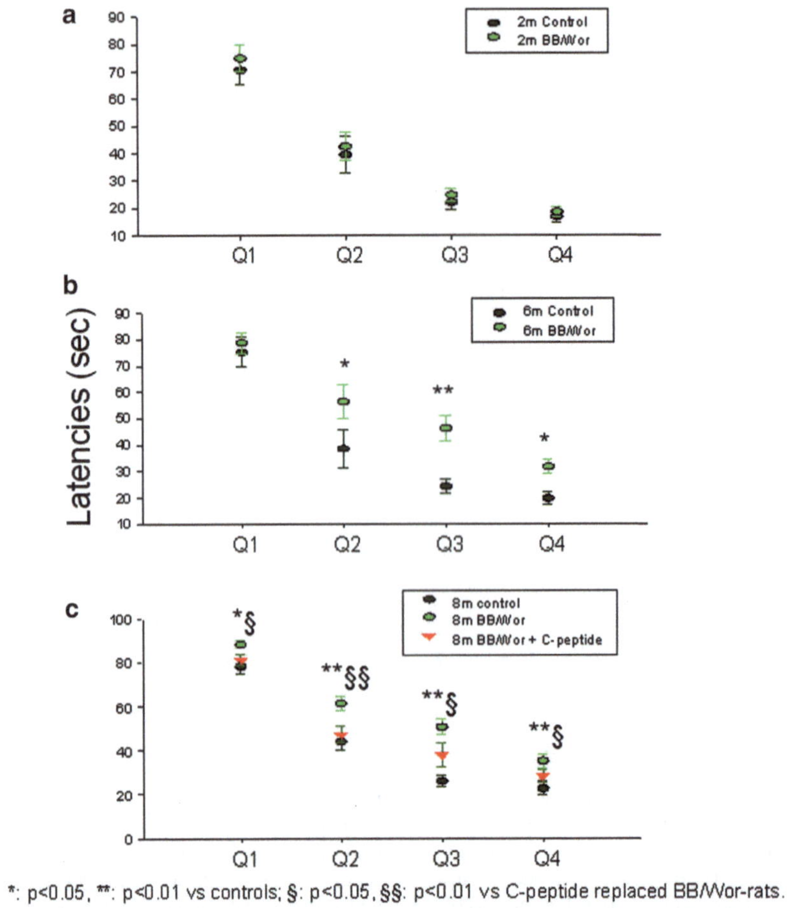

Fig. 9.2 Longitudinal neurobehavioral assessments using the Morris water maze method. In this paradigm, animals are released from four quadrants of a circular water pool and the time taken to reach a platform from each quadrant (Q1–Q4) is recorded. After 2 months of diabetes, no deficits were obtainable (**a**). Only after 6 months of untreated diabetes were there significant deficits in the latencies (**b**). Animals treated with C-peptide from onset of diabetes showed significant prevention of the behavioral deficits at 8 months of diabetes (**c**). The abnormalities of the Morris water maze reflect impaired spatial memory and long-term memory deficits. Original data obtained from ref. [22]

Insulin and C-Peptide Function, Neurotrophism, and Synaptic Alterations

As previously shown, the early neurobehavioral changes in both reference and working memories were associated with impaired expression of the IR in 2-month diabetic rats and impaired insulin-signaling as reflected by decreased expression of p-Akt and significantly increased p-GSK-3β [20, 22]. The decreased insulin-signaling activity was accompanied by decreased expression of both IGF-1 and IGF-2 as well as IGF-IR expression in 2-month diabetic hippocampi [20]. This was later followed by significantly decreased expression of NGF and NGF-R-TrK A evident in 8-month diabetic BB/Wor-rats. Abnormalities in the neurotrophic networking of hippocampus was significantly prevented by full C-peptide substitution from onset of diabetes [20, 22] (Fig. 9.3), presumably by preventing the defects in gene-regulation of neurotrophic factors and their receptors caused by impaired insulin-signaling [20, 22, 91, 92]. Both insulin and NGF lend potent neurotrophic

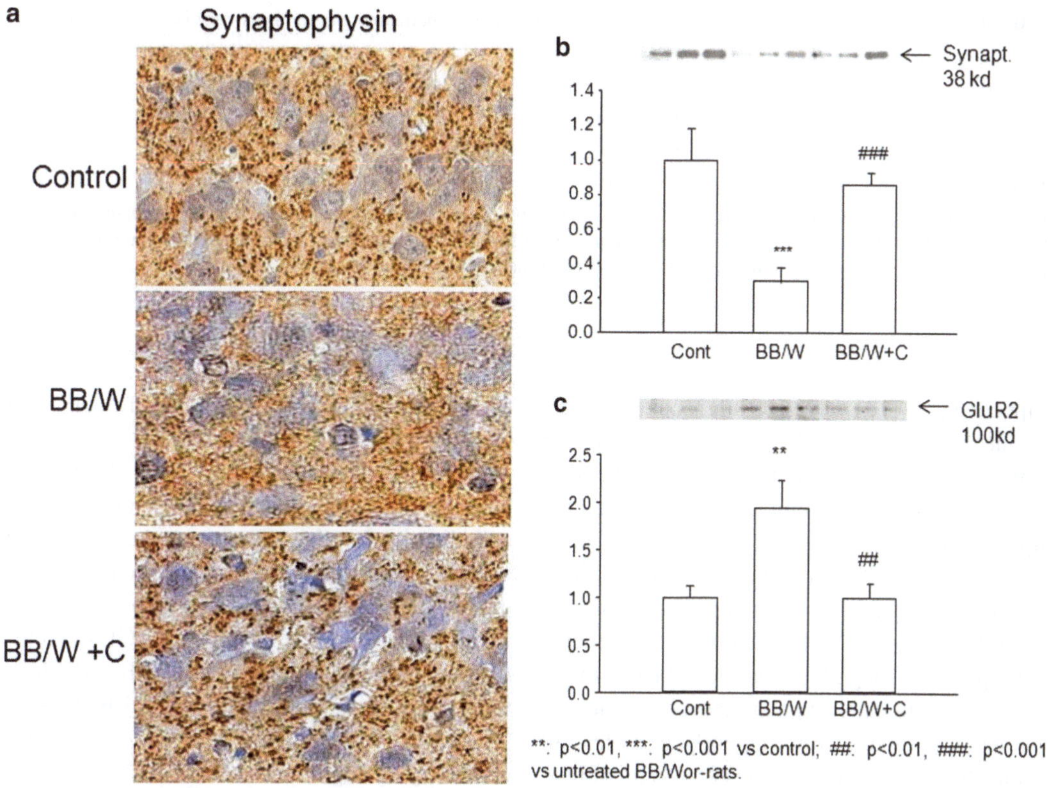

Fig. 9.3 Expression of presynaptic synaptophysin (**a, b**) and postsynaptic subunit GluR2 (**c**) in control, diabetic, and C-peptide replaced diabetic BB/Wor-rat. Immunostaining for synaptophysin in hippocampal CA_1 shows decreased stainability in diabetic as compared to control rats. This is fully prevented by replacement of C-peptide for 4 months (**a**). The corresponding immunoblot (**b**) shows approximately a 70% decrease in the expression of synaptophysin in diabetic rats, which is fully prevented by full substitution of C-peptide. The expression of the postsynaptic glutamate receptor GluR2 subunit was increased twofold in 7-month diabetic rats (**c**) which was fully ameliorated by C-peptide replacement from onset of diabetes. Data obtained from ref. [20]

support in hippocampus. Insulin is intimately involved in neurotransmitter synthesis including acetylcholin and glutamate [95] and NGF secretion provides protective effects on cholinergic neuronal populations [96, 97]. Interestingly, IGF-2, which was markedly suppressed in diabetic rats and was significantly abrogated by C-peptide, promotes hippocampal acetylcholin release, whereas IGF-1, which was mildly suppressed in diabetic animals and completely restored by C-peptide, has the opposite effect on hippocampal acetylcholine release [98, 99]. These neurotrophic factors together with brain-derived neurotrophic factor (BDNF) are known to modulate pre- and postsynaptic transmission and plasticity [100]. In the BB/Wor-rat, the early perturbation of trophic factor activities was accompanied by presynaptic degeneration in hippocampi of 4-month diabetic rats, as shown by decreased synaptophysin expression and decreased numbers of presynaptic terminals of pyramidal neurons of the Ammon's horn area 1 (CA_1) of hippocampus [20]. The suppression of synaptophysin and degeneration and loss of presynaptic terminal neurites were fully prevented by physiological C-peptide replacement [20] (Fig. 9.3). The described abnormalities were later followed by up-regulations of postsynaptic glutamate receptors subunits GluR2 and GluR4 [20]. GluR2 is the more prevalent in the forebrain and

Table 9.1 MicroPET data obtained from brains of 3-month male diabetic and age- and sex-matched control rats

	K-cplx (min)			rMRGlc (μmol/100 g/min)		
Region	Control	Diabetic	Δ (%)	Control	Diabetic	Δ (%)
Cortex	0.0164 (5)	0.0111 (8)	−32	17.95 (3)	51.12 (9)	283
Hippocampus	0.0173 (9)	0.0136 (6)	−22	19.08 (4)	62.15 (7)	326
Whole brain	0.0166 (5)	0.0123 (6)	−26	18.20 (3)	56.43 (9)	307

Uptakei rate constant for the tracer (K-cplx) was decreased by 22–32% in diabetic brains. On the other hand, the metabolic rate of glucose (rMRGlc) was increased by approximately threefold in diabetic rats as compared to control animals. Numbers in parenthesis indicate numbers of animals examined. Data obtained from ref. [20]

hippocampus [101, 102]. GluR2 controls Ca^{2+} permeability of the AMPA receptor and plays an important role in long-term synaptic modulation [103]. C-peptide replacement fully prevented the up-regulation of GluR2 (Fig. 9.3) and prevented partially that of GluR4 [20]. Future studies will reveal as to whether these changes relate to long-term depression and long-term memory deficits. It is apparent though that numerous factors originating from impaired insulin and C-peptide signaling and possibly from hyperglycemia lead to sequential perturbations in the expression of neurotrophic factors with aberrations of synaptic connectivity leading to sequential and progressive behavioral deficits.

Glucose Metabolism, RAGE, and Inflammatory Responses

Most animal models of type 1 diabetes, including the BB/Wor-rat, are maintained at high glycemic levels, but free of ketonuria. Blood glucose levels are not influenced by C-peptide replacement. MicroPet imaging of diabetic BB/Wor-rats has revealed a threefold increase in the regional metabolic rate of glucose (rMRG1c) in whole brain as well as similar regional levels in hippocampus and cerebral cortex (Table 9.1). However, the glucose uptake rate of ^{18}F-fluorodeoxyglucose showed an approximate 30% decrease [20]. These data are similar to those reported in humans [104]. Increased cerebral glucose was associated with an increased presence of RAGE (Fig. 9.4), which was colocalized with glial fibrillary acid protein (GFAP) in proliferating astrocytes, although the presence of RAGE was also seen to a lesser extent in hippocampal pyramidal cells and oligodendroglia cells of the white matter [68] in keeping with its distribution in human type 1 diabetes [48] and in the STZ-induced diabetic Swiss Weber mouse model [23]. RAGE is a multiligand receptor, stimulating NFκB, which is upregulated in hippocampus in the BB/Wor-rat. Up-regulation of RAGE and NFκB was accompanied by up-regulation of TNF-α, IL-1β, IL-2, and IL-6 (Fig. 9.4), whereas the anti-inflammatory interleukin IL-10 was downregulated [68]. Somewhat unexpectedly C-peptide replacement, which does not effect hyperglycemia, prevented the up-regulation of both RAGE and NFκB in hippocampus (Fig. 9.4). These data suggest that the up-regulation of RAGE and its response to C-peptide supplementation may be largely regulated by insulin-signaling activities rather than by a direct effect of hyperglycemia [69, 72, 90, 105]. It is known that NFκB is upregulated by impaired insulin-signaling and it is also known that it upregulates RAGE itself, hence providing a self-perpetuating loop [20]. Corrections of RAGE and NFκB by C-peptide resulted in prevention of the enhanced expression of TNF-α and the proinflammatory interleukins, whereas the suppressed expression of the anti-inflammatory IL-10 was abrogated (Fig. 9.4). The activation of inflammatory factors is likely to have multiple in part self-perpetuating effects on insulin-signaling itself as well as effects on oxidative stress and apoptotic activities [2, 20].

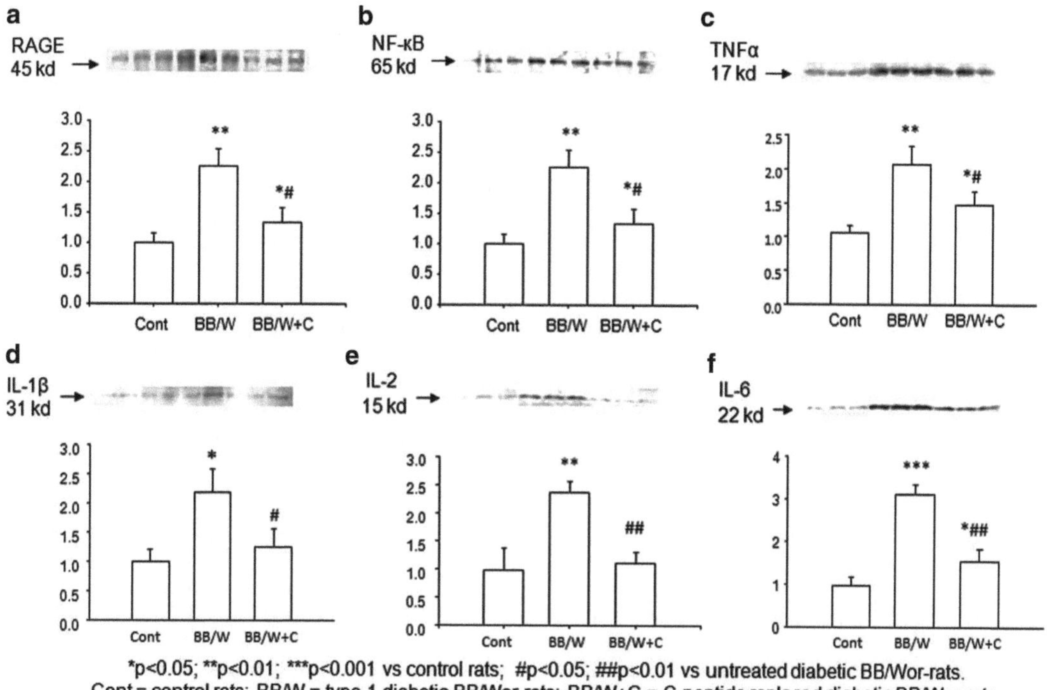

Fig. 9.4 The expressions of RAGE (**a**), NFκB (**b**), and TNF-α (**c**) were significantly increased in diabetic hippocampi of BB/W-rats. Full replacement of rat II C-peptide prevented significantly such up-regulations. As a consequence of these aberrations, the expressions of proinflammatory interleukins IL-1β (**d**), IL-2 (**e**), and IL-6 (**f**) were also markedly upregulated. This activation of proinflammatory interleukins in the hippocampus was significantly prevented by C-peptide replacement

Neurodegenerative Changes in Type 1 Diabetic Encephalopathy

As mentioned above, degenerative changes of presynaptic neurites occur early in experimental models of type 1 diabetes [20, 24]. There is growing evidence suggesting links between Alzheimer's disease and diabetes [1, 5]. This linkage appears to be more prevalent in patients with type 2 diabetes [2, 45] and has been linked to hyperinsulinemia and impaired insulin function due to insulin resistance [106–108]. However, insulin-signaling activities are also significantly compromised in the brain in type 1 diabetes [22, 48], suggesting an increased risk for AD also in type 1 diabetes [109, 110]. It has been shown that increased activity of GSK-3 is associated with behavioral and biochemical features of AD [111]. However, several possible mechanisms may underlie such relationships. It is well known that caveolin-1, which is upregulated in type 2 diabetes, induces up-regulation of amyloid precursor proteins (APP) as well as the enzymes BACE and γ-secretase which mediate the formation of amyloid-β (Aβ) [2, 107, 112, 113]. Furthermore, there appears to exist a reciprocal relationship between the scaffolding of caveolin signaling and that of insulin. The IR colocalizes with caveolin-1 in caveolae of cell membranes [114, 115]. In fact, in the type 1 BB/Wor-rat, caveolin-1, APP, and BACE are significantly upregulated together with Aβ, demonstrating the relationship between insulin and caveolin signaling (Fig. 9.5). It should be mentioned though that such relationships are more profound in the type 2 diabetic counterpart, the BBZDR/Wor-rat [107]. Nevertheless, even in type 1 diabetic BB/W-rats, there is a significantly increased accumulation of Aβ (Fig. 9.5), one of

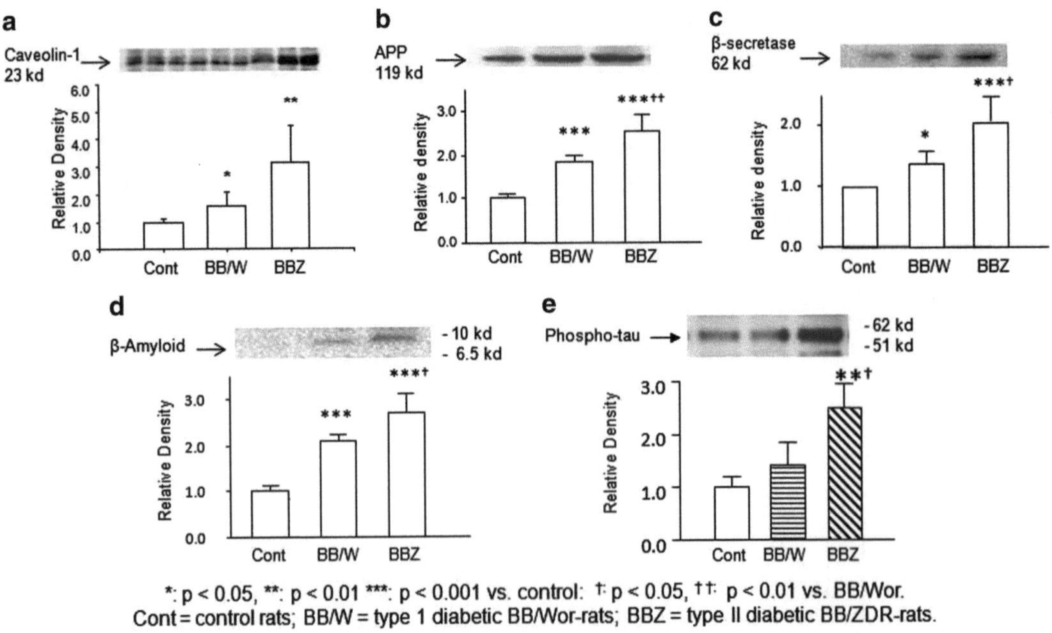

Fig. 9.5 Comparison of intermediaries of the amyloidogenic APP metabolism (**a–d**) and phospho-tau expression (**e**) in type 1 BB/Wor-rats as compared to the type 2 diabetic BBZDR-rats. Caveolin-1 is significantly increased in type 1 diabetic hippocampi (**a**). It should be noted that this up-regulation was twofold in type 2 diabetic rats. Similar differences were noted with respect to amyloid precursor protein (APP) (**b**), β-secretase (BACE) (**c**), and beta-amyloid (Aβ) (**d**). The expression of hyperphosphorylated tau was increased, but not significantly so in the type 1 BB/Wor-rat (**e**), whereas this was increased 2.5-fold in type 2 BBZDR/Wor-rats. Data partly obtained from ref. [108]

the hallmarks of human AD. The accumulation of spliced tau proteins and their subsequent hyperphosphorylation have been linked to caspase activation (see below) with splicing of the tau protein and the phosphorylation of the spliced products by predominantly GSK-3 [107, 110, 116]. Accumulation of hyperphosphorylated tau is also more profound in the type 2 BBZDR/Wor-rat [107]. Similar differences in the deposition of phosphorylated tau was recently demonstrated in type 2 diabetic db/db mice as compared to type 1 STZ-induced diabetic mice [117].

Both insulin and C-peptide demonstrate strong antiapoptotic effects. In previous studies, we have shown that insulinopenic diabetes is accompanied by up-regulation of a number of proapoptotic factors and those indicative of DNA damage. Hence, factors like NGFR-p75, Fax, Bax, and cleaved PARP are significantly upregulated together with caspase 12 and caspase 3 [22, 64, 69]. Also indicators of oxidative DNA damage such as 8-OH-dG are upregulated. Activation of oxidative and apoptotic stressors was accompanied by increased TUNEL staining of pyramidal cells in hippocampus, particularly of the sensitive CA_1 region, and by increased DNA laddering [22]. The end result of increased apoptotic activity is a significant decrease in hippocampal pyramidal cell numbers [20, 22]. Such perturbations along with decreased insulin activity per se are likely to contribute to the aberrations of tau handling (see above). Complete C-peptide replacement for the 8-month duration of diabetes, from which these data are obtained, prevented activation of proapoptotic factors, prevented activation of caspases, DNA laddering, and significantly decreased neuronal cell loss, effects which were accompanied by normalization of behavioral deficits [20, 22]. These findings underline the pivotal role of impaired insulin-signaling activities and which are almost completely abrogated by C-peptide substitution, in the progressive development of type 1 diabetic encephalopathy. This construct is supported by recent data describing the beneficial

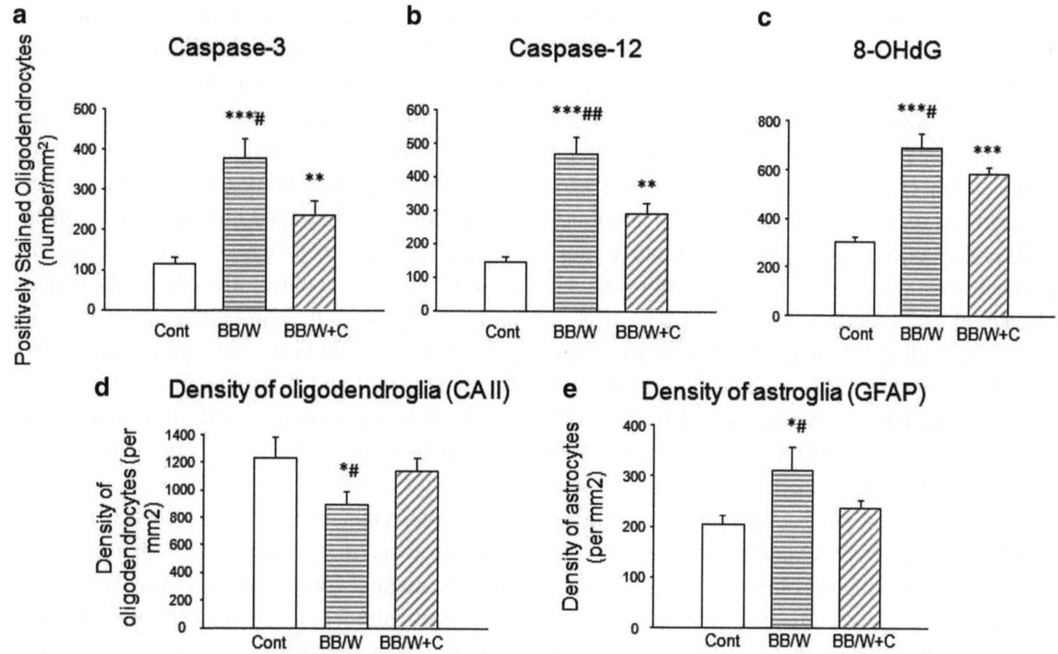

Fig. 9.6 Examination of cerebral white matter in the BB/W-rat. Already in 2-month diabetic rats, activation of caspase 3 (**a**), caspase 12 (**b**), and 8-OHdG (**c**) was evident, indicative of apoptotic stress and oxidative DNA damage. Matching immunocytochemical examination (not shown) confirmed localization to white matter oligodendroglia cells. Full C-peptide replacement started at the onset of diabetes significantly prevented these aberrations. Quantitative analyses of oligodendroglia (**d**) and astrocyte (**e**) densities in white matter showed decreased densities of myelinating oligodendroglia and increased densities of reactive astrocytes. These changes were almost completely prevented by C-peptide replacements

effects of intranasal insulin delivery on intracerebral insulin-signaling intermediaries, cerebral atrophy, and cognitive deficits in STZ-induced diabetic mice [24]. The experimental data are consistent with findings in long-standing and poorly controlled type 1 diabetes in patients, demonstrating impaired insulin and IGF-1 activities and severe neuronal loss in hippocampus and cerebral cortex [48].

White Matter Changes

White matter atrophy has repeatedly been described in human type 1 diabetic patients [12, 46, 47, 49]. Similar white matter changes occur in STZ-induced diabetic mice [23, 24], although this murine model does not display gray matter deficits even after long-standing diabetes [24]. Both in humans and in the diabetic mouse model, white matter changes have been associated with increased expression of RAGE and inflammation. These changes are consistent with those reported in the BB/Wor-rats in which the up-regulation of RAGE in the white matter is associated with significantly increased expression of TNF-α and proinflammatory IL-6 [20]. Changes of enhanced inflammation are associated with and preceded by increased expression of Bax and cleaved PARP already in 2-month diabetic rats. Further examination of the white matter in these subacutely diabetic rats revealed significantly increased expression of activated caspase 3 and 12, and as an indicator of oxidative DNA damage, a more than twofold increase in the expression of 8-OH-dG [68] (Fig. 9.6). Immunocytochemical studies confirmed the localization of caspase 3, caspase 12, and 8OH-dG to white matter oligodendrocytes. Changes reflective of increased inflammation as well as activation of caspases and 8-OH-dG were significantly prevented by full C-peptide replacement from onset of diabetes (Fig. 9.6), underlining the anti-inflammatory and antiapoptotic effects of C-peptide [68]. Quantitative morphometric analyses of the white matter showed already after 2 months of diabetes a 27% loss of oligodendroglial cells and a 55% increase in the density of white matter reactive astrocytes (Fig. 9.6), changes which worsened from 2 to 8 month's duration of diabetes. These degenerative changes of the white matter were almost fully prevented by complete C-peptide substitution [20, 68] and were partly but significantly reversed by C-peptide treatment commencing at 4 months of diabetes.

These data suggest that similar factors, such as inflammation, oxidative, and apoptotic stressors, are operable in the white matter as in gray matter structures. Importantly though, the white matter abnormalities such as loss of myelinating glia occur much earlier than the neuronal deficits described in hippocampus and cerebral cortex [2, 20–22, 64, 68]. As alluded to earlier, these discrepancies in the susceptibility to the metabolic insults caused by insulin- and C-peptide deficiencies may at least in part relate to the later occurring "growth-spurt" of the white matter coinciding with the onset of diabetes in this model [117]. The timing of these "growth spurts" in relation to onset of diabetes may explain the lack of neuronal loss in the STZ-induced mouse model [23, 24] and particular vulnerability of infants with early onset of diabetes as alluded to previously.

Summary and Conclusions

It is now well established that type 1 diabetes can result in intellectual and cognitive deficits. In this respect, the age of onset of diabetes seems to be critical in the sense that a developing brain is certainly more susceptible to the damaging effects of diabetes than is a developed brain. This is in part also reflected in animal models of type 1 diabetes, particularly with respect to the discrepancies of gray and white matter developmental growth spurts in relation to onset of diabetes.

As outlined in this chapter, it is apparent that the abnormalities responsible for type 1 diabetic encephalopathy are complex and not fully understood. However, they appear to occur in a sequential manner and to progress with duration and quality of diabetes control. Recently, it is increasingly recognized that impaired insulin action plays a pivotal role in the pathogenesis of type 1 encephalopathy and that C-peptide replacement has important ameliorating effects in that it corrects many of the aberrations caused by insulin deficiency.

The mechanisms by which C-peptide replacement corrects the abnormalities characterizing the neurological complications in type 1 diabetes have been alluded to in this chapter and has recently been repeatedly reviewed [2, 20, 69, 73, 85]. It is therefore evident that insulin replacement alone is not likely to normalize underlying pathobiological mechanisms. Instead, type 1 diabetes appears to be a defect in the interactions between two failing hormones ([73, 74, 92]; also see Chap. 3).

This is not to say that hyperglycemia per se and its consequences with respect to aberrant glucose handling and oxidative stress are not important, but may play secondary pathogenetic roles. Moreover, there are several mechanistic interactions between insulin deficiency and hyperglycemia.

As demonstrated here, diabetic encephalopathy evolves with duration of diabetes in a sequential manner. A construct of the progressive and interrelated abnormalities as we understand them at the moment is depicted in Fig. 9.7.

The major initiating event appears to be impaired insulin-signaling activity, caused by insulin and C-peptide deficiencies and their lack of interaction. These two hormones are potent neurotrophic factors in their own right, but also impart important regulatory functions on other neurotrophic factors and their receptors. Abnormalities of neurotrophic factors impact on neurotransmitter synthesis, the expression and phosphorylation of neuroskeletal proteins, and

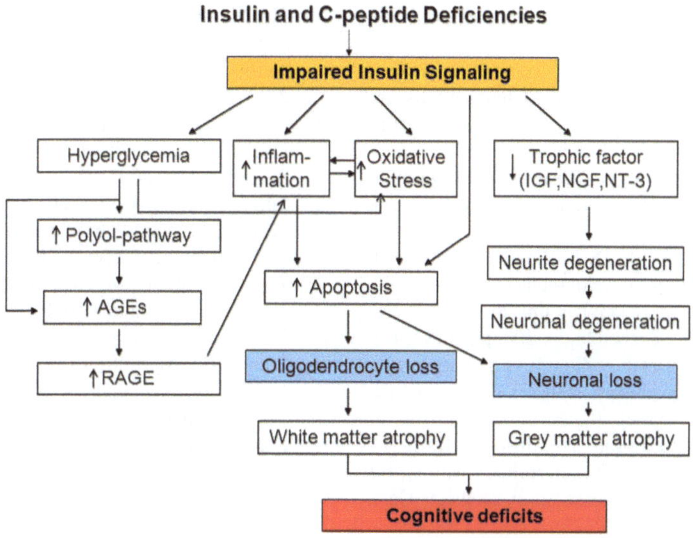

Fig. 9.7 Flow chart depicting the temporal relationships of metabolic and structural abnormalities in type 1 diabetic encephalopathy caused by insulin and C-peptide deficiencies. Impaired insulin signaling results in hyperglycemia with activation of the polyolpathway and formation of AGEs and up-regulation of RAGE. Suppressed insulin signaling leads to inflammation via up-regulation of NFκB and to oxidative stress, which is also caused by hyperglycemia. Insulin and C-peptide deficiencies impact on other neurotrophic factors like IGF's, NGF, and NT-3, resulting in impaired synthesis of neurotransmitters and early neurobehavioral deficits. Impaired neurotrophic support also results in neurite and neuronal degeneration and neuronal loss with impacts on interneuronal connectivity. Impaired insulin signaling together with oxidative stress and inflammation causes activation of caspases and oxidative DNA damage. Eventually such changes result in loss of white matter oligodendroglia cell and neuronal populations with atrophy of white and gray matters and ultimately progressive cognitive deficits

induce inflammation. It should be mentioned that inflammatory responses might also be induced by hyperglycemia (see Chap. 11). Somewhat surprisingly though, C-peptide which does not correct hyperglycemia corrects the up-regulation of RAGE and consequent up-regulation of inflammatory factors. These early perturbations, which may be reversible, have impelling effects on synaptic connectivity and underlie neurite degeneration. They are likely to underlie early functional neurobehavioral deficits like impaired reference and working memory and later occurring spatial and long-term memory. Insulin and C-peptide deficiencies and induction of inflammation have downstream effects on oxidative stress and apoptosis, compromising the survival of myelinating oligodendroglia in the white matter and gray matter neuronal populations such as those of hippocampus and frontal cortex. The resulting structural abnormalities inevitably lead to adverse effects on storage and retrieval of information and long-term memory. Under experimental conditions, the sequential abnormalities are largely prevented by full C-peptide replacement and in some instances reversed. In conclusion, therefore, information to date demonstrate highly significant effects of C-peptide replacement on type 1 diabetic encephalopathy, and other complications, suggesting that optimal treatment of type 1 diabetic patients should include replacement of both hormones.

References

1. Biessels GJ, Luchsinger JA, editors. Diabetes and the brain. New York: Humana Press; 2009.
2. Sima AAF. Encephalopathies: the emerging diabetic complications. Acta Diabetol. 2010;47:279–93.
3. Ott A, Stolk RP, van Harskamp F, et al. Diabetes mellitus and the risk of dementia: the Rotterdam study. Neurology. 1999;58:1937–41.
4. Arvanitakis Z, Wilson RS, Bienias JL, Evans DA, Bennett DA. Diabetes mellitus and risk of Alzheimer's

disease and decline in cognitive function. Arch Neurol. 2004;61:661–6.
5. Luchsinger JA, Tang MX, Stern Y, Shea S, Mayeux R. Diabetes mellitus and risk of Alzheimer's disease and dementia with stroke in a multiethnic cohort. Am J Epidemiol. 2001;154:635–41.
6. Erkinjuntti T, Ganthier S. The concept of vascular cognitive impairment. Front Neurol Neurosci. 2009;24:79–85.
7. Schoenle EJ, Schoenle D, Molinari L, Largo RH. Impaired intellectual development in children with type I diabetes: association with HbA(1c), age at diagnosis and sex. Diabetologia. 2002;45:108–14.
8. Ryan C, Vega A, Drash A. Cognitive deficits in adolescents who developed diabetes early in life. Pediatrics. 1985;75:921–7.
9. Northam EA, Anderson PJ, Jacobs R, et al. Neuropsychological profiles of children with type 1 diabetes 6 years after disease onset. Diabetes Care. 2001;24:1541–6.
10. Dahlquist G, Källén B. School performance in children with type 1 diabetes – a population-based register study. Diabetologia. 2007;50:957–64.
11. Northam EA, Rankins D, Lin A, et al. Central nervous system function in youth with type 1 diabetes 12 years after disease onset. Diabetes Care. 2009;32: 445–50.
12. Ho MS, Weller NJ, Ives FJ, et al. Prevalence of structural central nervous system abnormalities in early-onset type 1 diabetes mellitus. J Pediatr. 2008;153(3):385–90.
13. Musen G, Lyoo IK, Sparks CR, et al. Effects of type 1 diabetes on gray matter density as measured by voxel-based morphometry. Diabetes. 2006;55: 326–33.
14. Ryan CM. Why is cognitive dysfunction associated with the development of diabetes early in life? The diathesis hypothesis. Pediatr Diabetes. 2006;7:289–97.
15. McCarthy AM, Lindgren S, Mengeling MA, et al. Effects of diabetes on learning in children. Pediatrics. 2002;109:1–10.
16. Kramer L, Fasching P, Madl C, et al. Previous episodes of hypoglycemic coma are not associated with permanent cognitive brain dysfunction in IDDM patients on intensive insulin treatment. Diabetes. 1998;47:1909–14.
17. The Diabetes Control and Complications Trial/ Epidemiology of Diabetes Interventions and Complications (DCCT/EDIC) Study Research Group. Long-term effect of diabetes and its treatment on cognitive function. N Engl J Med. 2007; 356:1842–52.
18. Reichard P, Britz A, Rosenqvist U. Intensified conventional insulin treatment and neuropsychological impairment. BMJ. 1991;303:1439–42.
19. Reichard P, Phil M, Rosenqvist U, Sule J. Complications in IDDM are caused by elevated blood glucose level. The Stockholm Diabetes Intervention Study (SDIS) at 10 year follow-up. Diabetologia. 1996;39:1483–8.
20. Sima AAF, Zhang W, Muzik O, et al. Sequential abnormalities in type 1 diabetic encephalopathy and the effects of C-peptide. Rev Diabet Stud. 2009;6: 211–22.
21. Li Z-G, Zhang W, Sima AAF. The role of impaired insulin/IGF action in primary diabetic encephalopathy. Brain Res. 2005;1037:12–24.
22. Sima AAF, Li Z-G. The effect of C-peptide on cognitive dysfunction and hippocampal apoptosis in type 1 diabetes. Diabetes. 2005;54:1497–505.
23. Toth C, Schmidt AM, Tuor UI, et al. Diabetes, leukoencephalopathy and RAGE. Neurobiol Dis. 2006; 23:445–61.
24. Francis GJ, Martinez JA, Lin WQ, et al. Intranasal insulin prevents cognitive decline, cerebral atrophy and white matter changes in murine type 1 diabetic encephalopathy. Brain. 2008;131:3311–34.
25. Dobbing J, Sands J. Vulnerability of developing brain: IX The effect of nutritional growth retardation on the timing of brain growth spurt. Biol Neonate. 1971;19:363–78.
26. Sima AAF. Undernutrition and peripheral nerves. Kungälv, Sweden: Gotab Publ; 1974.
27. Winick M, Rosso T. The effect of severe early malnutrition on cellular growth of human brain. Pediatr Res. 1969;3:181–4.
28. Di Mario U, Morano S, Valle E, Pozzessere G. Electrophysiological alterations of the central nervous system in diabetes mellitus. Diabetes Metab Rev. 1995;11:259–78.
29. Pozzessere G, Rizzo PA, Valle E, et al. A longitudinal study of multimodal evoked potentials in diabetes mellitus. Diabetes Res. 1989;10:17–20.
30. Das T, Kundu S, Mazumdar AK, Mukhopadhyay SC. Studies on central nervous system function in diabetes mellitus. J Indian Med Assoc. 2001;99: 86–7.
31. Toth F, Varkonyi TT, Kiss JG, et al. Brainstem auditory-evoked potential examinations in diabetic patients. Scand Audiol Suppl. 2001;52:156–9.
32. Dejgaard A, Gade A, Larsson H, et al. Evidence for diabetic encephalopathy. Diabet Med. 1991;8: 795–801.
33. Collier A, Reid W, McInnes A, et al. Somatosensory and visual evoked potentials in insulin-dependent diabetics with mild peripheral neuropathy. Diabetes Res Clin Pract. 1988;5:171–5.
34. Pietravalle P, Morano S, Cristina G, et al. Early complications in type 1 diabetes: central nervous system alterations preceded kidney abnormalities. Diabetes Res Clin Pract. 1993;21:143–54.
35. Bax G, Lelli S, Grandis U, et al. Early involvement of central nervous system in type 1 diabetic patients. Diabetes Care. 1995;18:559–62.
36. Pozzessere G, Valle E, deCrignis S, et al. Abnormalities of cognitive function in IDDM revealed by P300 event related potential analysis. Comparison with short-latency evoked potentials and psychometric tests. Diabetes. 1991;40:952–8.
37. Pelich J, Howard L, Starr A. P300 latency correlates with digit span. Psychophysiology. 1983;20:665–9.

38. Ziegler O, Querci B, Algan M, et al. Improved visual evoked potential latencies in poorly controlled diabetic patients after short-term strict metabolic control. Diabetes Care. 1994;17:1141–7.
39. Reske-Nielsen E, Lundback K, Rafaelson OJ. Pathological changes in the central and peripheral nervous system of young long-term diabetics. Diabetologia. 1965;1:233–41.
40. Brands AMA, Biessels GJ, deHaan EHF, Kappelle LJ, Kessels RPC. The effects of type 1 diabetes on cognitive performance: a meta-analysis. Diabetes Care. 2005;28:726–35.
41. Park CR. Cognitive effects of insulin in the central nervous system. Neurosci Biobehav Res. 2001;25: 311–23.
42. Rovet J, Alvarez M. Attentional functioning in children and adolescents with IDDM. Diabetes Care. 1997;20:803–10.
43. Ryan CM. Cognition in children and adolescents with type 1 diabetes. In: Biessel GJ, Luchsinger JA, editors. Diabetes and the brain. New York: Humana Press; 2009. p. 251–75.
44. Ferguson SC, Blane A, Perros P, et al. Cognitive ability and brain structure in type 1 diabetes: relation to microangiopathy and preceding severe hypoglycemia. Diabetes. 2003;52:149–56.
45. Fox MA, Chen RS, Holmes CS. Gender differences in memory and learning in children with insulin-dependent diabetes mellitus (IDDM) over a 4-year follow-up interval. J Pediatr Psychol. 2003;28: 569–78.
46. Stiles MC, Seaquist ER. Cerebral structural and functional changes in type 1 diabetes. Minerva Med. 2010;101:105–14.
47. Hoffman WH, Artlett CM, Zhang W, et al. Receptor for advanced glycation end products and neuronal deficit in the fatal brain edema of diabetic ketoacidosis. Brain Res. 2008;1238:154–62.
48. Hoffman WH, Andjelkovic AV, Zhang W, Passmore GG, Sima AAF. Insulin and IGF-1 receptors, nitrotyrosin and cerebral neuronal deficits in two young patients with ketoacidosis and fatal brain edema. Brain Res. 2010;1343:168–77.
49. Sarac K, Akinci A, Alkan A, et al. Brain metabolites on proton magnetic spectroscopy in children with poorly controlled type 1 diabetes mellitus. Neuroradiology. 2005;47:562–5.
50. van Duinkerken E, Klein M, Schoonenboom NS, et al. Functional brain connectivity and neurocognitive functioning in patients with long-standing type 1 diabetes with and without microvascular complications: a magnetoencephalography study. Diabetes. 2009;58:2335–43.
51. Wessels AM, Simsek S, Remijnse PL, et al. Voxel-based morphometry demonstrates reduced grey matter density on brain MRI in patients with diabetic retinopathy. Diabetologia. 2006;49:2474–80.
52. Yau PI, Javier DC, Ryan CM, et al. Preliminary evidence for brain complications in obese adolescents with type 2 diabetes mellitus. Diabetologia. 2010;53:2298–306.
53. Ehehalt S, Blumenstock G, Willasch AM, DIARY-study Group Baden-Württemberg, et al. Continuous rise in incidence of childhood type 1 diabetes in Germany. Diabet Med. 2008;25:755–7.
54. Harjutsalo V, Sjöberg L, Tuomilehto J. Time trends in the incidence of type 1 diabetes in Finnish children: a cohort study. Lancet. 2008;371:1777–82.
55. Kumar P, Krishna P, Reddy SC, et al. Incidence of type 1 diabetes mellitus and associated complications among children and young adults: results from Karnataka Diabetes Registry 1995–2008. J Indian Med Assoc. 2008;106:708–11.
56. Bener A, Alsaied A, Al-Ali M, et al. Impact of lifestyle and dietary habits on hypovitaminosis D in type 1 diabetes mellitus and healthy children in Qatar, a sun-rich country. Ann Nutr Metab. 2008; 53:215–22.
57. Wilkins TJ. The accelerator hypothesis: weight gain as the missing link between type I and type II diabetes. Diabetologia. 2001;44:914–22.
58. Dabelea D. The accelerating epidemic of childhood diabetes. Lancet. 2009;372:1999–2000.
59. Chan JC, Malik V, Jia W, et al. Diabetes in Asia: epidemiology, risk factors, and pathophysiology. JAMA. 2009;301:2129–40.
60. Jakobsen J, Sidenius P, Gundersen HJ, Østerby R. Quantitative changes of cerebral neocortical structure in insulin treated long-term streptozotocin-induced diabetes in rats. Diabetes. 1987;36:597–601.
61. Biessels GJ, Kamal A, Ramakers GM, et al. Place learning and hippocampal synaptic plasticity in streptozotocin-induced diabetic rats. Diabetes. 1996;45:1259–66.
62. Biessels GJ, Kamal A, Urban IJ, et al. Water maze learning and hippocampal synaptic plasticity in streptozotocin-diabetic rats: effect of insulin treatment. Brain Res. 1998;800:125–35.
63. Kamal A, Biessels GJ, Gispen WH, Ramakers GM. Synaptic transmission changes in the pyramidal cells of the hippocampus in streptozotocin-induced diabetes mellitus in rats. Brain Res. 2006;1073:276–80.
64. Sima AAF, Kamiya H, Li Z-G. Insulin, C-peptide hyperglycemia and central nervous system complications in diabetes. Eur J Pharmacol. 2004;490: 187–97.
65. Hoyer S. Glucose metabolism and insulin receptor signal transduction in Alzheimer disease. Eur J Pharmacol. 2004;2004(490):115–25.
66. Porte Jr D, Baskin DG, Schwarz NW. Insulin signaling in the central nervous system. Diabetes. 2005;54: 1264–76.
67. Kamiya H, Zhang W, Sima AAF. Dynamic changes of neuroskeletal proteins underlie impaired axonal maturation and progressive degeneration in type 1 diabetes. Exp Diabesity Res. 2009;2009:793281.
68. Sima AAF, Zhang W, Kreipke CW, Rafols JA, Hoffman WH. Inflammation in diabetic encephalopathy is prevented by C-peptide. Rev Diabet Stud. 2009;6:37–42.
69. Li Z-G, Zhang W, Sima AAF. C-peptide enhances insulin-mediated cell growth and protection against

high glucose induced apoptosis in SH-SY5Y cells. Diabetes Metab Res Rev. 2003;19:375–85.
70. Sima AAF, Li Z-G, Zhang W. The IGF system and neurological complications in diabetes. Exp Diabesity Res. 2003;4:235–56.
71. Grunberger G, Qiang X, Li ZG, et al. Molecular basis for the insulinomimetic effects of C-peptide. Diabetologia. 2001;44:1247–57.
72. Jörnvall H, Lindahl E, Astorga-Wells J, et al. Oligomerization and insulin interactions of proinsulin C-peptide: three-fold relationships to properties of insulin. Biochem Biophys Res Commun. 2010; 391:1561–6.
73. Shafqat J, Melles E, Sigmundsson K, et al. Proinsulin C-peptide elicits disaggregation of insulin resulting in enhanced physiological insulin effects. Cell Mol Life Sci. 2006;63:1805–11.
74. Meyer JA, Subasinghe W, Sima AAF, et al. Hyperglycemia-induced phosphatidylserine translocation is associated with zink-activated C-peptide resistance in type 2 diabetic erythrocytes. Mol Biol Syst. 2009;5:1157–62.
75. Li Z-G, Qiang X, Sima AAF, Grunberger G. C-peptide attenuates protein tyrosine phosphatase activity and enhances glycogen synthesis in L6 myoblasts. Biochem Biophys Res Commun. 2001; 26:615–9.
76. Jägerbrink T, Lindahl E, Shafqat J, Jörnvall H. Proinsulin C-peptide interaction with protein tyrosine phosphatase 1B demonstrated with a labeling reaction. Biochem Biophys Res Commun. 2009;387:31–5.
77. Rigler R, Pramanik A, Jonasson P, et al. Specific binding of proinsulin C-peptide to human cell membranes. Proc Natl Acad Sci USA. 1999;96: 13318–23.
78. Lindahl E, Nyman U, Melles E, et al. Cellular internalization of proinsulin C-peptide. Cell Mol Life Sci. 2007;64:479–86.
79. Hills CE, Brunskill NJ. Cellular and physiological effects of C-peptide. Clin Sci (Lond). 2009;116: 565–74.
80. Ido Y, Vindigni A, Chang K, et al. Prevention of vascular and neural dysfunction in diabetic rats by C-peptide. Science. 1997;277:563–6.
81. Luppi P, Geng X, Cifarelli V, et al. C-peptide is internalized in human endothelial and vascular smooth muscle cells via early endosomes. Diabetologia. 2009;52:2218–28.
82. Lindahl E, Nyman U, Zanian F, et al. Proinsulin C-peptide regulates ribosomal RNA expression. J Biol Chem. 2010;286:3462–9.
83. Pierson CR, Zhang W, Murakawa Y, Sima AAF. Insulin deficiency rather than hyperglycemia account for impaired neurotrophic responses and nerve fiber regeneration in type 1 diabetic neuropathy. J Neuropathol Exp Neurol. 2003;62:260–71.
84. Sima AAF. Pathological mechanisms involved in diabetic neuropathy. Can we slow the process? Curr Opin Invest Drugs. 2006;7:324–37.
85. Kamiya H, Zhang W, Sima AAF. The beneficial effects of C-peptide on diabetic polyneuropathy. Rev Diabet Stud. 2009;6:187–202.
86. Haidet J, Cifarelli V, Trucco M, Luppi P. Anti-inflammatory properties of C-peptide. Rev Diabet Stud. 2009;6:168–79.
87. Yerneni KK, Bai W, Khan BV, et al. Hyperglycemia-induced activation of nuclear transcription factor kappaB in vascular smooth muscle cells. Diabetes. 1999;48:855–64.
88. Grunberger G, Sima AAF. The C-peptide signaling. Exp Diabesity Res. 2004;5:25–36.
89. Hayden MS, Shosh S. Signaling to NF-kappa B. Genes Dev. 2004;18:2195–224.
90. Ramasamy R, Vanucci SJ, Yau SD, et al. Advanced glycation end products and RAGE: a common thread in aging, diabetes, neurodegeneration and inflammation. Glycobiology. 2004;15:16R–28.
91. Kamiya H, Zhang W, Ekberg K, Wahren J, Sima AAF. C-peptide reverses nociceptive neuropathy in type 1 diabetic BB/Wor-rat. Diabetes. 2006;55:3581–7.
92. Sima AAF, Kamiya H. Is C-peptide replacement the missing link for successful treatment of neurological complications in type 1 diabetes? Curr Drug Targets. 2008;9:37–46.
93. Crusio WE, Schwegler H. Learning spatial orientation tasks in the radial-maze and structural variation in the hippocampus of inbred mice. Behav Brain Funct. 2005;1:3.
94. Morris R. Development of a water maze procedure for studying spatial learning in the rat. J Neurosci. 1984;11:47–60.
95. Balakrishnan S, Mathew J, Paulose CS. Cholinergic and glutamergic receptor functional regulation in long-term, low dose somatotropine and insulin treatment to aging rats: rejuvenation of brain function. Mol Cell Endocrinol. 2010;314:23–30.
96. Corner JM, Franks KM, Titterness AK, et al. NGF is essential for hippocampal plasticity and learning. J Neurosci. 2009;35:10883–9.
97. Moon E, Her Y, Lee JB, et al. The multi-herbal medicine Gongjin-dau enhances memory and learning tasks via NGF regulation. Neurosci Lett. 2009; 466(3):114–9.
98. Seto D, Zhang WH, McNicoll A, et al. Insulin-like growth factor I inhibits endogenous acetylcholin release from rat hippocampal formation: possible involvement of GABA in mediating the effects. Neuroscience. 2002;115:603–12.
99. Kar S, Seto D, Doré S, Hanisch U, Quirion R. Insulin-like growth factors-1 and -II differentially regulate endogenous acetylcholine release from the rat hippocampal formation. Proc Natl Acad Sci USA. 1997;94:14054–9.
100. Madara JC, Levine ES. Presynaptic and postsynaptic NMDA receptors mediate distinct effects of brain-derived neurotrophic factor on synaptic transmission. J Neurophysiol. 2008;100:3175–84.
101. Medvedev NI, Rodriquez-Arellano JJ, Popov VI, et al. The glutamate receptor 2 subunits controls

post-synaptic density complexity and spine shape in the dentate gyrus. Eur J Neurosci. 2008;27:315–25.
102. Tanaka H, Grooms SY, Bennett MV, Zukin RS. The AMPAR subunit GLUR2: still front and center stage. Brain Res. 2000;886:190–207.
103. Isaac JT, Asky M, McBain CJ. The role of the GluR2 subunit in AMPA receptor function and synaptic plasticity. Neuron. 2007;54:859–71.
104. Heikkilä O, Lundbom N, Timonen M, et al. Hyperglycemia is associated with changes in the regional concentrations of glucose and myo-inositol within the brain. Diabetologia. 2009;52:534–40.
105. Mukherjee TK, Mukhopadhyay S, Hoidal JR. The role of reactive oxygen species in TNF-alpha-dependent expression of the receptor for advanced glycation end products in human umbilical vein endothelial cells. Biochim Biophys Acta. 2005;1744:213–23.
106. Sima AAF, Li Z-G. Diabetes and Alzheimer's disease – is there a connection? Rev Diabet Stud. 2007;4:161–8.
107. Li Z-G, Zhang W, Sima AAF. Alzheimer-like changes in rat models of spontaneous diabetes. Diabetes. 2007;56:1817–24.
108. Tezapsidis N, Johnston JM, Smith MA, et al. Leptin: a novel therapeutic strategy for Alzheimer's disease. J Alzheimers Dis. 2009;16:731–40.
109. Burns JM, Donnelly JE, Anderson HS, et al. Peripheral insulin and brain structure in early Alzheimer's disease. Neurology. 2007;69:1094–104.
110. Jolivalt CG, Lee CA, Beiswenger KK, et al. Defective insulin signaling pathway and increased glycogen synthase kinase-3 activity in the brain of diabetic mice: parallels with Alzheimer's disease and correction by insulin. J Neurosci Res. 2008;86:3265–74.
111. Jolivalt CG, Hurford R, Lee CA, et al. Type 1 diabetes exaggerates features of Alzheimer's disease in APP transgenic mice. Exp Neurol. 2010;223:422–31.
112. Cordy JM, Hooper NM, Turner AJ. The involvement of lipid rafts in Alzheimer's disease. Mol Membr Biol. 2006;23:111–22.
113. Sima AAF, Zhang W. Caveolin 1 plays a central role in amyloidogenesis in type 2 diabetes (abstract). In: XXth Neurodiab. Stockholm: EASD; 2010.
114. Parton RG, Simons K. The multiple faces of caveolae. Nat Rev Mol Biol. 2007;8:185–94.
115. Chen J, Copozza F, Wu A, et al. Regulation of insulin receptor substrate-1 expression levels by caveolin-1. J Cell Physiol. 2008;217:281–9.
116. Uetsuki T, Takemoto K, Nishimura I, et al. Activation of neuronal caspase-3 by intracellular accumulation of wild-type Alzheimer amyloid precursor protein. J Neurosci. 1999;19:6955–64.
117. Kim B, Backus C, Oh S, Hayes JM, Feldman EL. Increased tau phosphorylation and cleavage in mouse models of type 1 and type 2 diabetes. Endocrinology. 2009;150:5294–301.

C-Peptide: A New Molecule with Anti-Inflammatory Properties

10

Jaime Haidet, Vincenza Cifarelli, Xuehui Geng, Massimo Trucco, and Patrizia Luppi

Keywords
C-peptide • Type 1 diabetes • Inflammation • Vascular disease

Introduction

C-peptide, once thought to be a biologically inactive molecule, has emerged as a new molecule with proven anti-inflammatory effects. C-peptide is a 31 amino acid peptide secreted in equimolar amounts with insulin from the pancreatic beta-cells. In healthy individuals, C-peptide circulates in nanomolar concentrations; however, in patients with Type 1 diabetes (T1D), C-peptide is decreased or absent. In type 1 diabetics, a group at increased risk of developing micro- and macrovascular complications, C-peptide replacement has ameliorated some of these complications as discussed in other chapters. As inflammatory mechanisms play a central role in vascular disease, strategies targeting inflammation are crucial to minimize the morbidity and mortality associated with T1D.

In this chapter, the anti-inflammatory properties of C-peptide on the vasculature and on other models of inflammation will be discussed. In addition, we will discuss C-peptide's binding to cellular membranes and internalization as well as intracellular signaling pathways affected by C-peptide in inflammatory responses.

C-Peptide and Vascular Dysfunction in Type 1 Diabetes

Inflammation and Endothelial Dysfunction in Type 1 Diabetes

T1D is a chronic disease defined by disruption of glucose homeostasis and by concurrent metabolic abnormalities as the result of insulin deficiency secondary to progressive autoimmune destruction of the insulin-producing pancreatic beta-cells [1]. In T1D, beta cell damage begins well before the development of impaired glucose tolerance (IGT) and clinical presentation and precedes declining insulin and C-peptide production [1]. At some point in the destruction of beta-cells and progression of T1D, insulin secretion is not sufficient to uphold metabolic stability due to the abnormalities of the dynamics of insulin release in response to

J. Haidet (✉)
Division of Endocrinology and Diabetes, Department of Pediatrics, Akron Children's Hospital, One Perkins Square, Akron, OH 44308, USA
e-mail: jhaidet@chmca.org

V. Cifarelli • X. Geng • M. Trucco • P. Luppi
Division of Immunogenetics, Department of Pediatrics, Children's Hospital of Pittsburgh of UPMC, Rangos Research Center, Pittsburgh, PA 15224, USA

A.A.F. Sima (ed.), *Diabetes & C-Peptide: Scientific and Clinical Aspects*, Contemporary Diabetes, DOI 10.1007/978-1-61779-391-2_10,

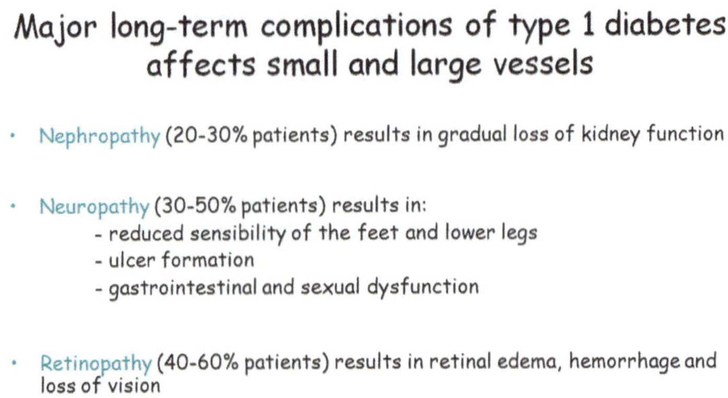

Fig. 10.1 Major long-term complications of type 1 diabetes (T1D) affects small and large vessels

stimulation and clinical signs and symptoms of diabetes such as polydipsia, polyuria, and weight loss arise.

Although T cells are identified as playing a central role in the autoimmune destruction of the insulin-producing beta-cells [2], recent studies indicate that components of the innate immune system (natural killer cells, monocytes, and inflammatory mediators) have a much larger role in the pathogenesis of T1D and associated vascular complications than previously recognized [3–6]. The principal role of monocytes in the early stages of T1D pathogenesis [7] has been demonstrated by showing that monocytes are the first to accumulate in the pancreatic islets of prediabetic BB rats [8]. Ensuing T and B lymphocyte infiltration is dependent upon prior monocyte invasion of the islets [8], suggesting monocytes and secreted inflammatory mediators may contribute to the early induction and augmentation of the autoimmune assault against the pancreatic beta-cells [9]. In the peripheral circulation of T1D patients, a more generalized inflammatory response with activation of monocytes and existence of oxidative stress has been found and is illustrated by the elevation of plasma levels of several inflammatory biomarkers, such as interleukin (IL)-1β, IL-6, IL-8, tumor necrosis factor (TNF)-α, and C-reactive protein. Not only have such inflammatory reactions been detected in children recently diagnosed with T1D, but also in adult T1D patients well after the onset of diabetes [10–15]. These inflammatory reactions have also been recognized in children with T1D during and shortly after hyperglycemia [16]. These findings indicate that a generalized inflammatory response is already present in the very early stages of diabetes [17, 18]. Furthermore, T1D patients with microvascular complications exhibit increased production of these inflammatory biomarkers over and above the levels detected in T1D patients without microvascular complications and healthy control subjects [13, 19–21]. A number of the inflammatory changes in T1D are detected at the level of monocytes. For example, up-regulation of the adhesion molecule CD11b (Mac-1) has been demonstrated [18] in addition to aberrant constitutive and lipopolysaccharide (LPS)-stimulated expression of cyclooxygenase (COX)-2, a defect which may predispose to a chronic inflammatory response in T1D [6, 22].

The vascular endothelium represents a likely target of this inflammatory response detected in patients with T1D. The inflammatory response induces endothelial cell activation, alters endothelial function, and monocyte adherence eventually leading to apparent vascular damage in the later stages of T1D. T1D is a well-established risk factor for vascular disease [23] (Fig. 10.1). During the course of diabetes, most T1D patients eventually develop one or several histopathological lesions affecting the vasculature of both small and large blood vessels, leading to micro- and macrovascular complications, respectively [23]. Microvascular complications, such as those affecting the small vessels of the eye, kidney, and retina, are associated and causative of the development of end-stage organ complications in T1D,

Fig. 10.2 Three components of vascular dysfunction in diabetes

Three components of vascular dysfunction in diabetes

- **Endothelial cell component:**
  - increased production of reactive oxygen species (ROS)
  - upregulation of cell adhesion molecules (e.g.,VCAM-1)
  - secretion of inflammatory cytokines (e.g., IL-8 and MCP-1)
- **Smooth muscle cell component:**
  - proliferation and migration of cells from the media to the intima of the vessel where the developing lesions are localized
- **Monocyte cell component**
  - accumulation of monocytes at sites of developing lesions

which contributes significantly to the morbidity associated with the disease [24] (Fig. 10.1). In addition, cardiovascular disease is a major cause of both morbidity and mortality in T1D; more specifically, by the age of 55, 35% of T1D patients die of coronary artery disease in comparison to 8 and 4% of nondiabetic men and women, respectively [23] and over 70% die of atherosclerosis-related disease [23] (Fig. 10.1). Since inflammation is critical in the development of T1D-associated vascular dysfunction [13, 19–21], it is important to understand the origin of the inflammatory response characterizing T1D. It is difficult to determine to what extent the inflammatory state is a primary pathogenic event and to what extent it is the response to a metabolic derangement such as hyperglycemia [25]. Regardless, therapeutic strategies to decrease inflammatory activity in T1D may improve endothelial function in this high-risk group.

Though the mechanisms of vascular disease in T1D are not definitively defined, it has been proposed that the diabetic milieu induces changes in the arterial wall that render the vessel more susceptible to premature vascular compromise [26]. One of these changes is represented by endothelial dysfunction, an early event in the pathogenesis of vascular complications in T1D, which is characterized by impaired flow-mediated vasodilation [27], a low-grade inflammation [28], and increased levels of endothelial cell adhesion molecules, including E-selectin, intercellular adhesion molecule-1 (ICAM-1), and vascular cell adhesion molecule-1 (VCAM-1) [19, 28–31] (Fig. 10.2). The up-regulation of adhesion molecules on endothelial cells allows attachment and migration of circulating monocytes into the vessel wall. Monocytes, which are pivotal cells in inflammatory responses as they serve as the principal reservoir of proinflammatory cytokines and are the first cells to be engaged in nonspecific immune responses (such as those triggered by environmental factors like hyperglycemia), play an integral role in the vascular compromise leading to atherosclerotic plaque formation. Following the expression of endothelial cell adhesion molecules at the cell surface, these molecules are shed as soluble forms and can be detected in the peripheral circulation. Thus, circulating endothelial cell adhesion molecule levels are considered biochemical markers of vascular dysfunction in high-risk individuals, i.e., T1D patients [19, 32–34]. In T1D patients, signs of endothelial dysfunction, with increased plasma concentrations of endothelial cell adhesion molecules, have been found shortly after clinical diagnosis of the disease, suggesting the presence of vascular compromise at an early stage of diabetes, when subjects are still free of any overt vascular symptoms [31, 35, 36]. Other studies also found signs of endothelial dysfunction in schoolchildren who tested positive for one or more diabetes-associated autoantibodies but who were not yet diabetic [31, 37–40]. As development of vascular damage is a consequence of endothelial dysfunction, this underscores the importance of early recognition and treatment of at-risk subjects in preventing the development of overt vascular complications.

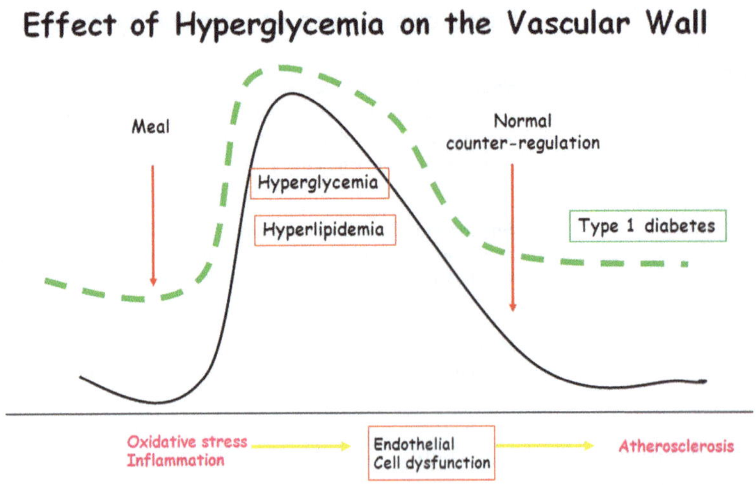

Fig. 10.3 Effect of hyperglycemia on the vascular wall. In T1D, high glucose is one proposed mechanism for the increased production of reactive oxygen species (ROS) in endothelial cells. Postprandial elevation of glucose may exert both short-term and long-term damaging effects on the vasculature. The hyperglycemic wave triggers inflammatory events in endothelial cells contributing to oxidative stress generation, cellular activation, and dysfunction. In a healthy subject, tight control of the postprandial hyperglycemic spikes minimizes the damaging effect of high glucose on the vascular endothelium by promptly reducing blood glucose levels to baseline, a situation that is not always achieved in diabetic patients

Oxidative stress is yet another component of inflammation and endothelial dysfunction. Accentuated oxidative stress is observed in TID patients with microvascular complications compared to T1D patients without microvascular complications as demonstrated by significantly elevated levels of nitrotyrosine, monocyte superoxide anion [13], DNA, and protein oxidation [41, 42]. In T1D, high glucose is one proposed mechanism for this increased production of reactive oxygen species (ROS) [43] (Fig. 10.3) as hyperglycemia-induced tissue damage occurs in susceptible cell types that are unable to reduce the transport of glucose inside the cell to maintain a constant internal glucose concentration in the face of hyperglycemia [44]. Postprandial elevation of glucose may exert both short-term and long-term damaging effects on the vasculature (Fig. 10.3). The hyperglycemic wave triggers inflammatory events in endothelial cells contributing to oxidative stress generation, cellular activation, and dysfunction. In a healthy subject, tight control of the postprandial hyperglycemic spikes minimizes the damaging effect of high glucose on the vascular endothelium by promptly reducing blood glucose levels to baseline, a situation that is not always achieved in diabetic patients. Endothelial cells suffer the damaging effects of ROS directly through cellular injury and indirectly through inactivation of nitric oxide or by serving as an endothelium-derived contracting factor [45, 46]. Increased ROS production leads to activation of the nuclear-factor (NF)-κB pathway at the molecular level [47, 48] and eventually to the production of inflammatory mediators [49]. Compared to diabetic patients without microvascular complications, T1D patients with microvascular complications have increased activation of the NF-κB pathway [13]. Because of the critical role the NF-κB pathway plays in inflammation, strategies targeting activation of this pathway are emerging in order to reduce inflammatory activity and prevent vascular dysfunction [50, 51].

A number of factors have been implicated in T1D-associated vascular disease. Since vascular disease is a major cause of morbidity and mortality associated with T1D, therapies targeting the causative factors are crucial to improving the quality and duration of life in this devastating disease. Next, we discuss the role of C-peptide in ameliorating inflammation and vascular dysfunction in the context of T1D.

C-Peptide and Endothelial Function

C-peptide, historically considered a biologically inactive peptide, has been shown to exert insulin-independent biological effects on a number of cells proving itself as a bioactive peptide with anti-inflammatory properties. The past decade has revealed the potential beneficial effects of C-peptide on dysfunctional endothelium as observed in several in vivo and in vitro models of inflammation-mediated vascular injury. In T1D, autoimmune attack on the pancreatic beta-cells eventually leads to C-peptide deficiency which has been considered an important factor in the development of vascular dysfunction. In support of this, higher fasting C-peptide levels in a clinic-based cohort of patients with T1D were found to have a protective effect on microvascular complications [52]. Furthermore, results from clinical trials of C-peptide replacement therapy to T1D patients with microvascular complications have revealed significant improvement in the signs and symptoms of peripheral neuropathy and kidney function [53, 54]. The mechanism(s) by which C-peptide employs its cytoprotective effects on the endothelium are not entirely understood; however, it has been reported that C-peptide can alter activation of different signaling pathways that subsequently modulate or shut down inflammatory responses. In the upcoming sections, the anti-inflammatory properties of C-peptide at the level of the vascular endothelium and vascular smooth muscle cells (VSMC) will be reviewed.

C-Peptide Effects on Endothelial Cells

The arterial endothelial cell layer is essential to maintaining vascular integrity, as one of the key events in the early stages of atherogenesis is adhesion and migration of circulating monocytes into the subendothelial space [55]. During physiologic conditions, the endothelial cell layer serves many functions. It acts as a barrier separating circulating factors and cells from the intima and media of the artery, it inhibits prolonged interaction with leukocytes, it serves as an anticoagulant and fibrinolytic surface, and it produces nitric oxide which is a vasodilator, inhibits VSMC migration and proliferation, and decreases leukocyte-endothelium interaction [55–57]. A number of circulating factors, such as hyperglycemia, may alter or damage the endothelial cells leading to their dysfunction [56]. Inflammatory stimuli and exposure to high glucose elicit up-regulation of cell adhesion molecules on endothelial cells [58–62] in addition to the release of chemotactic factors such as IL-8 and monocyte chemoattractant factor (MCP)-1 [61, 62]. IL-8 and MCP-1 are mediators which play a crucial role in leukocyte-endothelium interactions [63]. Selectins (L-selectin; or P-selectin; CD62L or CD62P) on the endothelium and carbohydrate moieties on the leukocytes are critical early in this process. Up-regulation of ICAM-1 (CD54) and VCAM-1 (CD106) on endothelial cells and activation of their specific counter-receptors on the leukocytes allows for tight binding of the leukocytes to the endothelium.

Evidence supports the concept that C-peptide may have atheroprotective properties (Fig. 10.4). C-peptide affects interactions of circulating monocytes and other leukocytes to endothelial cells by reducing the up-regulation of critical endothelial cell adhesion molecules typically observed under inflammatory conditions and exposure to high glucose. This was first demonstrated in rat mesenteric venules [64]. The inflammatory agents thrombin or N^G-nitro-l-l-arginine methyl ester (L-NAME), which cause acute endothelial dysfunction, were superfused into rat mesentery where they resulted in increased numbers of rolling, adhering, and transmigrating leukocytes. Pretreatment with C-peptide attenuated expression of the endothelial cell adhesion molecule ICAM-1 and P-selectin on the mesenteric microvascular endothelium, significantly reducing the leukocyte-endothelium interactions.

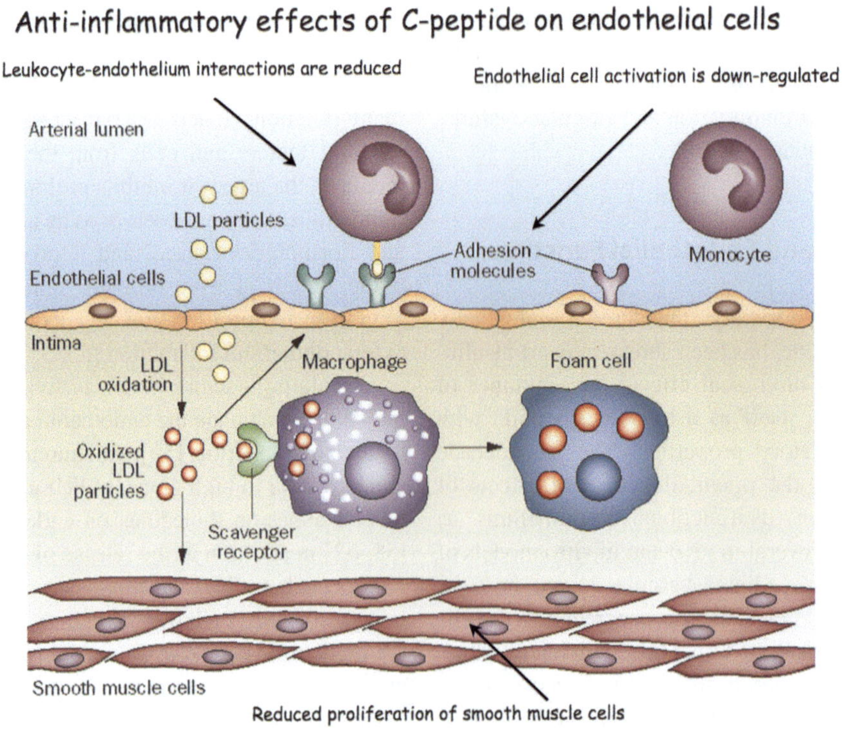

Fig. 10.4 Anti-inflammatory activity of C-peptide on endothelial cells. Exposure of endothelial cells to high glucose causes inflammatory changes culminating in the up-regulation of cell adhesion molecules (i.e., VCAM-1) and secretion of proinflammatory cytokines (i.e., IL-8 and MCP-1). As a consequence, monocytes and other circulating leukocytes adhere to the activated endothelial cells by interacting with the upregulated adhesion molecules. Subsequently, leukocytes migrate to the subendothelial space, phagocyte oxidize-LDL and become foam cells. Smooth muscle cells proliferate and migrate from the media to the intima of the vessel wall where the new atherosclerotic plaque is developing. C-peptide has been demonstrated to act as an anti-inflammatory molecule by reducing expression of endothelial cell adhesion molecules, leukocyte-endothelium interactions, and proliferation of smooth muscle cells. Adapted by permission from Macmillan Publishers Ltd. [110]

These findings have been recently confirmed in vitro in a model of high glucose-induced endothelial dysfunction [65]. In this model, adhesion of the monocytic cell line U-937 to high glucose-stimulated aortic endothelial cells (HAEC) decreased by 50% after addition of physiologic concentrations of C-peptide, an effect not detected when C-peptide was heat-inactivated [65] (Fig. 10.5). Decreased expression of the adhesion molecule VCAM-1 on HAEC by C-peptide, an effect demonstrated both at the level of mRNA and protein, was likely responsible. In addition, C-peptide was demonstrated to reduce high glucose-induced secretion of IL-8 and MCP-1 by HAEC to basal levels measured under normal glucose concentrations [65]. IL-8 and MCP-1 are two chemokines essential to bolstering leukocyte adhesion to endothelial cells. In contrast, under normal glucose conditions, C-peptide did not seem to have any apparent effect on endothelial cells, thus suggesting that the most meaningful biological effects of C-peptide on the endothelium materialize in conditions of vascular insult or damage.

In addition to decreasing leukocyte-endothelial cell interaction, recent data suggest C-peptide may also play a role in endothelial cell proliferation. The autologous saphenous vein is routinely used for revascularization procedures undertaken secondary to coronary artery disease; however, postbypass graft occlusions are common because of intimal hyperplasia [66]. An investigation into

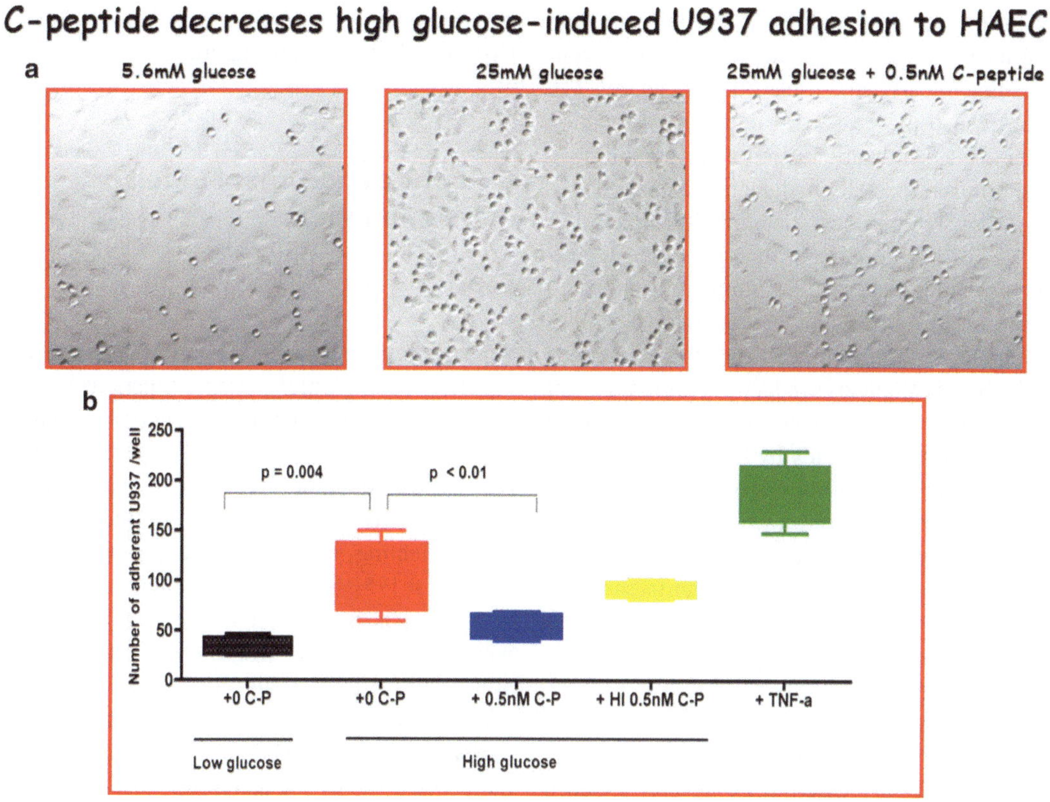

Fig. 10.5 C-peptide decreases high glucose-induced U937 adhesion to HAEC. HAEC were cultured in 25 mmol/L glucose in the presence or absence of physiologic C-peptide (C-P) for 4 h. U937 cells were added for 1 h and adherent cells counted under a microscope. In (**a**) photographic view of U937 monocytes adherent to HAEC under the different conditions; in (**b**) boxplot graphs showing the median values (limits are the 5th and 95th percentiles) of number of adherent U937 monocytes per well. High glucose increased the number of adherent U937 ($p = 0.0004$ vs. 5.6 mmol/L glucose). Addition of C-peptide reduced the number of adherent U937 monocytes ($p < 0.01$ vs. 25 mmol/L glucose alone). Heat-inactivated (HI) C-peptide did not significantly inhibit adherence of U-937. TNF-α (10 ng/mL) produced more than a fivefold increase in adherent U937 cells in comparison to high glucose and was used as positive control. Adapted with kind permission from Springer Science+Business Media [65]

insulin and C-peptide's roles in modulation of human saphenous vein neointima formation revealed that C-peptide increased endothelial cell number by about 40%, thus indicating C-peptide may promote reendothelialization and thus limit neointimal development [66].

C-Peptide Effects on Smooth Muscle Cells

VSMC are yet another cell type that play a critical role in vascular disease and atherosclerotic plaque formation. VSMC become directly intermixed in areas of inflammation when growth factors (such as platelet-derived growth factor [PDGF]) and inflammatory stimuli provoke VSMC to migrate and proliferate [67]. VSMC are crucial to the formation of an intermediate lesion; and with continued inflammation and remodeling, the formation of advanced, complicated lesions of macroangiopathy [67]. Increased proliferation, increased migration into the intima, altered matrix components, increased matrix degradation, and increased nonenzymatic collagen glycation of VSMC have all been implicated in diabetic macrovascular disease [68]. In high glucose circumstances, human, porcine, and rat VSMC have all been shown to proliferate and migrate from the media to the subendothelial space thus contributing to early atherosclerotic lesions [69–71]. VSMC also play a part in neointima formation after revascularization commonly leading to occlusions, especially in diabetic patients [66].

There are conflicting data on C-peptide's role in VSMC proliferation with some data suggesting a proatherogenic effect, while other data suggest an anti-atherogenic effect. In two studies imitating hyperglycemia in diabetes, C-peptide reduced high glucose-induced proliferation of VSMC thus suggesting an anti-atherogenic effect [72, 73]. In the first study by Kobayashi et al., rat aortic smooth muscle cells (AoSMCs) cultured in high-glucose conditions with 1–100 nmol/L of C-peptide showed a dose-dependent reduction in proliferation which was mediated through inhibited phosphorylation of p42/p44 MAP kinases and inhibited PDGF-β receptor expression [73]. In the second study by Cifarelli et al. using human umbilical artery smooth muscle cells (UASMC) and human AoSMCs, physiologic concentrations of C-peptide decreased high glucose-induced proliferation by reducing phosphorylation of IκBα [72]. In contrast to the aforementioned studies, a study by Walcher et al. revealed human and rat AoSMC proliferation upon stimulation with the respective C-peptide in a dose-dependent manner with a maximal induction at 10 nmol/L human C-peptide or 0.5 nmol/L rat C-peptide thus suggesting a proatherogenic effect [74] (Chap. 14). A very recent study investigating neointima formation in organ-cultured human saphenous veins revealed increased neointima formation in the presence of insulin, an effect ameliorated by C-peptide related to reduced insulin-induced *SREBF1* expression [66]. This same effect was not seen in internal mammary artery smooth muscle cells. This prompted further investigation using human AoSMCs, where the same authors found that C-peptide was proproliferative when cultured with human AoSMCs. Though the data are conflicting, these findings underscore a role of C-peptide in VSMC function. Source of smooth muscle cells, C-peptide concentration, and glucose concentration all need to be considered and further studies need to be pursued in order to delineate the exact role of C-peptide in VSMC proliferation.

C-Peptide and Other Models of Inflammation

Sepsis

Sepsis is defined as infection plus systemic manifestations of infection, severe sepsis as sepsis plus sepsis-induced organ dysfunction or tissue hypoperfusion, and septic shock as severe sepsis plus hypotension not reversed with fluid resuscitation [75]. These are common healthcare problems affecting millions of people worldwide every year [75]. Septic shock is highly lethal and severe sepsis is a frequently fatal condition as well, killing 30–70% with as many deaths annually as those from acute myocardial infarction (MI) [76, 77]. Overall, sepsis accounts for 9.3% of deaths in the United States annually [77]. The incidence is increasing and is especially common in the elderly, thus it is likely to increase further as the population ages [75, 76]. In addition, survivors of sepsis consistently demonstrate impaired quality of life and have ongoing mortality beyond short-term endpoints [78].

Systemic inflammation, with increased circulatory levels of inflammatory cytokines, is a component of severe sepsis and of other critical illnesses which is usually necessary for recovery [79]. In addition to the beneficial effects of proinflammatory cytokines, their excessive production may also become more dangerous than the initial infection or trauma by causing capillary leakage, tissue injury, and lethal multiple organ failure [77]. To date, the conventional therapies, combined with circulatory and respiratory support, are not always adequate to reverse the systemic inflammation [80, 81]; and despite advances in medicine, sepsis continues to carry a high morbidity and mortality rate. In this setting, anti-inflammatory strategies may be life-saving.

A report using an animal model of endotoxic shock showed that injections of C-peptide in vivo to LPS-treated mice drastically improved survival rate of the animals compared to vehicle-treated mice, an effect associated with reduced plasma levels of the proinflammatory cytokines TNF-α and MCP-1 and a decreased overall inflammatory response in the lung [80]. C-peptide inhibited phosphorylation of extracellular signal-regulated kinase (ERK)1/2 followed by up-regulation of nuclear expression and DNA binding of the nuclear transcription factor proliferator-activated-receptor(PPAR)-γ (which plays an important role in the modulation of inflammation) in the lungs of these endotoxin-treated mice [80].

Ischemia/Reperfusion

There are >1 million MIs each year in the United States with an average of 1 American dying every 38 s from cardiovascular disease [82]. Furthermore, approximately 700,000 patients undergo cardioplegic arrest for various cardiac surgeries each year in the United States with the total number of inpatient cardiovascular operations and procedures increasing [82, 83]. Along with the ischemic injury related to MIs and cardioplegic arrest comes reperfusion injury. The pathophysiologic mechanisms underlying ischemia-reperfusion injury are complex with the neutrophil taking on a prominent role in the inflammatory component of postischemic injury [84]. Ischemia-reperfusion prompts a series of events which eventually lead to the adherence of neutrophils to the vascular endothelium, followed by transendothelial migration and direct interaction with myocytes [84]. This is a prerequisite to typical reperfusion injury which includes endothelial dysfunction, microvascular collapse and blood flow defects, MI, and apoptosis [84]. Polymorphonuclear leukocyte (PMN) infiltration actuates endothelial and myocardial injury by releasing cytotoxic substances such as oxygen-derived free radicals, inflammatory cytokines, and proteolytic enzymes [85]. In neutrophil-depleted animals undergoing reperfused MI, the infarct size was significantly decreased suggesting a significant amount of myocardial injury may be induced by neutrophil-associated mechanisms [86]. Given the aforementioned data, strategies targeting ischemia-reperfusion injury and PMN infiltration are of utmost importance.

In a study by Young et al., the effect of C-peptide on cardiac contractile function in the isolated perfused rat heart following PMN-induced ischemia-reperfusion injury was examined [85]. PMN adherence to the vascular endothelium was decreased in rats administered C-peptide. By reducing PMN infiltration to the myocardium, systemic administration of C-peptide restored cardiac contractile function and postreperfusion coronary heart flow.

Encephalopathy

C-peptide has also been found to play an important role in intracellular signaling and inflammation in the central nervous system. This is particularly important in T1D patients who, in addition to possibly having impairments in learning, memory, problem solving, and mental and motor speed, may also suffer from primary diabetic encephalopathy as a late complication of T1D [87]. In the rat model of human T1D, the type 1 BB/Wor rat, cognitive impairment is associated with apoptosis-induced neuronal loss in the hippocampus [88]. In this model, C-peptide replacement reduced several apoptotic mechanisms significantly reducing the cognitive dysfunction and hippocampal neuronal loss [89]. Furthermore, in diabetic hippocampi the expression of NF-κB was significantly increased which was associated with increased expression of RAGE and the downstream activation of proinflammatory TNF-α, IL-1β, IL-2, and IL-6 [87]. When the diabetic rats received C-peptide replacement, the up-regulation of RAGE and activation of NF-κB, TNF-α, IL-1β, IL-2, and IL-6 were decreased which was also associated with the prevention of astrocyte proliferation [87]. Other preliminary studies have also revealed deficits in temporal white matter with increased RAGE expression and proinflammatory cytokines, which were significantly prevented by C-peptide replacement [90]. For further details of C-peptide's role in encephalopathy, please see Chap. 9.

Internalization of C-Peptide in Vascular Cells

The cell biology of C-peptide is for the most part unknown, in particular regarding how C-peptide achieves its intracellular activities in target cells. A specific C-peptide receptor has not been identified yet, although it is often suggested to be a G-protein-coupled receptor as deduced from effects of pertussis toxin [91, 92]. In a recently published paper, we investigated the pathway the peptide uses to cross the cellular membrane and possible subcellular destinations in vascular cells. By using confocal laser scanner microscopy, we followed the dynamics of internalization of AlexaFluor-labeled C-peptide probes applied to live human HAEC and VSMC [93]. We found that C-peptide internalizes to punctate structures localized at the level of the cellular membrane and in the cytoplasm in both cell types [93] (Fig. 10.6). Internalization of C-peptide was minimal after 5 min, clearly detectable after 10 min, resulted in bright staining after 30 min, and was completed by 1 h [93]. By using specific organelle reporter dyes, it was established that the punctate structures identify with the specific endocytic organelles early endosomes. C-peptide eventually trafficked to lysosomes in live HAEC and UASMC [93]. Other groups, working with HEK-293 cells and fibroblasts, found nuclear localization of C-peptide [92]. Specifically, C-peptide can be detected in the nucleoli where it promotes transcription of genes encoding for ribosomal RNA [94]. Identification of the subcellular compartments in which C-peptide localizes upon its entry into target cells is important as these compartments likely represent the sites of intracellular signaling activity of C-peptide.

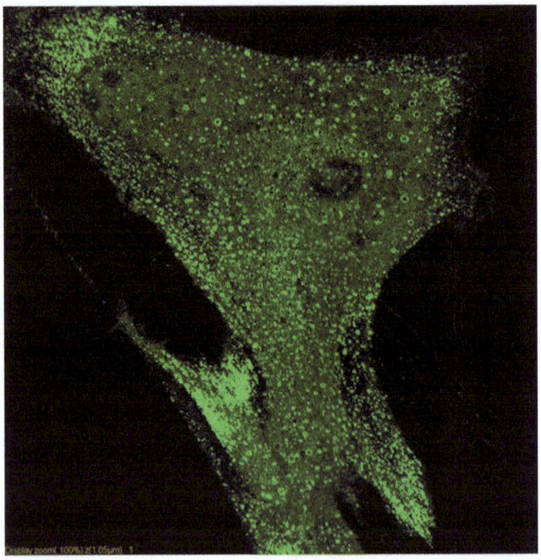

Fig. 10.6 C-peptide internalizes in human vascular endothelial cells as punctate structures. Internalization of C-peptide has been studied by using AlexaFluor488-labeled C-peptide probe in live-cell imaging using a laser scanning confocal microscopy [93]. The *green* punctate-staining corresponds to the C-peptide probe localized at the periphery of the cell and in the cytoplasm

In one potential scenario, it can be hypothesized that C-peptide binds to its receptor at the level of the plasma membrane, gets activated, and the complex begins the signaling activity. In this scenario, the activated C-peptide/C-peptide receptor complex is quickly internalized into early endosomes where it continues to signal (Fig. 10.7). Receptor internalization, in this case, serves not only to modulate receptor density at the plasma membrane, but also to generate intracellular signaling endosomes that confer signal specificity and diversity in the different cell types. Early endosomes are, in fact, emerging as important sites for intracellular signaling events of ligands associated with their specific receptor [95]. Localization of C-peptide to early endosomes does not exclude trafficking of C-peptide to other subcellular sites upon its entry into target cells. As an alternative potential scenario, the signaling activity of the activated C-peptide-receptor complex is exclusively localized at the plasma membrane and endosomal localization represents a sorting station toward recycling or lysosomal degradation. In this last scenario, internalization of the C-peptide/C-peptide receptor complex to early endosomes serves as a mechanism to control receptor density at the cell surface and attenuate signal duration and strength. For example, downregulation of C-peptide receptors at the cell surface may happen in response to high extracellular C-peptide concentration (Fig. 10.8).

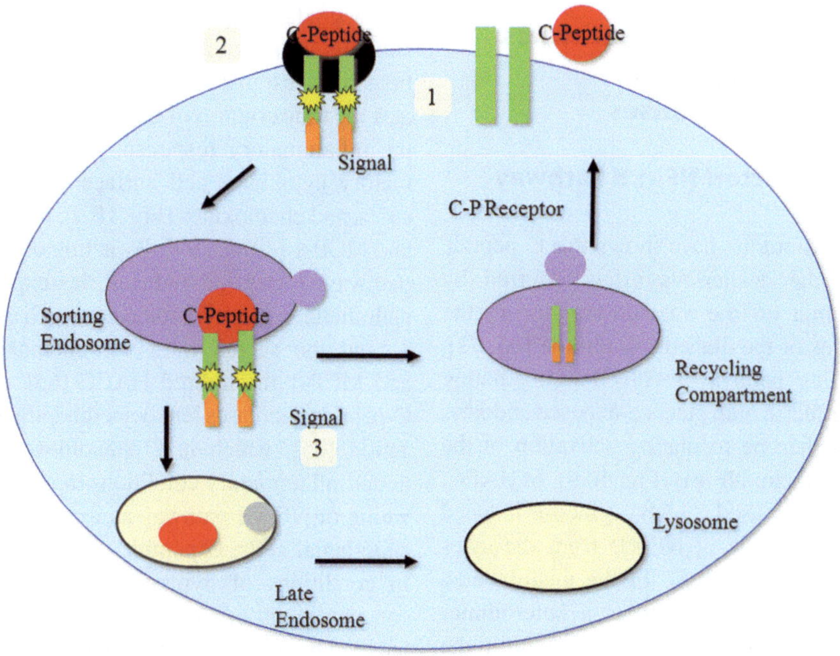

Fig. 10.7 Proposed model for C-peptide/C-peptide-receptor complex signaling from early endosomes. We propose a potential model for C-peptide internalization and intracellular signaling activity in which C-peptide after its binding to its specific receptor at the plasma membrane (*1*) gets activated (*2*), begins the signaling activity, and is quickly internalized into early endosomes (*3*) where it continues to signal

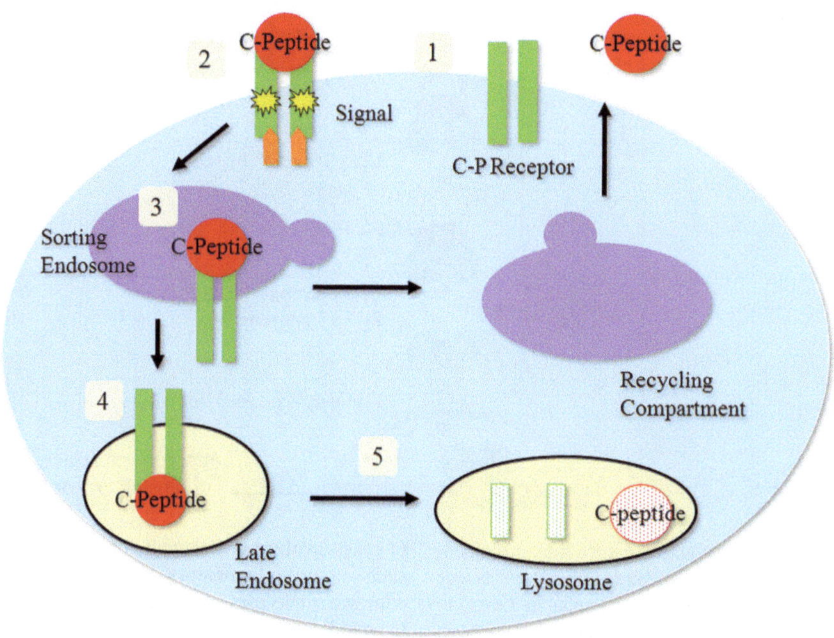

Fig. 10.8 Proposed model for C-peptide/C-peptide-receptor complex signaling from the plasma membrane. We propose an alternate potential model to explain C-peptide signaling activity in which C-peptide binds to its specific receptor at the level of the plasma membrane (*1*) and begins its signaling activity (*2*). Internalization of the C-peptide-receptor complex via endocytic pathway to early endosomes terminates the intracellular signaling activity and internalized activated receptor–peptide complexes gets degraded in the lysosomal compartment

Intracellular Signaling Pathways Affected by C-Peptide in Inflammatory Responses

The Nuclear Factor(NF)-κB Pathway

Recent in vitro studies have shown that C-peptide neutralizes the deleterious effect inferred by hyperglycemia on the vasculature during the earlier stages of the diabetic syndrome [65, 72]. One signaling pathway involved in mediating C-peptide effect in high glucose-exposed endothelial cells is the one mediating activation of the transcription factor NF-κB (Fig. 10.9). In HAEC, C-peptide decreased high glucose-induced nuclear translocation of NF-κB from the cytoplasm to the nucleus [65]. In the unstimulated state, in fact, NF-κB exists as a heterodimer composed of p50 and p65 subunits bound to the inhibitor protein IκB in the cytoplasm. A key event in NF-κB activation requires IκB phosphorylation and degradation, causing the release of p50/p65 subunits [96] from IκB. The active p50/p65 heterodimer translocates to the nucleus and initiates the transcription of several genes involved in the inflammatory response, such as proinflammatory cytokines, cell surface adhesion molecules, and chemokines (Fig. 10.9), including IL-8 and MCP-1 [49, 62, 97]. By acting on the NF-κB pathway, C-peptide reduces the expression of endothelial adhesion molecules, such as VCAM-1, and the secretion of the chemokines IL-8 and MCP-1 in cultured HAEC [65]. Moreover, C-peptide decreases leukocyte-endothelium interaction [65], which is a phenomenon observed under inflammatory conditions that requires activation of NF-κB pathway as well. In addition to endothelial cells, C-peptide targets VSMC [73]. In conditions of hyperglycemia, physiological concentrations of C-peptide attenuated glucose-induced hyperproliferation of VSMC, a phenomenon associated with a specific inhibitory effect on NF-κB [72].

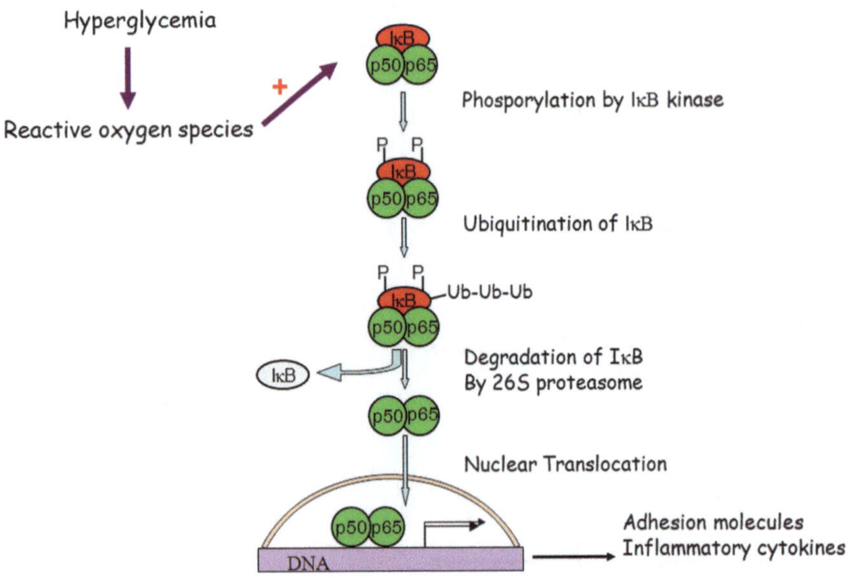

Fig. 10.9 NF-κB is a potential target for the anti-inflammatory activity displayed by C-peptide. NF-κB exists as a heterodimer composed of p50 and p65 subunits bound to IKB in the unstimulated state. Upon cellular activation, such as after exposure of endothelial cells to high glucose, increased production of ROS mediates phosphorylation and degradation of IKB, thus causing the release of p50/p65 components of NF-κB. The active p50/p65 heterodimer translocates to the nucleus and initiates the transcription of genes involved in the regulation of leukocyte responses, such as proinflammatory cytokines and cell-surface adhesion molecules expression. It has been shown that C-peptide decreases nuclear translocation of p65/p50 subunits in high glucose-activated endothelial cells. C-peptide might act at different levels along the NF-κB pathway, such as regulating ROS production, or modulating IKB phosphorylation, or even physically interacting with the p65/p50 subunits in the nucleus preventing their DNA binding

Although the NF-κB pathway has been identified as a critical target of C-peptide in reducing inflammation in the vasculature, the mechanistic events of C-peptide action in reducing NF-κB activation remain unrevealed. C-peptide can reduce NF-κB translocation to the nucleus by using different strategies. One possible mechanism is that C-peptide turns off the cascade of phosphorylation events ultimately leading to the activation of kinase proteins involved in the phosphorylation of the inhibitor protein IκB. By shutting down the phosphorylation cascade, C-peptide might interfere with the dissociation of IκB:NF-κB complex in the cytoplasm, limiting the migration of p65/p50 subunits to the nucleus thus reducing the activation of genes involved in inflammatory processes. The phosphorylation cascade is carried through recruitment of several kinase proteins such as IκB, IKKα, and IKKβ and it is initiated at the level of the plasma membrane after the binding of a ligand to a membrane receptor (e.g., Toll-like receptor). At which level of the phosphorylation cascade C-peptide might act is unknown. To date, a specific C-peptide receptor or a membrane receptor through which C-peptide might function has not been identified. As discussed previously, recent evidence demonstrates that C-peptide localizes at the level of early endosomes after its uptake from the plasma membrane of endothelial cells [93]. Endosome localization of C-peptide might represent a site from which C-peptide/C-peptide receptor complex affects the activation of the NF-κB pathway, as it has been demonstrated for certain Toll-like receptor pathways [98]. Another possible mechanism of C-peptide action is that C-peptide limits the degradation of cytoplasmic IκB, usually carried on by degradative machinery called proteasome. By affecting the activation of the proteasome and eventually avoiding the degradation of IκB, C-peptide might limit the translocation of NF-κB from the cytoplasm to the nucleus. Another possible scenario is that C-peptide controls the transcriptional activity of NF-κB by physically binding to the p65/p50 subunits in the cytoplasm, thus reducing both their nuclear translocation and their DNA-binding ability. C-peptide might also reduce high glucose-induced ROS production, one of the first events required for the activation of NF-κB pathway during inflammation. Further studies are required to investigate the molecular mechanism(s) by which C-peptide affects the NF-κB pathway.

The Peroxisome-Proliferator-Activated Receptor γ (PPAR-γ) Pathway

It has been shown that C-peptide affects the activity of peroxisome-proliferator-activated receptor γ (PPAR-γ) [99], a ligand-dependent nuclear transcription factor that plays a critical role in the modulation of lipid and glucose metabolism as well as of inflammation [100]. In vitro *studies* conducted in kidney proximal tubular cells have shown that C-peptide increases PPAR-γ phosphorylation by activation of PI3K. In the same study, it has been demonstrated that C-peptide triggers expression of the PPAR-γ-regulated gene CD36, which is a scavenger receptor for ox-LDL uptake, in the THP-1 monocytic cell line [99]. PPAR-γ has direct actions at the vascular level [101] acting as a key modulator in endothelial biology, vascular smooth muscle function, and macrophage activity [102]. PPAR-γ regulates the expression of several genes involved in inflammation and vascular disorders such as atherosclerosis [103] by either controlling the gene transcriptional machinery [101, 104, 105] or interacting with other transcription factors such as activator protein (AP)-1, STAT (signal transducers and activators of transcription) and NF-κB [106]. NF-κB is a major target of PPAR-γ [107] in the endothelium, smooth muscle, and macrophages [108]. It has been shown that PPAR-γ inhibits the activity of NF-κB by suppressing its promoter activity and, moreover, PPAR-γ agonists are able to prevent phosphorylation of NF-κB p65 subunit as well [109]. It is not clear which is the mechanism(s) by which C-peptide affects PPAR-γ activation, but studies on opossum kidney tubular epithelial cells demonstrated that it is via a ligand-independent mechanism [99]. A similar effect has been reported in lung epithelial cells of LPS-treated mice, an animal model of endotoxic shock [80]. In this latter study, C-peptide improves survival of LPS-treated mice and reduces lung and systemic inflammatory responses, with reduction of plasma levels of proinflammatory cytokines [80]. In these mice, the mechanism of PPAR-γ up-regulation by C-peptide appeared to be mediated through an inhibitory effect on LPS-induced phosphorylation of extracellular signal-regulated kinase (ERK)1/2 in the lung, a pathway-mediating transduction of oxidative signals to the nucleus.

Conclusions

Increasing evidence suggests that C-peptide exerts cytoprotective effects to cells exposed to a variety of stressful events by modulating major intracellular pathways involved in inflammation. Several investigators have demonstrated that C-peptide acts on key events in the inflammatory response underlying vascular dysfunction, such as reducing proinflammatory cytokine secretion, cell adhesion molecule expression, and leukocyte-endothelium interaction. Internalization of C-peptide in vascular cells has also been demonstrated and activity at the level of the NF-κB and PPAR-γ pathways has been showed by different groups. Although there is still much to learn about the cell biology and specific mechanism(s) of action of C-peptide, there is no doubt that C-peptide is emerging as a new molecule with therapeutic potential in the treatment of diseases with a strong inflammatory component, such as sepsis, T1D, and diabetes-associated vascular complications. In this regard, results from small clinical trials have already demonstrated the beneficial effect of C-peptide replacement in preventing or treating kidney and neural dysfunction in T1D patients.

References

1. Eisenbarth GS. Type I diabetes mellitus. A chronic autoimmune disease. N Engl J Med. 1986;314(21):1360–8.
2. Conrad B, Weidmann E, Trucco G, et al. Evidence for superantigen involvement in insulin-dependent diabetes mellitus aetiology. Nature. 1994;371(6495):351–5.
3. Goodier MR, Nawroly N, Beyan H, et al. Identical twins discordant for type 1 diabetes show a different pattern of in vitro CD56+ cell activation. Diabetes Metab Res Rev. 2006;22(5):367–75.
4. Wilson SB, Kent SC, Patton KT, et al. Extreme Th1 bias of invariant Valpha24JalphaQ T cells in type 1 diabetes. Nature. 1998;391(6663):177–81.
5. Adler T, Akiyama H, Herder C, et al. Heat shock protein 60 elicits abnormal response in macrophages of diabetes-prone non-obese diabetic mice. Biochem Biophys Res Commun. 2002;294(3):592–6.
6. Beyan H, Goodier MR, Nawroly NS, et al. Altered monocyte cyclooxygenase response to lipopolysaccharide in type 1 diabetes. Diabetes. 2006;55(12):3439–45.
7. Kolb-Bachofen V, Kolb H. A role for macrophages in the pathogenesis of type 1 diabetes. Autoimmunity. 1989;3(2):145–54.
8. Hanenberg H, Kolb-Bachofen V, Kantwerk-Funke G, et al. Macrophage infiltration precedes and is a prerequisite for lymphocytic insulitis in pancreatic islets of pre-diabetic BB rats. Diabetologia. 1989;32(2):126–34.
9. Eizirik DL, Colli ML, Ortis F. The role of inflammation in insulitis and beta-cell loss in type 1 diabetes. Nat Rev Endocrinol. 2009;5(4):219–26.
10. Schalkwijk CG, Poland DC, van Dijk W, et al. Plasma concentration of C-reactive protein is increased in type I diabetic patients without clinical macroangiopathy and correlates with markers of endothelial dysfunction: evidence for chronic inflammation. Diabetologia. 1999;42(3):351–7.
11. Kilpatrick ES, Keevil BG, Jagger C, et al. Determinants of raised C-reactive protein concentration in type 1 diabetes. QJM. 2000;93(4):231–6.
12. Lechleitner M, Koch T, Herold M, et al. Tumour necrosis factor-alpha plasma level in patients with type 1 diabetes mellitus and its association with glycaemic control and cardiovascular risk factors. J Intern Med. 2000;248(1):67–76.
13. Devaraj S, Cheung AT, Jialal I, et al. Evidence of increased inflammation and microcirculatory abnormalities in patients with type 1 diabetes and their role in microvascular complications. Diabetes. 2007;56(11):2790–6.
14. Devaraj S, Glaser N, Griffen S, et al. Increased monocytic activity and biomarkers of inflammation in patients with type 1 diabetes. Diabetes. 2006;55(3):774–9.
15. Plesner A, Greenbaum CJ, Gaur LK, et al. Macrophages from high-risk HLA-DQB1*0201/*0302 type 1 diabetes mellitus patients are hypersensitive to lipopolysaccharide stimulation. Scand J Immunol. 2002;56(5):522–9.
16. Rosa JS, Flores RL, Oliver SR, et al. Sustained IL-1alpha, IL-4, and IL-6 elevations following correction of hyperglycemia in children with type 1 diabetes mellitus. Pediatr Diabetes. 2008;9(1):9–16.
17. Erbagci AB, Tarakcioglu M, Coskun Y, et al. Mediators of inflammation in children with type I

diabetes mellitus: cytokines in type I diabetic children. Clin Biochem. 2001;34(8):645–50.
18. Cifarelli V, Libman IM, Deluca A, et al. Increased expression of monocyte CD11b (Mac-1) in overweight recent-onset type 1 diabetic children. Rev Diabet Stud. 2007;4(2):112–17.
19. Schram MT, Chaturvedi N, Schalkwijk C, et al. Vascular risk factors and markers of endothelial function as determinants of inflammatory markers in type 1 diabetes: the EURODIAB Prospective Complications Study. Diabetes Care. 2003;26(7):2165–73.
20. Saraheimo M, Teppo AM, Forsblom C, et al. Diabetic nephropathy is associated with low-grade inflammation in type 1 diabetic patients. Diabetologia. 2003;46(10):1402–7.
21. Schalkwijk CG, Ter Wee PM, Stehouwer CD. Plasma levels of AGE peptides in type 1 diabetic patients are associated with serum creatinine and not with albumin excretion rate: possible role of AGE peptide-associated endothelial dysfunction. Ann N Y Acad Sci. 2005;1043:662–70.
22. Litherland SA, Xie XT, Hutson AD, et al. Aberrant prostaglandin synthase 2 expression defines an antigen-presenting cell defect for insulin-dependent diabetes mellitus. J Clin Invest. 1999;104(4):515–23.
23. Libby P, Nathan DM, Abraham K, et al. Report of the National Heart, Lung, and Blood Institute-National Institute of Diabetes and Digestive and Kidney Diseases Working Group on cardiovascular complications of type 1 diabetes mellitus. Circulation. 2005;111(25):3489–93.
24. Zatz R, Brenner BM. Pathogenesis of diabetic microangiopathy. The hemodynamic view. Am J Med. 1986;80(3):443–53.
25. Zimmerman MA, Flores SC. Autoimmune-mediated oxidative stress and endothelial dysfunction: implications of accelerated vascular injury in type I diabetes. J Surg Res. 2009;155(1):173–8.
26. Andresen JL, Rasmussen LM, Ledet T. Diabetic macroangiopathy and atherosclerosis. Diabetes. 1996;45 Suppl 3:S91–4.
27. Jarvisalo MJ, Raitakari M, Toikka JO, et al. Endothelial dysfunction and increased arterial intima-media thickness in children with type 1 diabetes. Circulation. 2004;109(14):1750–5.
28. Yngen M, Ostenson CG, Hu H, et al. Enhanced P-selectin expression and increased soluble CD40 ligand in patients with type 1 diabetes mellitus and microangiopathy: evidence for platelet hyperactivity and chronic inflammation. Diabetologia. 2004;47(3):537–40.
29. Clausen P, Jacobsen P, Rossing K, et al. Plasma concentrations of VCAM-1 and ICAM-1 are elevated in patients with type 1 diabetes mellitus with microalbuminuria and overt nephropathy. Diabet Med. 2000;17(9):644–9.
30. Jude EB, Douglas JT, Anderson SG, et al. Circulating cellular adhesion molecules ICAM-1, VCAM-1, P- and E-selectin in the prediction of cardiovascular disease in diabetes mellitus. Eur J Intern Med. 2002;13(3):185–9.
31. Lampeter ER, Kishimoto TK, Rothlein R, et al. Elevated levels of circulating adhesion molecules in IDDM patients and in subjects at risk for IDDM. Diabetes. 1992;41(12):1668–71.
32. Ribau JC, Hadcock SJ, Teoh K, et al. Endothelial adhesion molecule expression is enhanced in the aorta and internal mammary artery of diabetic patients. J Surg Res. 1999;85(2):225–33.
33. Schmidt AM, Crandall J, Hori O, et al. Elevated plasma levels of vascular cell adhesion molecule-1 (VCAM-1) in diabetic patients with microalbuminuria: a marker of vascular dysfunction and progressive vascular disease. Br J Haematol. 1996;92(3):747–50.
34. Huo Y, Ley K. Adhesion molecules and atherogenesis. Acta Physiol Scand. 2001;173(1):35–43.
35. Elhadd TA, Kennedy G, Hill A, et al. Abnormal markers of endothelial cell activation and oxidative stress in children, adolescents and young adults with type 1 diabetes with no clinical vascular disease. Diabetes Metab Res Rev. 1999;15(6):405–11.
36. Dogruel N, Kirel B, Akgun Y, et al. Serum soluble endothelial-cell specific adhesion molecules in children with insulin-dependent diabetes mellitus. J Pediatr Endocrinol Metab. 2001;14(3):287–93.
37. Toivonen A, Kulmala P, Rahko J, et al. Soluble adhesion molecules in Finnish schoolchildren with signs of preclinical type 1 diabetes. Diabetes Metab Res Rev. 2004;20(1):48–54.
38. Toivonen A, Kulmala P, Savola K, et al. Soluble adhesion molecules in preclinical type 1 diabetes. The Childhood Diabetes in Finland Study Group. Pediatr Res. 2001;49(1):24–9.
39. Toivonen AM, Kimpimaki T, Kupila A, et al. Soluble adhesion molecules in young children with signs of beta-cell autoimmunity – prospective follow-up from birth. Diabetes Metab Res Rev. 2006;22(3):176–83.
40. Toivonen AM, Kulmala P, Savola K, et al. Soluble adhesion molecules in pre-clinical type 1 diabetes: a prospective study. Diabetologia. 2003;46(4):492–5.
41. Martin-Gallan P, Carrascosa A, Gussinye M, et al. Biomarkers of diabetes-associated oxidative stress and antioxidant status in young diabetic patients with or without subclinical complications. Free Radic Biol Med. 2003;34(12):1563–74.
42. Dandona P, Thusu K, Cook S, et al. Oxidative damage to DNA in diabetes mellitus. Lancet. 1996;347(8999):444–5.
43. Sivitz WI, Yorek MA. Mitochondrial dysfunction in diabetes: from molecular mechanisms to functional significance and therapeutic opportunities. Antioxid Redox Signal. 2010;12(4):537–77.
44. Brownlee M. The pathobiology of diabetic complications: a unifying mechanism. Diabetes. 2005;54(6):1615–25.
45. Katusic ZS, Vanhoutte PM. Superoxide anion is an endothelium-derived contracting factor. Am J Physiol. 1989;257(1 Pt 2):H33–7.

46. Rubanyi GM, Vanhoutte PM. Superoxide anions and hyperoxia inactivate endothelium-derived relaxing factor. Am J Physiol. 1986;250(5 Pt 2):H822–7.
47. Nishikawa T, Edelstein D, Du XL, et al. Normalizing mitochondrial superoxide production blocks three pathways of hyperglycaemic damage. Nature. 2000; 404(6779):787–90.
48. Janssen-Heininger YM, Poynter ME, Baeuerle PA. Recent advances towards understanding redox mechanisms in the activation of nuclear factor kappaB. Free Radic Biol Med. 2000;28(9):1317–27.
49. Soares MP, Muniappan A, Kaczmarek E, et al. Adenovirus-mediated expression of a dominant negative mutant of p65/RelA inhibits proinflammatory gene expression in endothelial cells without sensitizing to apoptosis. J Immunol. 1998;161(9):4572–82.
50. Zuckerbraun BS, McCloskey CA, Mahidhara RS, et al. Overexpression of mutated IkappaBalpha inhibits vascular smooth muscle cell proliferation and intimal hyperplasia formation. J Vasc Surg. 2003;38(4):812–19.
51. Morishita R, Sugimoto T, Aoki M, et al. In vivo transfection of cis element "decoy" against nuclear factor-kappaB binding site prevents myocardial infarction. Nat Med. 1997;3(8):894–9.
52. Panero F, Novelli G, Zucco C, et al. Fasting plasma C-peptide and micro- and macrovascular complications in a large clinic-based cohort of type 1 diabetic patients. Diabetes Care. 2009;32(2):301–5.
53. Ekberg K, Brismar T, Johansson BL, et al. C-peptide replacement therapy and sensory nerve function in type 1 diabetic neuropathy. Diabetes Care. 2007; 30(1):71–6.
54. Johansson BL, Borg K, Fernqvist-Forbes E, et al. Beneficial effects of C-peptide on incipient nephropathy and neuropathy in patients with type 1 diabetes mellitus. Diabet Med. 2000;17(3):181–9.
55. Libby P. Inflammation in atherosclerosis. Nature. 2002;420(6917):868–74.
56. Eckel RH, Wassef M, Chait A, et al. Prevention conference VI: diabetes and cardiovascular disease: Writing Group II: pathogenesis of atherosclerosis in diabetes. Circulation. 2002;105(18):e138–43.
57. Hickey MJ, Kubes P. Role of nitric oxide in regulation of leucocyte-endothelial cell interactions. Exp Physiol. 1997;82(2):339–48.
58. Kado S, Wakatsuki T, Yamamoto M, et al. Expression of intercellular adhesion molecule-1 induced by high glucose concentrations in human aortic endothelial cells. Life Sci. 2001;68(7):727–37.
59. Kim JA, Berliner JA, Natarajan RD, et al. Evidence that glucose increases monocyte binding to human aortic endothelial cells. Diabetes. 1994;43(9):1103–7.
60. Morigi M, Angioletti S, Imberti B, et al. Leukocyte-endothelial interaction is augmented by high glucose concentrations and hyperglycemia in a NF-kB-dependent fashion. J Clin Invest. 1998;101(9): 1905–15.
61. Haubner F, Lehle K, Munzel D, et al. Hyperglycemia increases the levels of vascular cellular adhesion molecule-1 and monocyte-chemoattractant-protein-1 in the diabetic endothelial cell. Biochem Biophys Res Commun. 2007;360(3):560–5.
62. Piga R, Naito Y, Kokura S, et al. Short-term high glucose exposure induces monocyte-endothelial cells adhesion and transmigration by increasing VCAM-1 and MCP-1 expression in human aortic endothelial cells. Atherosclerosis. 2007;193(2):328–34.
63. Gerszten RE, Garcia-Zepeda EA, Lim YC, et al. MCP-1 and IL-8 trigger firm adhesion of monocytes to vascular endothelium under flow conditions. Nature. 1999;398(6729):718–23.
64. Scalia R, Coyle KM, Levine BJ, et al. C-peptide inhibits leukocyte-endothelium interaction in the microcirculation during acute endothelial dysfunction. FASEB J. 2000;14(14):2357–64.
65. Luppi P, Cifarelli V, Tse H, et al. Human C-peptide antagonises high glucose-induced endothelial dysfunction through the nuclear factor-kappaB pathway. Diabetologia. 2008;51(8):1534–43.
66. Mughal RS, Scragg JL, Lister P, et al. Cellular mechanisms by which proinsulin C-peptide prevents insulin-induced neointima formation in human saphenous vein. Diabetologia. 2010;53(8):1761–71.
67. Ross R. Atherosclerosis – an inflammatory disease. N Engl J Med. 1999;340(2):115–26.
68. Orasanu G, Plutzky J. The pathologic continuum of diabetic vascular disease. J Am Coll Cardiol. 2009;53(5 Suppl):S35–42.
69. Nakamura J, Kasuya Y, Hamada Y, et al. Glucose-induced hyperproliferation of cultured rat aortic smooth muscle cells through polyol pathway hyperactivity. Diabetologia. 2001;44(4):480–7.
70. Natarajan R, Gonzales N, Xu L, et al. Vascular smooth muscle cells exhibit increased growth in response to elevated glucose. Biochem Biophys Res Commun. 1992;187(1):552–60.
71. Yamamoto M, Acevedo-Duncan M, Chalfant CE, et al. Acute glucose-induced downregulation of PKC-betaII accelerates cultured VSMC proliferation. Am J Physiol Cell Physiol. 2000;279(3):C587–95.
72. Cifarelli V, Luppi P, Tse HM, et al. Human proinsulin C-peptide reduces high glucose-induced proliferation and NF-kappaB activation in vascular smooth muscle cells. Atherosclerosis. 2008;201(2):248–57.
73. Kobayashi Y, Naruse K, Hamada Y, et al. Human proinsulin C-peptide prevents proliferation of rat aortic smooth muscle cells cultured in high-glucose conditions. Diabetologia. 2005;48(11):2396–401.
74. Walcher D, Babiak C, Poletek P, et al. C-peptide induces vascular smooth muscle cell proliferation: involvement of SRC-kinase, phosphatidylinositol 3-kinase, and extracellular signal-regulated kinase 1/2. Circ Res. 2006;99(11):1181–7.
75. Dellinger RP, Levy MM, Carlet JM, et al. Surviving Sepsis Campaign: international guidelines for management of severe sepsis and septic shock: 2008. Intensive Care Med. 2008;34(1):17–60.
76. Angus DC, Linde-Zwirble WT, Lidicker J, et al. Epidemiology of severe sepsis in the United States:

analysis of incidence, outcome, and associated costs of care. Crit Care Med. 2001;29(7):1303–10.
77. Cai B, Deitch EA, Ulloa L. Novel insights for systemic inflammation in sepsis and hemorrhage. Mediators Inflamm. 2010;2010:642462.
78. Winters BD, Eberlein M, Leung J, et al. Long-term mortality and quality of life in sepsis: a systematic review. Crit Care Med. 2010;38(5):1276–83.
79. Bone RC. Toward an epidemiology and natural history of SIRS (systemic inflammatory response syndrome). JAMA. 1992;268(24):3452–5.
80. Vish MG, Mangeshkar P, Piraino G, et al. Proinsulin C-peptide exerts beneficial effects in endotoxic shock in mice. Crit Care Med. 2007;35(5):1348–55.
81. Dellinger RP, Carlet JM, Masur H, et al. Surviving Sepsis Campaign guidelines for management of severe sepsis and septic shock. Crit Care Med. 2004;32(3):858–73.
82. Lloyd-Jones D, Adams RJ, Brown TM, et al. Heart disease and stroke statistics – 2010 update: a report from the American Heart Association. Circulation. 2011;121(7):e46–215.
83. Turer AT, Hill JA. Pathogenesis of myocardial ischemia-reperfusion injury and rationale for therapy. Am J Cardiol. 2010;106(3):360–8.
84. Jordan JE, Zhao ZQ, Vinten-Johansen J. The role of neutrophils in myocardial ischemia-reperfusion injury. Cardiovasc Res. 1999;43(4):860–78.
85. Young LH, Ikeda Y, Scalia R, et al. C-peptide exerts cardioprotective effects in myocardial ischemia-reperfusion. Am J Physiol Heart Circ Physiol. 2000; 279(4):H1453–9.
86. Nah DY, Rhee MY. The inflammatory response and cardiac repair after myocardial infarction. Korean Circ J. 2009;39(10):393–8.
87. Sima AA, Zhang W, Kreipke CW, et al. Inflammation in diabetic encephalopathy is prevented by C-peptide. Rev Diabet Stud. 2009;6(1):37–42.
88. Li ZG, Zhang W, Grunberger G, et al. Hippocampal neuronal apoptosis in type 1 diabetes. Brain Res. 2002;946(2):221–31.
89. Sima AA, Li ZG. The effect of C-peptide on cognitive dysfunction and hippocampal apoptosis in type 1 diabetic rats. Diabetes. 2005;54(5):1497–505.
90. Sima AA, Zhang W, Muzik O, et al. Sequential abnormalities in type 1 diabetic encephalopathy and the effects of C-peptide. Rev Diabet Stud. 2009;6(3): 211–22.
91. Rigler R, Pramanik A, Jonasson P, et al. Specific binding of proinsulin C-peptide to human cell membranes. Proc Natl Acad Sci USA. 1999;96(23):13318–23.
92. Lindahl E, Nyman U, Melles E, et al. Cellular internalization of proinsulin C-peptide. Cell Mol Life Sci. 2007;64(4):479–86.
93. Luppi P, Geng X, Cifarelli V, et al. C-peptide is internalised in human endothelial and vascular smooth muscle cells via early endosomes. Diabetologia. 2009;52(10):2218–28.
94. Lindahl E, Nyman U, Zaman F, et al. Proinsulin C-peptide regulates ribosomal RNA expression. J Biol Chem. 2010;285(5):3462–9.
95. Miaczynska M, Pelkmans L, Zerial M. Not just a sink: endosomes in control of signal transduction. Curr Opin Cell Biol. 2004;16(4):400–6.
96. Viatour P, Merville MP, Bours V, et al. Phosphorylation of NF-kappaB and IkappaB proteins: implications in cancer and inflammation. Trends Biochem Sci. 2005;30(1):43–52.
97. Tak PP, Firestein GS. NF-kappaB: a key role in inflammatory diseases. J Clin Invest. 2001;107(1): 7–11.
98. Husebye H, Halaas O, Stenmark H, et al. Endocytic pathways regulate Toll-like receptor 4 signaling and link innate and adaptive immunity. EMBO J. 2006; 25(4):683–92.
99. Al-Rasheed NM, Chana RS, Baines RJ, et al. Ligand-independent activation of peroxisome proliferator-activated receptor-gamma by insulin and C-peptide in kidney proximal tubular cells: dependent on phosphatidylinositol 3-kinase activity. J Biol Chem. 2004;279(48):49747–54.
100. Kliewer SA, Umesono K, Noonan DJ, et al. Convergence of 9-cis retinoic acid and peroxisome proliferator signalling pathways through heterodimer formation of their receptors. Nature. 1992; 358(6389):771–4.
101. Berger JP, Akiyama TE, Meinke PT. PPARs: therapeutic targets for metabolic disease. Trends Pharmacol Sci. 2005;26(5):244–51.
102. Duan SZ, Usher MG, Mortensen RM. Peroxisome proliferator-activated receptor-gamma-mediated effects in the vasculature. Circ Res. 2008;102(3): 283–94.
103. Pasceri V, Wu HD, Willerson JT, et al. Modulation of vascular inflammation in vitro and in vivo by peroxisome proliferator-activated receptor-gamma activators. Circulation. 2000;101(3):235–8.
104. Lee CH, Olson P, Evans RM. Minireview: lipid metabolism, metabolic diseases, and peroxisome proliferator-activated receptors. Endocrinology. 2003;144(6):2201–7.
105. Rosen ED, Spiegelman BM. PPARgamma: a nuclear regulator of metabolism, differentiation, and cell growth. J Biol Chem. 2001;276(41):37731–4.
106. Lehrke M, Lazar MA. The many faces of PPARgamma. Cell. 2005;123(6):993–9.
107. De Bosscher K, Vanden Berghe W, Haegeman G. Cross-talk between nuclear receptors and nuclear factor kappaB. Oncogene. 2006;25(51): 6868–86.
108. De Martin R, Hoeth M, Hofer-Warbinek R, et al. The transcription factor NF-kappa B and the regulation of vascular cell function. Arterioscler Thromb Vasc Biol. 2000;20(11):E83–8.
109. Sasaki M, Jordan P, Welbourne T, et al. Troglitazone, a PPAR-gamma activator prevents endothelial cell adhesion molecule expression and lymphocyte adhesion mediated by TNF-alpha. BMC Physiol. 2005;5(1):3.
110. Rocha VZ, Libby P. Obesity, inflammation, and atherosclerosis. Nat Rev Cardiol. 2009;6(6): 399–409.

11 C-Peptide: Connecting Diabetes with Macrovascular Complications

Karen E. Porter and Romana S. Mughal

Keywords

Coronary heart disease • Revascularisation • Smooth muscle cell • Endothelial cell • Mechanisms

Introduction

The incidence of diabetes is increasing globally; the estimated prevalence in 2010 being 285 million worldwide (www.http://diabetes.org.uk). In the UK alone, the number of people diagnosed with diabetes has increased from 1.4 to 2.6 million since 1996 (www.http://diabetes.org.uk). These individuals are at high risk of cardiovascular disease and in this population coronary artery disease (CAD) is common, regularly manifesting itself earlier in life than in individuals without diabetes [1]. While strategies that maintain tight glucose control have been reported to ameliorate some of the microvascular complications of diabetes (retinopathy, nephropathy, neuropathy) [2], this approach appears to have little or no benefit in the macrovasculature [3]. A greater understanding of the complexity of the diabetic milieu may therefore be invaluable in exposing therapeutic targets to reduce the incidence of macrovascular diseases in diabetes.

Revascularisation in Patients with Diabetes

The predisposition to CAD and higher rates of myocardial infarction in diabetic individuals underlie the key cause of morbidity and mortality in this population [4, 5]. The pattern of CAD in diabetic patients is generally multivessel in nature [6, 7] and accounts for up to 80% of diabetes-related mortality [8]. The multiplicity and diffuse nature of atherosclerotic lesions is often complex in these patients, resulting in more difficult revascularisation procedures than in their non-diabetic counterparts [9]. Despite improvements in coronary interventional techniques, the risk of complications in diabetic patients remains, with considerably higher morbidity and inferior short- and long-term prognosis [10, 11]; yet patients with diabetes represent around twenty five percent of all those presenting for coronary revascularisation [12, 13]. In the general population, restenosis is the principal limiting factor that influences the

K.E. Porter (✉) • R.S. Mughal
Division of Cardiovascular and Neuronal Remodelling, Leeds Institute of Genetics, Health and Therapeutics, University of Leeds, Leeds, West Yorkshire, UK
e-mail: k.e.porter@leeds.ac.uk

A.A.F. Sima (ed.), *Diabetes & C-Peptide: Scientific and Clinical Aspects*, Contemporary Diabetes, DOI 10.1007/978-1-61779-391-2_11,

success of revascularisation procedures, and this pathology is characterised by enhanced intimal hyperplasia (IH) and impaired compensatory remodelling [9, 14]. However, irrespective of the technique employed, angioplasty, stenting or coronary artery bypass grafting (CABG) [15–17], the significantly inferior long-term outcomes in diabetic individuals are a key concern.

In spite of the limitations of revascularisation procedures, CABG appears to be a preferred strategy in patients with diabetes [18–20]. By necessity, this method invariably utilises the patient's own long saphenous vein (SV) as a bypass conduit due to ease of harvesting and ready availability. Alternatively, the internal mammary artery (IMA) is a more robust graft in both diabetic and non-diabetic patients alike [21]. However, its significantly smaller size is a major restriction to its more frequent use; perhaps more so in diabetic patients in whom multiple grafts are routinely required [7]. In patients with diabetes, the native SV wall has been shown to display marked intimal irregularities when compared with non-diabetic SV, the extent of which appears to be related to the degree of metabolic abnormality [22]. Interestingly, the same study demonstrated that the IMA was structurally preserved in diabetic and non-diabetic patients alike.

Implantation of venous bypass grafts has immediate effects on smooth muscle cell (SMC) and endothelial cell (EC) biology; removal from their normal anatomical location of low flow, pressure and shear stress exposes them to an arterial environment to which they are not adapted. Inevitable EC damage during harvesting and surgical grafting contributes to loss of homeostatic mechanisms, promoting SMC proliferation and migration that culminate in IH and ultimately graft occlusion and failure [23]. Diabetic patients undergoing CABG generally have accompanying complications of hyperglycaemia and hyperlipidaemia together with hypercoagulable tendency, all of which may impart vulnerability to complications [16]. However, even when good glycaemic control can be achieved, IH remains prevalent in SV bypass grafts of diabetic patients, suggesting that there are additional contributing factors to their poor outcome [24].

Role of Insulin

Clinical Studies

Among patients with diabetes, some early studies indicated that insulin levels per se may predict adverse macrovascular outcomes. For example, over 20 years ago, a Finnish study presented data that suggested an association between hyperinsulinaemia and the occurrence of vascular disease, concluding that greater clarification of the role of insulin as a risk factor was required [25]. Around the same time, a relationship between dose of exogenous insulin and extent of macrovascular disease was demonstrated [26] and the same authors further concluded that diabetic patients who developed CAD had a requirement for higher doses of insulin than those without incident disease [27]. However, during the 1990s, opinion as to whether insulin itself predisposed to cardiovascular risk was contradictory. A meta-analysis study claimed that elevated insulin was an independent risk factor [28], while other studies did not support such a view (reviewed in [29]).

Exogenous insulin replacement results in elevated serum levels [30, 31] and the prognostic importance of this is exemplified by a small observational study wherein insulin-treated adults with diabetes had a higher incidence of coronary heart disease [32]. In the same period, it was reported that excessive neointimal formation in patients with diabetes was likely to be a consequence of the complexity of the diabetic hormonal and biochemical milieu, but was associated with insulin treatment in particular [33], supporting the notion that insulin was potentially detrimental.

A more recent clinical study investigated the impact of diabetes and its co-morbidities on long-term survival of patients undergoing CABG [34]. Cardiac-related events were found to be similar in non-diabetic and diabetic patients, but, in accordance with the previous studies, survival was adversely affected in those patients who were insulin-treated. Taken together, these data suggest that the requirement for insulin therapy has a strong negative impact on long-term cardiac-specific survival.

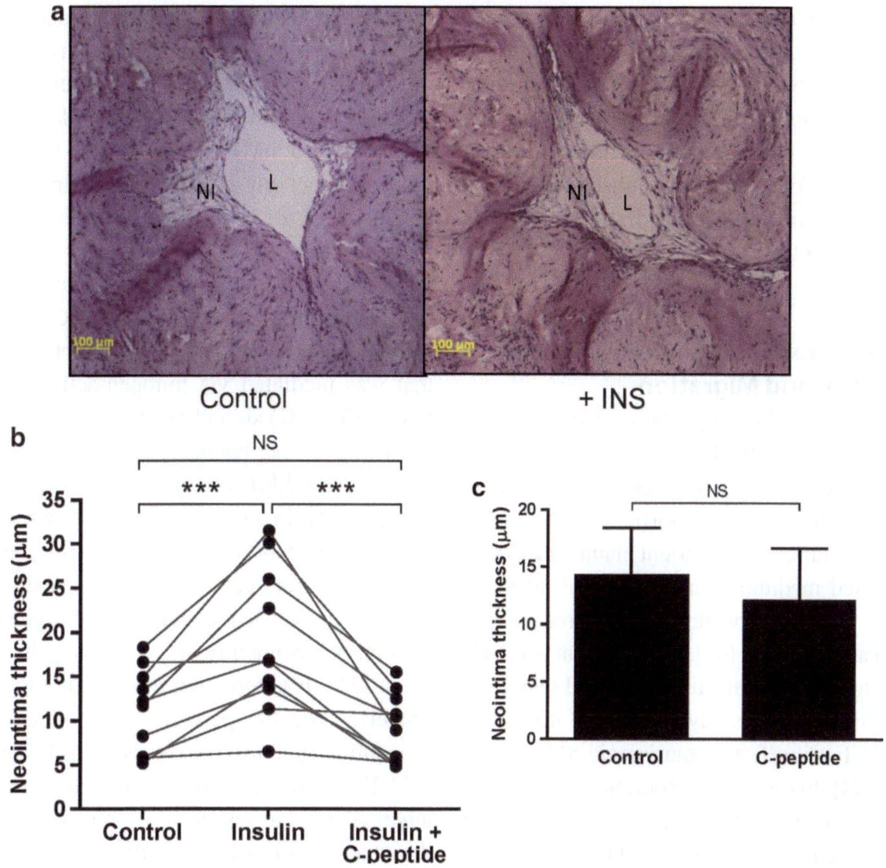

Fig. 11.1 (**a**) Representative histological cross-sections of saphenous vein (SV) rings cultured in the absence (control) or presence (+INS) of 100 nM insulin for 14 days. Insulin promotes increased neointimal (NI) formation and reduced lumen (L) size. (**b**) Image analysis of full length SV sections to calculate mean neointima thickness. Scatter plot shows individual values from different patients, with data from the same patients linked. ***$p<0.001$, *NS* not statistically significant ($n=10$). Adapted from [42]. (**c**) C-peptide treatment alone (10 nM) has no modulatory effect on NI thickness, *NS* not statistically significant ($n=4$)

Experimental Studies

Neointima Formation In Vivo and In Vitro

Insulin, while effectively controlling blood glucose in insulin-dependent diabetes, has been shown to exacerbate IH in vivo in laboratory animals. Following arterial balloon injury, insulin administration increased neointima formation in normal [35] and diabetic [36, 37] rats. Chronic insulin treatment in cholesterol-fed rabbits aggravated atherosclerosis [38], although another similar study claimed no effect [39]. In contrast, recent evidence in a rat arterial injury model reported that insulin treatment decreased neointimal thickness, suggesting a vasculoprotective effect [40]. These discrepant results may be due to differences in the dose of insulin, timescale of treatment and/or follow-up and cell-type or species specificity.

While there are no data from human in vivo studies, insulin enhanced neointima formation in organ-cultured human SV and IMA in vitro [41]. Our own recent studies clearly demonstrated insulin treatment of SV organ cultures from multiple patients without diabetes led to a significant augmentation of neointimal thickening compared with paired, untreated segments from the same patient (Fig. 11.1a, b [42]). Moreover, we also noted that the magnitude of effect in response to insulin was variable between patient samples. Since increased SMC proliferation and migration are critical events leading to vascular neointima formation, it is possible that insulin acting on SMC may therefore impact upon the pathogenesis of IH in insulin-dependent diabetic patients discussed below.

Vascular Smooth Muscle Cell Proliferation and Migration

Vascular SMC are known to be responsive to the growth-stimulatory effects of insulin and insulin-like growth factors (IGF). Stout et al. demonstrated that insulin induced primate aortic SMC proliferation in a concentration-dependent manner in serum-supplemented medium over a period of up to 10 days [43]. Similarly, insulin induced proliferation of human arterial SMC [44], an effect that was later proposed to be due to insulin-stimulated release of IGF-1 [45]. Another study showed a mitogenic effect of IGF-1 itself on human aortic SMC (measured by ^{3}[H] thymidine incorporation) albeit with lower potency than the classical SMC mitogen platelet-derived growth factor (PDGF-BB) [46]. In our own recent study, to avoid the confounding issue of undefined growth factors contained in serum, we utilised a "basal" medium containing minimal serum (0.2% v/v) combined with PDGF. In accordance with previous reports, we discovered that supplementation with insulin increased SV-SMC proliferation concentration – dependently yet interestingly, IMA-SMC cultured from the *same* patients were entirely resistant to insulin's growth-promoting effects [42]. Clearly the pathogenesis of graft IH is multifactorial; however, this lack of mitogenic effect of insulin on IMA-SMC may offer an explanation for the superior patency rates of IMA grafts, even in diabetic patients.

In addition to insulin, glucose has been reported to increase proliferation of cultured human infragenicular SMC and together they are synergistic [47]. However, that particular study was performed using SMC from patients with diabetes; cells from non-diabetic subjects were not investigated. Some other studies have reported a growth-promoting effect of high glucose alone on vascular SMC; in human aorta and umbilical artery (25 mM) [48], and rat aorta (20 mM) [49, 50]. In contrast, our own studies using SMC cultured from multiple patients under conditions of normal (5.5 mM) and elevated (25 mM) glucose did not detect any growth-modulating properties of glucose itself in cells of either non-diabetic or diabetic origin [51].

As well as its demonstrable effects on proliferation, insulin can influence SMC migration. In bovine aortic SMC, insulin promoted migration that was mediated via mitogen-activated protein kinase (MAPK) signalling [52]. In our laboratory, we demonstrated that insulin promotes chemotaxis of human SV-SMC of non-diabetic origin [42, 51]. Interestingly, in a separate study we observed that cells of diabetic origin consistently exhibited higher migratory capacities than those of non-diabetic origin when maintained in the presence of insulin, independently of its role as a chemotactic agent [51]. It is tempting to speculate that in the diabetic state the perceived "beneficial" effects of insulin signalling via phosphoinositide 3-kinase (PI3-K) are impaired, while the "detrimental" (pro-atherogenic, pro-restenosis) pathways may predominate via preserved MAPK signalling.

Proinsulin C-Peptide

The 31-amino acid human proinsulin C-peptide links the A and B chains of proinsulin and ensures correct protein folding. C-peptide is cleaved from proinsulin during insulin biosynthesis and is subsequently released as a by-product into the circulation with insulin [53, 54]. Patients with Type 1 diabetes have low or absent C-peptide due to impaired proinsulin synthesis. In contrast, C-peptide levels are initially elevated in Type 2 diabetic patients, but they also eventually become insulin-dependent. Early studies to address any physiological roles for C-peptide concluded that it performed no biological functions (reviewed in [55]), inferred from the lack of conservation of the C-peptide sequence across species both in terms of chain length and amino acid composition. Hence, relatively little further interest was shown until the early 1990s when administration of the peptide to patients with Type 1 diabetes demonstrated surprising findings that provoked renewed enthusiasm.

It was found that patients with low but sustained plasma concentrations of C-peptide were less prone to the long-term diabetic microvascular complications than those totally C-peptide-deficient [56–58]. Importantly, chronic administration of *replacement* doses of C-peptide has been shown to be effective in the microvasculature in both animal models and patients with Type 1 diabetes (reviewed in [59–61]). Conversely, C-peptide infusion into healthy individuals had no demonstrable effects, suggesting that at normal plasma concentrations (0.5–1.5 nM) [60] saturation of C-peptide-binding sites is achieved and that further increasing levels of C-peptide imparts no benefit [62]. Indeed, saturation of C-peptide binding has been shown to occur at a concentration of 0.9 nM in membranes of renal tubular cells [61].

In summary, in the last 15 years, there has been a wealth of new studies reporting the impact of C-peptide on a variety of cell types and cell functions, with the general perception that C-peptide is beneficial (reviewed in [63, 64]). Its effects in the microvessels have generated intense interest and activity, although less is known of its role in the coronary and peripheral circulation. The role of C-peptide deficiency as a risk factor for CAD and its accompanying complications certainly deserves further study. Current opinion in this area will now be discussed.

Cellular Effects of C-Peptide

Vascular Endothelial Cells

In health, physiological concentrations of nitric oxide (NO) are synthesised by the endothelium through the expression and activity of nitric oxide synthase (eNOS), thus maintaining vascular tone and endothelial homeostasis (reviewed in [65]). A key mediator of endothelial dysfunction and a major hallmark of diabetes is hyperglycaemia, leading to impaired NO synthesis and subsequent endothelial dysfunction that precedes the onset of atherosclerosis [66]. Observations of cultured EC in high glucose concentrations have also shown increased apoptosis, suggesting another mechanism of endothelial damage inflicted by hyperglycaemia in diabetic patients [67]. Further, it has been reported that intermittent cycles of hyperglycaemia are more damaging than steady high glucose levels [68], suggesting that poor glycaemic control is deleterious.

Around two decades ago, EC dysfunction and reduced response to endothelial NO was demonstrated in isolated blood vessels from diabetic patients [69] and confirmed in vivo by studies of forearm blood flow in diabetic individuals [70]. Another study conducted in exercising diabetic patients using the same technique produced the first report of increased vasodilatation as a result of acute C-peptide infusion [71], effects that were also apparent at rest [72]. Interestingly, this C-peptide-induced vasodilatation was not observed in non-diabetic individuals, a result explained by more recent reports that demonstrated "saturability" at physiological levels of C-peptide.

Multiple studies have suggested that, at least in the microvessels, vascular dysfunction in diabetes is associated with decreased levels of circulating C-peptide (reviewed in [61, 73]), leading to the hypothesis that normalising circulating levels of C-peptide may improve vascular function. Support for this concept is the fact that whole pancreas [74] or islet [75] transplantation reduces diabetic nephropathy and improves renal function following a period of normoglycaemia compared to treatment with insulin alone. It is therefore conceivable that the approach of C-peptide replacement might also be applicable to alleviating macrovascular disease such as atherosclerosis and its resultant complications.

In the absence of diabetes, NO secretion maintains endothelial integrity and function, but in the presence of risk factors the endothelium can be activated to express adhesion molecules, cytokines and chemotactic factors that contribute to an inflammatory state in arterial walls and promote atherosclerosis [76]. In vitro, exposure of human umbilical vein EC to elevated (30 mM) glucose selectively induced expression of ICAM-1 within 24 h that was maintained for up to 2 weeks [77]. Similarly, a more recent study of cultured human

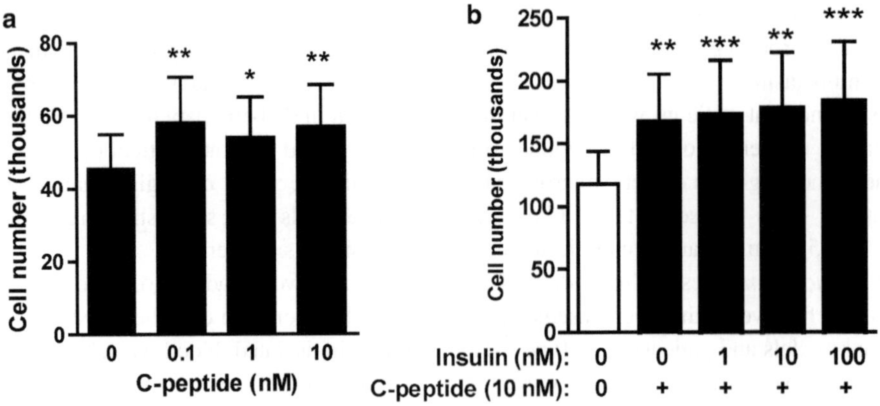

Fig. 11.2 (**a**) C-peptide increases human SV-EC proliferation over a 5-day period. A modest but consistent (~40%) increase in cell number is observed at all concentrations of C-peptide. ANOVA $p<0.001$ for the effect of C-peptide $**p<0.01$, $*p<0.05$ vs. control ($n=6$) [42]. (**b**) Co-supplementation of C-peptide-treated SV-EC (10 nM) with 0–100 nM insulin for 5 days does not modulate the effect of C-peptide alone. $***p<0.001$, $**p<0.01$ ($n=5$). Adapted from [42]

aortic endothelium demonstrated that short-term exposure to high (25 mM), but not normal (5.6 mM), glucose levels induced expression of endothelial VCAM-1, increased monocyte adherence and increased secretion of IL-8 and MCP-1 [78]. Interestingly, co-incubation with physiological levels of C-peptide abolished all these effects, leading the authors to speculate that C-peptide administration to insulin-dependent patients might ameliorate the pro-inflammatory state induced by hyperglycaemia at the level of both endothelial and immune cell function. In support of these data, two previous studies of vascular injury demonstrated that C-peptide could attenuate the expression of P-selectin and ICAM-1 in rat microvascular endothelium in vivo [79]. Furthermore, reduced leukocyte infiltration into perfused hearts taken from C-peptide-treated animals was shown to be due to enhanced NO release [80]. Direct evidence for the ability of C-peptide to increase NO production through enhanced eNOS expression has also been reported in cultured aortic EC [81]. The potential limitations of that study were the use of *human* C-peptide to stimulate *rat* EC, although some homology is reported [82]. The levels of glucose used in those studies are also not stated.

Taken together, the above reports suggest that C-peptide at replacement concentrations has potential to recover EC dysfunction in diabetic macrovascular complications. However, in all these studies the effect of insulin itself was not investigated yet; in healthy individuals C-peptide is only ever present with insulin. In our own laboratory, we recently explored the effects of insulin and C-peptide, alone and in combination, on human SV EC proliferation and migration [42]. Using cells cultured from multiple non-diabetic patients, neither C-peptide nor insulin, alone or combined, had any discernible effect on EC migration over a 24-h period. Conversely, we revealed that physiological levels of C-peptide (0.1–10 nM) induced an increase in EC number of ~40% over a 5-day period, a maximum growth-promoting effect being observed at the lowest concentration and maintained at higher concentrations (Fig. 11.2a [42]). Exposure of EC to insulin alone (1–100 nM) had no effect, but importantly, neither synergism nor modulation of C-peptide effects by insulin was apparent (Fig. 11.2b). Our data suggest that the pro-proliferative capacity of C-peptide on SV EC may impart benefits by accelerating re-endothelialisation which is known to inhibit neo-IH [83].

A few studies have suggested that, under certain circumstances, there may be synergism between insulin and C-peptide, although such a relationship has not been reported in human vascular cells. A study performed in rat L6 and 3T3 fibroblasts showed that physiological concentrations of C-peptide can mimic the effect of insulin, with their effects being additive, although only at submaximal concentrations of each [84]. In human neuroblastoma SH-SY5Y cells, C-peptide in the presence of insulin enhanced cell growth and protected against high glucose-induced apoptosis [85]. Insulin and C-peptide separately induced dose-dependent arteriolar dilatation in the rat, although the response to insulin was significantly depressed in diabetic animals [59]. The authors further demonstrated that pre-treatment with a low dose of C-peptide restored the dilator response to insulin in the diabetic animals, proposing a role for synergistic interaction between them.

Vascular Smooth Muscle Cells

Proliferation and migration of vascular SMC and resultant neointima formation are central to the development and progression of atherosclerosis and restenosis [86], events that are augmented in patients with diabetes [33]. Previously mentioned studies [43, 44, 46, 47, 50] reported that hyperglycaemia and hyperinsulinaemia, alone or in combination, can accelerate SMC proliferation, although C-peptide has only been investigated in more recent years.

Kobayashi et al. reported that high glucose-induced rat aortic SMC proliferation was inhibited by human C-peptide [49]; the opposite effect to that reported for insulin. However, limitations of that study were that insulin was not investigated and that supra-physiological levels of C-peptide (~100-fold) over a prolonged period (3 weeks) were required to observe an effect. Although substantial homology between rat and human C-peptide has been demonstrated [82], species and cell-type specific effects may explain these data. A more recent publication that used human C-peptide and two different arterial sources of human SMC showed that acute high glucose-induced proliferation was inhibited by C-peptide [48]. In that study, although replacement levels of C-peptide were utilised and inhibitory effects on SMC proliferation were apparent, as in the previous study, the effects of insulin itself were not explored.

It has been frequently documented that positive effects of C-peptide cannot be detected in healthy individuals, but are only observed in animal models and diabetic patients that exhibit low or absent C-peptide [59–61]. Therefore, any potential adverse vascular effects of endogenous insulin in non-diabetic patients may well be counteracted by the concomitant secretion of C-peptide. As discussed earlier in this chapter, the outcomes of CABG in patients with diabetes are significantly poorer than in their non-diabetic counterparts, particularly after SV grafting. Therefore, we explored the effects of insulin and C-peptide, alone and in combination, on human SV neointima formation and SV-SMC proliferation and migration. One of the key findings of our study was that neointima formation in organ-cultured SV was increased by insulin (Fig. 11.1a, b) and consistently abolished by co-incubation with C-peptide (Fig. 11.1b [42]). Surprisingly, C-peptide alone had no discernible effect and neointimal thickness was comparable with vehicle-treated vein segments (Fig. 11.1c). These effects were mirrored in SV-SMC proliferation and migration assays and, taken together, would support the notion that whilst insulin treatment provides metabolic control in the diabetic individual, concomitant treatment with replacement levels of C-peptide may negate the potential adverse effects of insulin on SV-SMC. The cell-type specific effects of both insulin and C-peptide were underscored by our observation that, in paired IMA-SMC, neither insulin nor C-peptide-induced proliferation and, perhaps not surprisingly, no modulatory or synergistic effects were apparent [42]. To summarise, our own work adds another element to the repertoire of C-peptide as a multifunctional peptide whose replacement in insulin-dependent diabetes may improve outcomes following SV bypass grafting.

Mechanisms of C-Peptide's Functional Effects

An examination of the literature indicates that the functional influences of C-peptide and associated underlying mechanisms are by no means universal or straightforward. Mechanisms that have been proposed for its beneficial effects are diverse yet often related and include increasing intracellular Ca^{2+}, phosphorylation of MAPK pathways, stimulation of Na^+ K^+-ATPase and increasing release of NO via upregulated eNOS expression and regulating expression and nuclear translocation of NF-κB (reviewed in [87]). C-peptide-induced suppression of pro-inflammatory NF-κB signalling has also been ascribed to correction of human aortic EC dysfunction [78].

Despite the reported diversity of biological effects, a target receptor for C-peptide has not been identified; nor does C-peptide bind to other peptide hormone receptors such as the insulin or IGF receptor [88]. Our own recent studies support this view since we demonstrated robust phosphorylation of Akt by insulin in SV-SMC, but no effect of C-peptide, and importantly, no evidence of modulation or synergism between them [42]. A similar pattern of effects was evident in respect of the MAPK-signalling pathway. On the contrary, previous studies have shown that several components of the PI3-K pathway are regulated by physiological concentrations of C-peptide, although these reports relate to cells of non-cardiovascular origin (reviewed in [87]).

In direct contrast to our own data, other studies in cardiovascular cell types have shown that the *antiproliferative* effect of C-peptide is mediated via *increased* phosphorylation of MAPK in rat aortic SMC [49], and another study showed that C-peptide-induced up-regulation of eNOS in rat aortic EC is also MAPK-dependent [81]. Through activation of p38 MAPK signalling, C-peptide was shown to activate cAMP response element (CRE) binding proteins in murine capillary EC, suggesting that CRE-dependent gene expression was important for its function in these cells [89].

Crucially, it appears therefore that the effects of C-peptide are species, tissue and cell-type-specific [90], emphasising the need to select relevant models to explore specific pathologies.

Binding and Cellular Internalisation of C-Peptide

Specific binding of C-peptide to human cell membranes appears to exhibit tissue specificity. Using Scatchard analysis, Rigler et al. found that a high affinity binding process was evident in human renal tubular cells with an association constant (K_{ass}) of 3.3×10^{9} M^{-1}. In the same study, human SV endothelium was shown to bind C-peptide with a K_{ass} of 2.0×10^{9} M^{-1}, yet in umbilical vein endothelial membranes there was a complete absence of binding [88]. The authors remarked that these findings were consistent with the observation that C-peptide was able to stimulate NO synthesis in aortic, but not umbilical vein EC [88]. Another report indicated that C-peptide was able to bind and cross plasma membranes in two different cell lines, HEK293 and Swiss 3T3 fibroblasts, localising in both the cytoplasm and the cell nucleus [91]. Moreover, specific nucleolar localisation was recently demonstrated that resulted in transcriptional effects on genes encoding for ribosomal RNA [92].

Upon localisation in the cytoplasm, it is also possible that C-peptide's functional effects are achieved through interaction with other subcellular components. Indeed, a recent study in human vascular EC and SMC revealed that, upon internalisation from the plasma membrane, fluorescent-labelled C-peptide co-localises with early endosomes [93]. The authors hypothesised that endosomes may therefore be a signalling "station" via which C-peptide mediates its functional activity in target cells.

SREBP-1 as a Novel Mediator in Vascular SMC?

In the absence of any clear modulatory effects of C-peptide, either alone or on insulin-mediated PI3-K and MAPK signalling, we progressed our studies by implementing a focused PCR array approach to identify potential molecular targets of insulin and investigate any modulation by C-peptide. Based on changes in transcript levels and statistical significance, we found that sterol regulatory element (SRE)-binding transcription factor-1 (SREBF1) and insulin-like growth factor receptor (IGF-1R) mRNA expression were increased in response to insulin, changes confirmed by real-time RT-PCR. Crucially, insulin-induced SREBF1 expression was fully prevented by co-incubation with C-peptide, whereas the effect of insulin on IGF-1R expression was not modulated by C-peptide (Fig. 11.3a, b [42]).

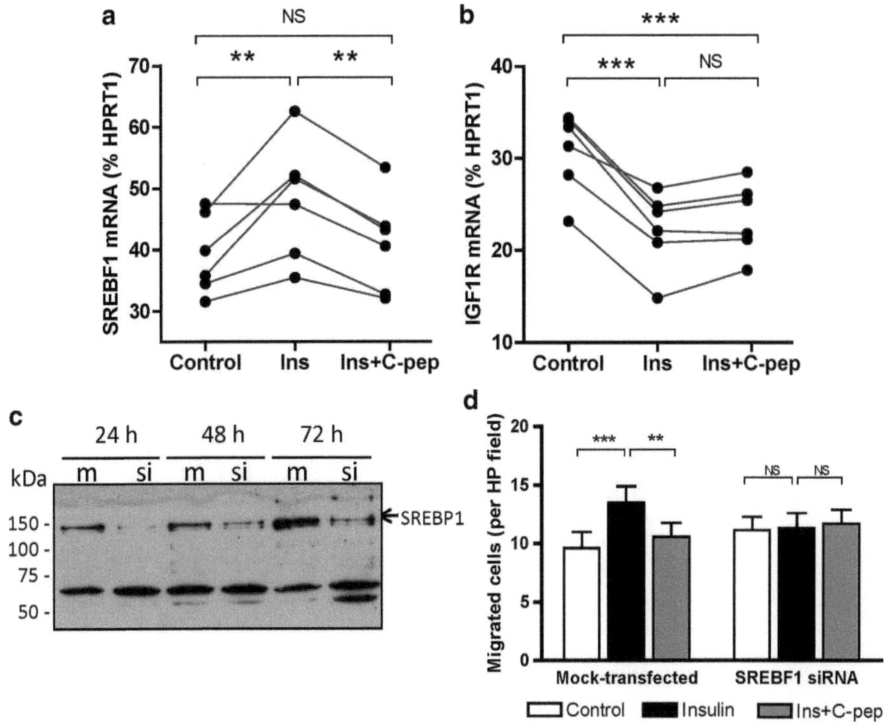

Fig. 11.3 Real-time RT-PCR data showing mRNA levels of SREBF1 (**a**) and IGF-1R (**b**) as percentage of HPRT1 housekeeping gene mRNA levels after 6-h treatment with 100 nM insulin alone or combined with 10 nM C-peptide. $^{***}p<0.001$, $^{**}p<0.01$, *NS* not statistically significant ($n=6$) [42]. (**c**) Western blot showing the effect of SREBF1 silencing on SREBP1 (125 kDa) expression between 24 and 72 h following siRNA transfection. m=mock transfected; si=SREBF1 siRNA transfected. (**d**) Migration assay performed 36 h after siRNA transfection, showing abolition of insulin's chemotactic effect in SREBF1-silenced cells

We therefore considered whether SREBF1 gene silencing would have any functional effect in SV-SMC and, to this end, cells were transfected with SREBF1 siRNA. Having confirmed significant knockdown of SREBP1 (the protein product of SREBF1) over a 72-h period (Fig. 11.3c), we performed SV-SMC migration assays. SREBF1 gene-silencing did not affect basal motility, but specifically abolished the additional migration observed in response to insulin. The level of inhibition achieved by SREBF-1 gene silencing was comparable to that observed with C-peptide (Fig. 11.3d [42]). One could therefore hypothesise that the ability of C-peptide to prevent insulin-mediated SV-SMC migration is through reduced SREBP1 expression, although this still remains to be verified.

SREBP1 belongs to a family of the basic helix-loop-helix-leucine zipper transcription factors that control lipid and carbohydrate metabolism and are therefore critical regulators of cellular membrane structure and function [94]. There are two isoforms of SREBP1, of which the 1c isoform is considered important in insulin-dependent functions due to its abundance in metabolic tissue. SREBPs are synthesised in the endoplasmic reticulum where they are retained as inactive precursors by SREB cleavage-activating protein (SCAP). In turn, the SREBP1/SCAP complex is held in the ER by binding of SCAP to the Insig proteins 1 and 2. In response to cellular demand for cholesterol, SCAP serves to escort SREBP1 from the ER to the Golgi [95] where sequential site-specific processing by two proteases S1P and S2P liberates the mature form of SREBP1 [96]. This mature form then translocates to the cell nucleus where its specific binding to SRE is able to regulate target gene expression [97]. Our studies in SV-SMC demonstrated a robust insulin-induced phosphorylation of Akt (via PI3-K)

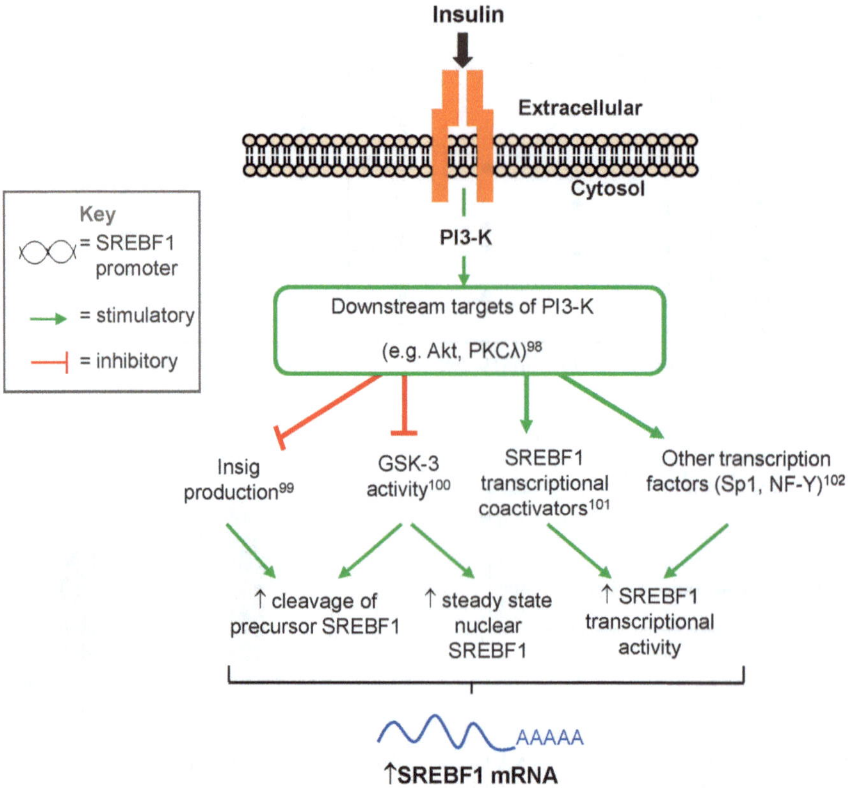

Fig. 11.4 Potential mediators of insulin-induced SREBF1. Shown are intermediary targets that lead to enhanced SREBP1 precursor cleavage, increased nuclear SREBP1 concentration and SREBP1 transcriptional activity, ultimately resulting in increased SREBF1 transcription. *Green arrows* represent a stimulatory action on PI3-K, Akt, PKCλ, SREBF1 transcriptional activity and other transcription factors (e.g. Sp1, NF-Y). *Red* pathways indicate inhibitory effect on Insig production and GSK-3 activity

leading to an increase in SREBF1 mRNA [42]. Other published work, although in non-vascular tissues, has elucidated some of the intermediary elements in this pathway. For example, insulin-induced SREBF1 transcription was shown to be dependent on activation of the downstream effector protein kinase C lambda (PKCλ) [98]. In other studies, insulin was shown to downregulate Insig proteins [99], inhibit activity of GSK-3 [100], or increase SREBF1 transcriptional activity through interaction with coactivators [101]. In rat primary hepatocytes, it was reported that the combined action of several transcription factors is required for activation of the SREBF1 promoter by insulin, including Sp1, NF-Y (nuclear factor Y) and SREBP1 itself [102]. It is feasible that any of these mechanisms are actively involved in insulin-induced SREBF1 expression as we observed in SV-SMC.

Figure 11.4 provides a summary of these data.

Potential Future Directions

An interesting recent study reported that SREBP1 is enhanced in murine aortic SMC after in vivo vascular injury, and in vitro in response to mitogenic stimulation, co-localising with α-smooth muscle actin [103]. SREBP1 is known to control many genes required for cellular lipid homeostasis, thereby regulating the plasma membrane [104]; its enhancement could therefore increase plasma membrane synthesis of cholesterol and other lipids and modulate properties necessary for cell

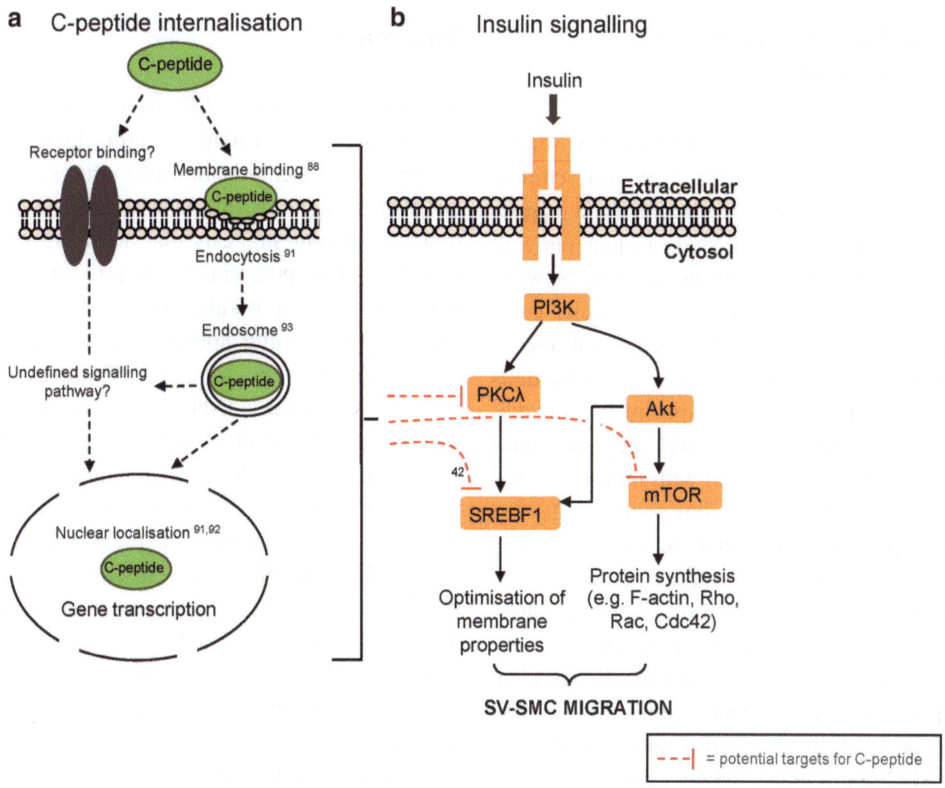

Fig. 11.5 Illustration of C-peptide internalisation and suggested targets for the opposing action of C-peptide on insulin-induced SV-SMC migration. (**a**) We propose that C-peptide binds to SV-SMC membranes, is internalised via endocytosis and subsequently transported through the cell via endosomes. We have previously shown transcriptional effects of C-peptide, therefore it is possible that C-peptide is localising within the nucleus. Classical ligand-receptor binding of C-peptide to an unknown receptor with subsequent downstream signalling cannot be ruled out. (**b**) Insulin binding to its receptor activates PI3-K and Akt. SREBF1 and mTOR are both downstream components of PI3-K signalling and are required for cell migration. Opposing actions of C-peptide on insulin-induced migration may occur in the cytosol with direct effects on target molecules downstream of Akt (PKCλ, SREBP1, mTOR) or via an endosome "signalling station". Additionally, transcriptional effects of C-peptide on associated target genes may occur following nuclear localisation

proliferation in response to mitogenic stimuli. Correspondingly, insulin-induced SREBP1 expression as we observed in our study [42] most likely optimises membrane properties to facilitate SMC migration, and notably, SREBF1 gene silencing effectively abolished insulin-induced migration. Whether the attenuated migratory response observed with C-peptide is directly attributable to its ability to suppress insulin-induced SREBP1 expression requires further study.

Recent evidence has suggested that irregularities in mTOR (mammalian target of rapamycin) function may contribute to certain disease states (e.g. cancer, diabetes) [105]. mTOR is a key regulator of cell growth and proliferation, acting downstream of PI3-K signalling and is involved in modulating protein synthesis in response to insulin [106]. mTOR has also been shown to be an important regulator of cell migration through its ability to stimulate F-actin and activate Rho family GTPases including Cdc42, Rac1 and RhoA, all of which are necessary for cell migration [107]. It is therefore intriguing to consider a role for mTOR in insulin-induced SV-SMC migration and the potential for C-peptide to suppress mTOR itself or prevent activation of its targets. An illustration of C-peptide internalisation and intracellular localisation is depicted in Fig. 11.5, together with proposed targets for C-peptide's capacity to prevent insulin-induced SV-SMC migration.

Does C-Peptide Contribute to Atherogenesis?

While many clinical and experimental studies would support the notion that C-peptide confers beneficial effects in the vasculature, a few oppose this view. A small clinical study in patients with type 2 diabetes reported an association between serum C-peptide levels and macrovascular complications (coronary artery and peripheral arterial disease), but not microvascular complications [108]. In another study, aortic specimens from diabetic subjects displayed elevated C-peptide immunoreactivity that co-localised with monocytes and lymphocytes [109, 110], leading to the suggestion that C-peptide is detrimental. In vitro, the same studies observed that C-peptide concentration dependently stimulated chemotaxis and a subsequent study by the same group reported similar functional effects on cultured rat aortic SMC [111]. It is possible therefore that chronically elevated C-peptide levels as observed in insulin resistance and early Type 2 diabetes may contribute to and accelerate atherogenesis [112]. It is notable that these studies were performed in the presence of C-peptide alone; insulin was not investigated and therefore the possibility exists that modulatory or synergistic interaction between insulin and C-peptide might occur. In vivo, insulin without C-peptide would be found in insulin-treated diabetic individuals, while C-peptide is only ever present together with insulin in healthy individuals. However, in the clinical setting of Type 2 diabetes, elevated C-peptide would inevitably also be accompanied by raised levels of insulin, which itself may be a contributing factor to observed functional effects. This is exemplified by our own recent work in which, in contrast to SV-SMC, C-peptide in isolation (a scenario that would not exist in vivo) was observed to *increase* proliferation of human aortic SMC to a level comparable with that of insulin alone. But of perhaps greater relevance, when administered together there was no further modulation, i.e. in the presence of insulin, C-peptide had *no* additional effect [42]. Further clarification is therefore needed in this respect. The evidence for C-peptide as an atherogenic molecule is reviewed fully in Chap. 13.

Summary

The impaired ability of ECs to regenerate and/or regain function is a major limiting factor to the success of revascularisation procedures, particularly in patients with diabetes. The evidence reviewed herein suggests that administration of C-peptide has potential to restore endothelial homeostasis at a number of functional levels including preventing apoptosis, promoting proliferation and ameliorating inflammation through reduced adhesion molecule expression. Moreover, the stimulatory effect of hyperglycaemia and/or insulin on vascular SMC proliferation and migration, important contributors to neointima formation, can be abrogated by C-peptide in laboratory studies. If these effects are reproducible in man in vivo, then co-administration of replacement doses of C-peptide in insulin-dependent diabetic patients holds potential to reduce failure of vascular reconstructions. Clinical trials will be required to test this hypothesis.

In conclusion, C-peptide therapy holds tremendous promise in treating or preventing a diversity of vascular complications in diabetes. On a cautionary note, the possibility of C-peptide being pro-atherogenic cannot be ignored. However, with robust evidence of species, tissue and cell-type-specific effects, together with a multiplicity of reported mechanisms, it may ultimately be feasible to exploit this diversity and design "pathway-targeted" approaches.

References

1. Flaherty JD, Davidson CJ. Diabetes and coronary revascularization. JAMA. 2005;293(12):1501–8.
2. Nathan DM, Cleary PA, Backlund JY, et al. Intensive diabetes treatment and cardiovascular disease in patients with type 1 diabetes. N Engl J Med. 2005; 353(25):2643–53.
3. Duckworth W, Abraira C, Moritz T, et al. Glucose control and vascular complications in veterans with type 2 diabetes. N Engl J Med. 2009;360(2): 129–39.
4. Kannel WB, McGee DL. Diabetes and cardiovascular risk factors: the Framingham study. Circulation. 1979;59(1):8–13.
5. Lee CD, Folsom AR, Pankow JS, Brancati FL. Cardiovascular events in diabetic and nondiabetic

adults with or without history of myocardial infarction. Circulation. 2004;109(7):855–60.
6. Goraya TY, Leibson CL, Palumbo PJ, et al. Coronary atherosclerosis in diabetes mellitus: a population-based autopsy study. J Am Coll Cardiol. 2002; 40(5):946–53.
7. Vlietstra RE, Kronmal RA, Frye RL, Seth AK, Tristani FE, Killip III T. Factors affecting the extent and severity of coronary artery disease in patients enrolled in the coronary artery surgery study. Arteriosclerosis. 1982;2(3):208–15.
8. Moreno PR, Fuster V. New aspects in the pathogenesis of diabetic atherothrombosis. J Am Coll Cardiol. 2004;44(12):2293–300.
9. Nicholls SJ, Tuzcu EM, Kalidindi S, et al. Effect of diabetes on progression of coronary atherosclerosis and arterial remodeling: a pooled analysis of 5 intravascular ultrasound trials. J Am Coll Cardiol. 2008;52(4):255–62.
10. Berry C, Tardif JC, Bourassa MG. Coronary heart disease in patients with diabetes: part II: recent advances in coronary revascularization. J Am Coll Cardiol. 2007;49(6):643–56.
11. Kubal C, Srinivasan AK, Grayson AD, Fabri BM, Chalmers JA. Effect of risk-adjusted diabetes on mortality and morbidity after coronary artery bypass surgery. Ann Thorac Surg. 2005;79(5):1570–6.
12. Daemen J, Kuck KH, Macaya C, et al. Multivessel coronary revascularization in patients with and without diabetes mellitus: 3-year follow-up of the ARTS-II (Arterial Revascularization Therapies Study-Part II) trial. J Am Coll Cardiol. 2008;52(24): 1957–67.
13. Hammoud T, Tanguay JF, Bourassa MG. Management of coronary artery disease: therapeutic options in patients with diabetes. J Am Coll Cardiol. 2000;36(2): 355–65.
14. Lexis CP, Rahel BM, Meeder JG, Zijlstra F, van der Horst IC. The role of glucose lowering agents on restenosis after percutaneous coronary intervention in patients with diabetes mellitus. Cardiovasc Diabetol. 2009;8:41.
15. Cutlip DE, Chauhan MS, Baim DS, et al. Clinical restenosis after coronary stenting: perspectives from multicenter clinical trials. J Am Coll Cardiol. 2002;40(12):2082–9.
16. Hakala T, Pitkanen O, Halonen P, Mustonen J, Turpeinen A, Hippelainen M. Early and late outcome after coronary artery bypass surgery in diabetic patients. Scand Cardiovasc J. 2005;39(3):177–81.
17. Kornowski R, Mintz GS, Kent KM, et al. Increased restenosis in diabetes mellitus after coronary interventions is due to exaggerated intimal hyperplasia. A serial intravascular ultrasound study. Circulation. 1997;95(6):1366–9.
18. The Bypass Angioplasty Revascularization Investigation (BARI) Investigators. Comparison of coronary bypass surgery with angioplasty in patients with multivessel disease. N Engl J Med. 1996;335(4): 217–25.
19. Kapur A, Hall RJ, Malik IS, et al. Randomized comparison of percutaneous coronary intervention with coronary artery bypass grafting in diabetic patients. 1-year results of the CARDia (Coronary Artery Revascularization in Diabetes) trial. J Am Coll Cardiol. 2010;55(5):432–40.
20. Niles NW, McGrath PD, Malenka D, et al. Survival of patients with diabetes and multivessel coronary artery disease after surgical or percutaneous coronary revascularization: results of a large regional prospective study. Northern New England Cardiovascular Disease Study Group. J Am Coll Cardiol. 2001;37(4):1008–15.
21. The BARI Investigators. Influence of diabetes on 5-year mortality and morbidity in a randomized trial comparing CABG and PTCA in patients with multivessel disease: the Bypass Angioplasty Revascularization Investigation (BARI). Circulation. 1997;96(6):1761–9.
22. Lorusso R, Pentiricci S, Raddino R, et al. Influence of type 2 diabetes on functional and structural properties of coronary artery bypass conduits. Diabetes. 2003;52(11):2814–20.
23. Wallitt EJ, Jevon M, Hornick PI. Therapeutics of vein graft intimal hyperplasia: 100 years on. Ann Thorac Surg. 2007;84(1):317–23.
24. Nathan DM. Long-term complications of diabetes mellitus. N Engl J Med. 1993;328(23):1676–85.
25. Pyorala K, Uusitupa M, Laakso M, Siitonen O, Niskanen L, Ronnemaa T. Macrovascular complications in relation to hyperinsulinaemia in non-insulin-dependent diabetes mellitus. Diabete Metab. 1987; 13(3 Pt 2):345–9.
26. Janka HU, Ziegler AG, Standl E, Mehnert H. Daily insulin dose as a predictor of macrovascular disease in insulin treated non-insulin-dependent diabetics. Diabete Metab. 1987;13(3 Pt 2):359–64.
27. Standl E, Janka HU. High serum insulin concentrations in relation to other cardiovascular risk factors in macrovascular disease of type 2 diabetes. Horm Metab Res Suppl. 1985;15:46–51.
28. Ruige JB, Assendelft WJ, Dekker JM, Kostense PJ, Heine RJ, Bouter LM. Insulin and risk of cardiovascular disease: a meta-analysis. Circulation. 1998; 97(10):996–1001.
29. Laakso M. Insulin resistance and coronary heart disease. Curr Opin Lipidol. 1996;7(4):217–26.
30. Ginsberg S, Block MB, Mako ME, Rubenstein AH. Serum insulin levels following administration of exogenous insulin. J Clin Endocrinol Metab. 1973; 36(6):1175–9.
31. Mudaliar SR, Lindberg FA, Joyce M, et al. Insulin aspart (B28 asp-insulin): a fast-acting analog of human insulin: absorption kinetics and action profile compared with regular human insulin in healthy nondiabetic subjects. Diabetes Care. 1999;22(9): 1501–6.
32. Kronmal RA, Barzilay JI, Tracy RP, Savage PJ, Orchard TJ, Burke GL. The relationship of fasting serum radioimmune insulin levels to incident coronary

heart disease in an insulin-treated diabetic cohort. J Clin Endocrinol Metab. 2004;89(6):2852–8.
33. Aronson D, Bloomgarden Z, Rayfield EJ. Potential mechanisms promoting restenosis in diabetic patients. J Am Coll Cardiol. 1996;27(3):528–35.
34. Mohammadi S, Dagenais F, Mathieu P, et al. Long-term impact of diabetes and its comorbidities in patients undergoing isolated primary coronary artery bypass graft surgery. Circulation. 2007;116(11 Suppl): I220–5.
35. Foster E, Zhang S, Kahn AM. Insulin stimulates arterial neointima formation in normal rats after balloon injury. Diabetes Obes Metab. 2006;8(3): 348–51.
36. Indolfi C, Torella D, Cavuto L, et al. Effects of balloon injury on neointimal hyperplasia in streptozotocin-induced diabetes and in hyperinsulinemic nondiabetic pancreatic islet-transplanted rats. Circulation. 2001;103(24):2980–6.
37. Park SH, Marso SP, Zhou Z, Foroudi F, Topol EJ, Lincoff AM. Neointimal hyperplasia after arterial injury is increased in a rat model of non-insulin-dependent diabetes mellitus. Circulation. 2001;104(7): 815–9.
38. Marquie G. Effect of insulin in the induction and regression of experimental cholesterol atherosclerosis in the rabbit. Postgrad Med J. 1978;54(628): 80–5.
39. Nordestgaard BG, gerholm-Larsen B, Stender S. Effect of exogenous hyperinsulinaemia on atherogenesis in cholesterol-fed rabbits. Diabetologia. 1997;40(5):512–20.
40. Breen DM, Chan KK, Dhaliwall JK, et al. Insulin increases reendothelialization and inhibits cell migration and neointimal growth after arterial injury. Arterioscler Thromb Vasc Biol. 2009;29(7):1060–6.
41. Huang B, Dreyer T, Heidt M, et al. Insulin and local growth factor PDGF induce intimal hyperplasia in bypass graft culture models of saphenous vein and internal mammary artery. Eur J Cardiothorac Surg. 2002;21(6):1002–8.
42. Mughal RS, Scragg JL, Lister P, et al. Cellular mechanisms by which proinsulin C-peptide prevents insulin-induced neointima formation in human saphenous vein. Diabetologia. 2010;53:1761–71.
43. Stout RW, Bierman EL, Ross R. Effect of insulin on the proliferation of cultured primate arterial smooth muscle cells. Circ Res. 1975;36(2):319–27.
44. Pfeifle B, Ditschuneit H. Effect of insulin on growth of cultured human arterial smooth muscle cells. Diabetologia. 1981;20(2):155–8.
45. Pfeifle B, Hamann H, Fussganger R, Ditschuneit H. Insulin as a growth regulator of arterial smooth muscle cells: effect of insulin of I.G.F.I. Diabete Metab. 1987;13(3 Pt 2):326–30.
46. Bornfeldt KE, Raines EW, Nakano T, Graves LM, Krebs EG, Ross R. Insulin-like growth factor-I and platelet-derived growth factor-BB induce directed migration of human arterial smooth muscle cells via signaling pathways that are distinct from those of proliferation. J Clin Invest. 1994;93(3):1266–74.
47. Avena R, Mitchell ME, Neville RF, Sidawy AN. The additive effects of glucose and insulin on the proliferation of infragenicular vascular smooth muscle cells. J Vasc Surg. 1998;28(6):1033–8.
48. Cifarelli V, Luppi P, Tse HM, He J, Piganelli J, Trucco M. Human proinsulin C-peptide reduces high glucose-induced proliferation and NF-kappaB activation in vascular smooth muscle cells. Atherosclerosis. 2008;201(2):248–57.
49. Kobayashi Y, Naruse K, Hamada Y, et al. Human proinsulin C-peptide prevents proliferation of rat aortic smooth muscle cells cultured in high-glucose conditions. Diabetologia. 2005;48(11):2396–401.
50. Nakamura J, Kasuya Y, Hamada Y, et al. Glucose-induced hyperproliferation of cultured rat aortic smooth muscle cells through polyol pathway hyperactivity. Diabetologia. 2001;44(4):480–7.
51. Madi HA, Riches K, Warburton P, O'Regan DJ, Turner NA, Porter KE. Inherent differences in morphology, proliferation, and migration in saphenous vein smooth muscle cells cultured from nondiabetic and Type 2 diabetic patients. Am J Physiol Cell Physiol. 2009;297(5):C1307–17.
52. Wang CC, Gurevich I, Draznin B. Insulin affects vascular smooth muscle cell phenotype and migration via distinct signaling pathways. Diabetes. 2003; 52(10):2562–9.
53. Clark JL, Cho S, Rubenstein AH, Steiner DF. Isolation of a proinsulin connecting peptide fragment (C-peptide) from bovine and human pancreas. Biochem Biophys Res Commun. 1969;35(4): 456–61.
54. Steiner DF, Cunningham D, Spigelman L, Aten B. Insulin biosynthesis: evidence for a precursor. Science. 1967;157(789):697–700.
55. Kitabchi AE. Proinsulin and C-peptide: a review. Metabolism. 1977;26(5):547–87.
56. Sjoberg S, Gunnarsson R, Gjotterberg M, Lefvert AK, Persson A, Ostman J. Residual insulin production, glycaemic control and prevalence of microvascular lesions and polyneuropathy in long-term type 1 (insulin-dependent) diabetes mellitus. Diabetologia. 1987;30(4):208–13.
57. Sjoberg S, Gjotterberg M, Berglund L, Moller E, Ostman J. Residual C-peptide excretion is associated with a better long-term glycemic control and slower progress of retinopathy in type I (insulin-dependent) diabetes mellitus. J Diabet Complications. 1991;5(1): 18–22.
58. Zerbini G, Mangili R, Luzi L. Higher post-absorptive C-peptide levels in type 1 diabetic patients without renal complications. Diabet Med. 1999; 16(12):1048.
59. Joshua IG, Zhang Q, Falcone JC, Bratcher AP, Rodriguez WE, Tyagi SC. Mechanisms of endothelial dysfunction with development of type 1 diabetes mellitus: role of insulin and C-peptide. J Cell Biochem. 2005;96(6):1149–56.
60. Wahren J. C-peptide: new findings and therapeutic implications in diabetes. Clin Physiol Funct Imaging. 2004;24(4):180–9.

61. Wahren J, Shafqat J, Johansson J, Chibalin A, Ekberg K, Jornvall H. Molecular and cellular effects of C-peptide – new perspectives on an old peptide. Exp Diabesity Res. 2004;5(1):15–23.
62. Hoogwerf BJ, Bantle JP, Gaenslen HE, et al. Infusion of synthetic human C-peptide does not affect plasma glucose, serum insulin, or plasma glucagon in healthy subjects. Metabolism. 1986;35(2):122–5.
63. Hills CE, Brunskill NJ. Cellular and physiological effects of C-peptide. Clin Sci (Lond). 2009;116(7): 565–74.
64. Nordquist L, Wahren J. C-peptide: the missing link in diabetic nephropathy? Rev Diabet Stud. 2009; 6(3):203–10.
65. Yetik-Anacak G, Catravas JD. Nitric oxide and the endothelium: history and impact on cardiovascular disease. Vascul Pharmacol. 2006;45(5):268–76.
66. Honing ML, Morrison PJ, Banga JD, Stroes ES, Rabelink TJ. Nitric oxide availability in diabetes mellitus. Diabetes Metab Rev. 1998;14(3):241–9.
67. Baumgartner-Parzer SM, Wagner L, Pettermann M, Grillari J, Gessl A, Waldhausl W. High-glucose – triggered apoptosis in cultured endothelial cells. Diabetes. 1995;44(11):1323–7.
68. Risso A, Mercuri F, Quagliaro L, Damante G, Ceriello A. Intermittent high glucose enhances apoptosis in human umbilical vein endothelial cells in culture. Am J Physiol Endocrinol Metab. 2001; 281(5):E924–30.
69. Cohen RA. The role of nitric oxide and other endothelium-derived vasoactive substances in vascular disease. Prog Cardiovasc Dis. 1995;38(2): 105–28.
70. Halkin A, Benjamin N, Doktor HS, Todd SD, Viberti G, Ritter JM. Vascular responsiveness and cation exchange in insulin-dependent diabetes. Clin Sci (Lond). 1991;81(2):223–32.
71. Johansson BL, Linde B, Wahren J. Effects of C-peptide on blood flow, capillary diffusion capacity and glucose utilization in the exercising forearm of type 1 (insulin-dependent) diabetic patients. Diabetologia. 1992;35(12):1151–8.
72. Johansson BL, Pernow J. C-peptide potentiates the vasoconstrictor effect of neuropeptide Y in insulin-dependent diabetic patients. Acta Physiol Scand. 1999;165(1):39–44.
73. Nordquist L, Johansson M. Proinsulin C-peptide: friend or foe in the development of diabetes-associated complications? Vasc Health Risk Manag. 2008; 4(6):1283–8.
74. Fioretto P, Steffes MW, Sutherland DE, Goetz FC, Mauer M. Reversal of lesions of diabetic nephropathy after pancreas transplantation. N Engl J Med. 1998; 339(2):69–75.
75. Fiorina P, Folli F, Zerbini G, et al. Islet transplantation is associated with improvement of renal function among uremic patients with type I diabetes mellitus and kidney transplants. J Am Soc Nephrol. 2003; 14(8):2150–8.
76. Libby P, Ridker PM, Maseri A. Inflammation and atherosclerosis. Circulation. 2002;105(9):1135–43.
77. Baumgartner-Parzer SM, Wagner L, Pettermann M, Gessl A, Waldhausl W. Modulation by high glucose of adhesion molecule expression in cultured endothelial cells. Diabetologia. 1995;38(11):1367–70.
78. Luppi P, Cifarelli V, Tse H, Piganelli J, Trucco M. Human C-peptide antagonises high glucose-induced endothelial dysfunction through the nuclear factor-kappaB pathway. Diabetologia. 2008;51(8): 1534–43.
79. Scalia R, Coyle KM, Levine BJ, Booth G, Lefer AM. C-peptide inhibits leukocyte-endothelium interaction in the microcirculation during acute endothelial dysfunction. FASEB J. 2000;14(14):2357–64.
80. Young LH, Ikeda Y, Scalia R, Lefer AM. C-peptide exerts cardioprotective effects in myocardial ischemia-reperfusion. Am J Physiol Heart Circ Physiol. 2000;279(4):H1453–9.
81. Kitamura T, Kimura K, Makondo K, et al. Proinsulin C-peptide increases nitric oxide production by enhancing mitogen-activated protein-kinase-dependent transcription of endothelial nitric oxide synthase in aortic endothelial cells of Wistar rats. Diabetologia. 2003;46(12):1698–705.
82. Ido Y, Vindigni A, Chang K, et al. Prevention of vascular and neural dysfunction in diabetic rats by C-peptide. Science. 1997;277(5325):563–6.
83. Tanous D, Brasen JH, Choy K, et al. Probucol inhibits in-stent thrombosis and neointimal hyperplasia by promoting re-endothelialization. Atherosclerosis. 2006;189(2):342–9.
84. Grunberger G, Qiang X, Li Z, et al. Molecular basis for the insulinomimetic effects of C-peptide. Diabetologia. 2001;44(10):1247–57.
85. Li ZG, Zhang W, Sima AA. C-peptide enhances insulin-mediated cell growth and protection against high glucose-induced apoptosis in SH-SY5Y cells. Diabetes Metab Res Rev. 2003;19(5):375–85.
86. Ross R. The pathogenesis of atherosclerosis: a perspective for the 1990s. Nature. 1993;362(6423): 801–9.
87. Hills CE, Brunskill NJ. Intracellular signalling by C-peptide. Exp Diabetes Res. 2008;2008:635158.
88. Rigler R, Pramanik A, Jonasson P, et al. Specific binding of proinsulin C-peptide to human cell membranes. Proc Natl Acad Sci USA. 1999;96(23): 13318–23.
89. Kitamura T, Kimura K, Jung BD, et al. Proinsulin C-peptide activates cAMP response element-binding proteins through the p38 mitogen-activated protein kinase pathway in mouse lung capillary endothelial cells. Biochem J. 2002;366(Pt 3):737–44.
90. Wahren J, Sima AA. C-peptide is relevant in type 1 diabetes and its complications: summary and conclusions to the special issue. Rev Diabet Stud. 2009; 6(3):223–4.
91. Lindahl E, Nyman U, Melles E, et al. Cellular internalization of proinsulin C-peptide. Cell Mol Life Sci. 2007;64(4):479–86.
92. Lindahl E, Nyman U, Zaman F, et al. Proinsulin C-peptide regulates ribosomal RNA expression. J Biol Chem. 2010;285(5):3462–9.

93. Luppi P, Geng X, Cifarelli V, Drain P, Trucco M. C-peptide is internalised in human endothelial and vascular smooth muscle cells via early endosomes. Diabetologia. 2009;52(10):2218–28.
94. Raghow R, Yellaturu C, Deng X, Park EA, Elam MB. SREBPs: the crossroads of physiological and pathological lipid homeostasis. Trends Endocrinol Metab. 2008;19(2):65–73.
95. Kallin A, Johannessen LE, Cani PD, et al. SREBP-1 regulates the expression of heme oxygenase 1 and the phosphatidylinositol-3 kinase regulatory subunit p55 gamma. J Lipid Res. 2007;48(7):1628–36.
96. Sakai J, Rawson RB. The sterol regulatory element-binding protein pathway: control of lipid homeostasis through regulated intracellular transport. Curr Opin Lipidol. 2001;12(3):261–6.
97. Osborne TF, Espenshade PJ. Evolutionary conservation and adaptation in the mechanism that regulates SREBP action: what a long, strange tRIP it's been. Genes Dev. 2009;23(22):2578–91.
98. Matsumoto M, Ogawa W, Akimoto K, et al. PKClambda in liver mediates insulin-induced SREBP-1c expression and determines both hepatic lipid content and overall insulin sensitivity. J Clin Invest. 2003;112(6):935–44.
99. Yellaturu CR, Deng X, Park EA, Raghow R, Elam MB. Insulin enhances the biogenesis of nuclear sterol regulatory element-binding protein (SREBP)-1c by posttranscriptional down-regulation of Insig-2A and its dissociation from SREBP cleavage-activating protein (SCAP).SREBP-1c complex. J Biol Chem. 2009;284(46):31726–34.
100. Sundqvist A, Bengoechea-Alonso MT, Ye X, et al. Control of lipid metabolism by phosphorylation-dependent degradation of the SREBP family of transcription factors by SCF(Fbw7). Cell Metab. 2005; 1(6):379–91.
101. Giandomenico V, Simonsson M, Gronroos E, Ericsson J. Coactivator-dependent acetylation stabilizes members of the SREBP family of transcription factors. Mol Cell Biol. 2003;23(7):2587–99.
102. Cagen LM, Deng X, Wilcox HG, Park EA, Raghow R, Elam MB. Insulin activates the rat sterol-regulatory-element-binding protein 1c (SREBP-1c) promoter through the combinatorial actions of SREBP, LXR, Sp-1 and NF-Y cis-acting elements. Biochem J. 2005;385(Pt 1):207–16.
103. Zhou RH, Pesant S, Cohn HI, Eckhart AD. Enhanced sterol response element-binding protein in postintervention restenotic blood vessels plays an important role in vascular smooth muscle proliferation. Life Sci. 2008;82(3–4):174–81.
104. Thewke D, Kramer M, Sinensky MS. Transcriptional homeostatic control of membrane lipid composition. Biochem Biophys Res Commun. 2000; 273(1):1–4.
105. Sarbassov DD, Ali SM, Sabatini DM. Growing roles for the mTOR pathway. Curr Opin Cell Biol. 2005;17(6):596–603.
106. Sarbassov DD, Ali SM, Kim DH, et al. Rictor, a novel binding partner of mTOR, defines a rapamycin-insensitive and raptor-independent pathway that regulates the cytoskeleton. Curr Biol. 2004;14(14): 1296–302.
107. Jacinto E, Loewith R, Schmidt A, et al. Mammalian TOR complex 2 controls the actin cytoskeleton and is rapamycin insensitive. Nat Cell Biol. 2004;6(11): 1122–8.
108. Sari R, Balci MK. Relationship between C peptide and chronic complications in type-2 diabetes mellitus. J Natl Med Assoc. 2005;97(8):1113–8.
109. Marx N, Walcher D, Raichle C, et al. C-peptide colocalizes with macrophages in early arteriosclerotic lesions of diabetic subjects and induces monocyte chemotaxis in vitro. Arterioscler Thromb Vasc Biol. 2004;24(3):540–5.
110. Walcher D, Aleksic M, Jerg V, et al. C-peptide induces chemotaxis of human CD4-positive cells: involvement of pertussis toxin-sensitive G-proteins and phosphoinositide 3-kinase. Diabetes. 2004;53(7): 1664–70.
111. Walcher D, Babiak C, Poletek P, et al. C-peptide induces vascular smooth muscle cell proliferation: involvement of SRC-kinase, phosphatidylinositol 3-kinase, and extracellular signal-regulated kinase 1/2. Circ Res. 2006;99(11):1181–7.
112. Marx N, Walcher D. C-peptide and atherogenesis: C-peptide as a mediator of lesion development in patients with type 2 diabetes mellitus? Exp Diabetes Res. 2008;2008:385108.

C-Peptide and Diabetic Neuropathy in Patients with Type 1 Diabetes

12

Karin Ekberg and John Wahren

Keywords
C-peptide • Type 1 diabetes • Sural nerve • Nerve conduction velocity

Introduction

Neuropathy is one of the most common long-term complications accompanying diabetes mellitus. It affects patients with both type 1 and type 2 diabetes, but it progresses more rapidly and its manifestations are more severe in type 1 diabetes [1, 2]. Diabetic neuropathy is defined by the presence of detectable sensory, motor, and autonomic nerve abnormalities on clinical examination, with or without the presence of symptoms [3, 4]. As many as 50% of the patients may be asymptomatic; diagnosis may only be made on examination or, in some cases, when the patient presents with a painless foot ulcer [5]. Other patients may not report symptoms, but admit on inquiry that their feet feel numb. A careful neurological examination of the lower limb usually reveals sensory loss as reflected by abnormal vibration, pressure, pain, or temperature perception, mediated by small and large fibers, as well as absence of ankle reflexes. Signs of autonomic neuropathy may include manifestations of, for example, impaired cardiovascular and gastrointestinal functions. Moreover, signs of peripheral sympathetic autonomic dysfunction are also frequently seen in patients with diabetes and may include a warm or cold foot, sometimes with distended dorsal foot veins, dry skin, and the presence of calluses under pressure-bearing areas. Diabetic neuropathies may present as a rapidly reversible effect of hyperglycemia and focal or multifocal neuropathies, but the most prevalent clinical form is the persistent distal symmetric polyneuropathy (DSPN) [4].

DSPN is characterized by a gradual progression of nerve structural changes comprising distal axonal degeneration of the "dying-back" type [6, 7], most prominent in the lower limbs in the early course of the disorder, but as the condition progresses the upper limbs also become affected. DSPN involves also small fiber sensory dysfunction [7]. The prevalence of DSPN is approximately 30% for diabetes patients in general [8], but the number varies greatly in the literature related to the definition chosen for presence of diabetic neuropathy and the methodology for assessment of its presence. Clinical examinations and patients' symptom assessment are considered important tools in the evaluation of neuropathy status, but both techniques rely greatly on subjective components and the cooperation of the

K. Ekberg • J. Wahren (✉)
Department of Molecular Medicine and Surgery, Karolinska Institutet, Fogdevreten 2, 171 77 Stockholm, Sweden
e-mail: john.wahren@ki.se

A.A.F. Sima (ed.), *Diabetes & C-Peptide: Scientific and Clinical Aspects*, Contemporary Diabetes, DOI 10.1007/978-1-61779-391-2_12, © Springer Science+Business Media, LLC 2012

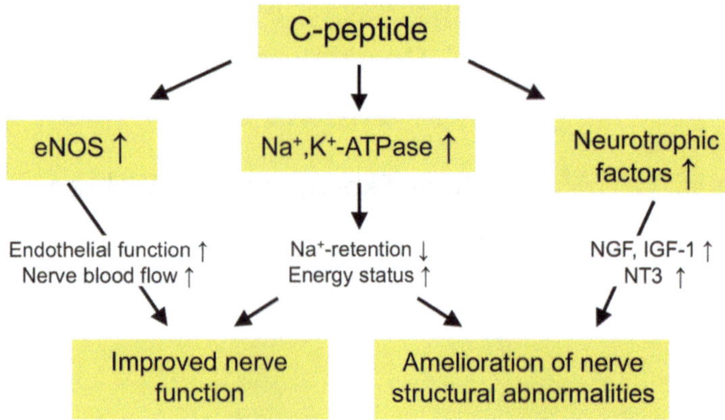

Fig. 12.1 Schematic presentation of C-peptide's potential effects on peripheral nerve function and structure

patient. Hence, the assessments typically have poor reproducibility and specificity. Assessments using more objective markers of polyneuropathy, especially nerve conduction velocity (NCV), may serve not only as reliable method for detection of neuropathy, but it is also useful for the prediction of prognosis and survival in diabetic patients [9, 10].

The pathogenesis of diabetic neuropathy involves metabolic effects mediated directly and indirectly by hyperglycemia, resulting in oxidative stress, accelerated polyol pathway metabolism, and generation of advanced glycation end-products [11–13]. Furthermore, diabetic neuropathy is accompanied by reduced nerve Na^+,K^+-ATPase activity, and microvascular abnormalities (e.g. reduced endoneurial perfusion) [14], and in type 1 diabetes, specific structural nerve abnormalities occur that are not frequent in type 2 diabetes. These abnormalities include axonal atrophy and characteristic nodal and paranodal changes that contribute to the progressive deterioration of NCV [15–17]. In contrast, in type 2 diabetes the axonal degeneration is milder and there are minimal nodal and paranodal abnormalities, if any [17, 18]. However, after several years, type 2 diabetes patients often become insulin and C-peptide deficient, and at this stage, it is most likely that the type 2 DSPN will present itself with characteristics similar to that of type 1 neuropathy.

In the case of type 1 diabetes, available data suggest that C-peptide deficiency is an important contributing factor to the characteristic functional and structural abnormalities of the peripheral nerves [19]. In conformity with this hypothesis, several studies have demonstrated that it is possible to retard the progression of diabetic complications by intensified insulin treatment and improved metabolic control, but development of neuropathy cannot be prevented [20–22]. Thus, other factors, such as C-peptide deficiency, are likely to be of importance for the progression of diabetic neuropathy in type 1 diabetes. Evidence documenting physiological effects of C-peptide has been presented during the latest decades. It shows that C-peptide, in contrast to previous belief, possesses the characteristics of a bioactive peptide. C-peptide binds specifically to various cell membranes, including endothelial, renal, and nerve cells [23], with subsequent activation of an intracellular signaling cascade resulting in stimulation of endothelial nitric oxide synthase (eNOS) and Na^+,K^+-ATPase [24]. Moreover, recent data indicate that C-peptide stimulates several transcriptional factors, as well as several neurotrophic factors [25]. Thus, it has been demonstrated that exogenous administration of C-peptide in replacement dose to patients lacking endogenous C-peptide results in restoration of reduced blood flow in several tissues [26–29] and improvement of renal [30] and nerve function; a schematic presentation of the several ways by which C-peptide exerts its beneficial effects on nerve function is given in Fig. 12.1. Indirect support for the formulation that C-peptide is of importance in connection with neuropathy in type 1 diabetes is obtained from the long-standing clinical observation that type 1 diabetes patients who retain a low but preserved endogenous C-peptide and insulin secretion are less prone to develop microvascular complications involving the kidneys, the eyes, or the nervous system than the majority of patients in whom beta-cell secretion ceases totally [31–33].

Clinical Studies on C-Peptide and Nerve Function

Several preclinical studies indicate significant effects by C-peptide on diabetes-induced nerve dysfunction and structural abnormalities [34–36], but as of yet the clinical experience regarding C-peptide's effects on nerve function is limited. The available clinical findings indicate, however, consistently beneficial effects of C-peptide on both peripheral and autonomic nerve function in type 1 diabetes patients. Thus, in a double-blind, placebo-controlled study including 46 type 1 diabetes patients in an early stage of nerve dysfunction (average age of 29 years, approximately 10 years diabetes duration), but presenting with reduced sensory and motor NCVs but no other signs or symptoms of neuropathy, C-peptide replacement (1.8 mg/day) or placebo was given for 3 months together with the patients' regular insulin therapy [37]. Sensory NCV assessed in the sural nerve bilaterally, but not motor NCV (peroneal nerve), increased gradually during the study. The increase after 3 months amounted to 2.7 m/s, corresponding to an 80% correction of the initial conduction velocity deficit in these patients (Fig. 12.2). This was accompanied by a simultaneous improvement in vibration perception assessed on the dorsum of the feet, even though these patients had only a mild reduction of vibration perception at baseline. These findings are consistent with an improved sural nerve function since vibration perception in this anatomic region is primarily mediated via the large fibers of the sural nerve.

A second clinical trial included a patient population with manifest neuropathy and type 1 diabetes [38]. This study was also a double-blind,

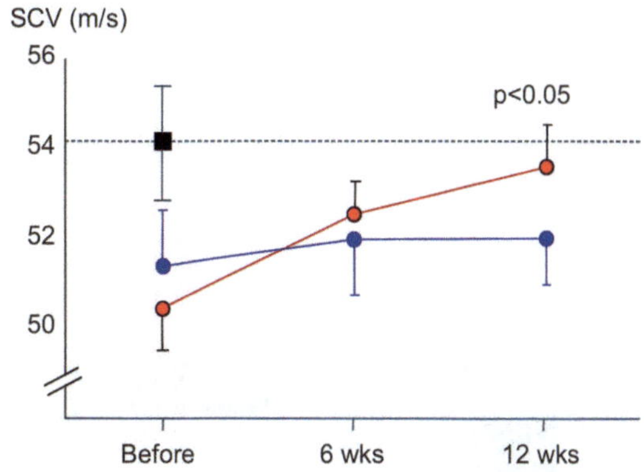

Fig. 12.2 Change in sural nerve conduction velocity (SCV) after 6 and 12 weeks of C-peptide therapy (*red symbols*) or placebo administration (*blue symbols*) in type 1 diabetes patients. The increase in SCV above baseline in the C-peptide group was 2.7 m/s ($p<0.01$) and the difference between the C-peptide and placebo groups after 12 weeks was 1.8 m/s ($p<0.05$). Data from ref. [19]

placebo-controlled, randomized multicenter study and included 161 type 1 diabetes patients with an average age of 44 and 29 years of diabetes duration, defined DSPN according to the San Antonio criteria [3] and measurable sural nerve action potentials. At baseline, these patients presented with sensory NCV in the sural nerve (SCV) that was on average 2.6 SD below normal after correction for body height. Following 6 months of C-peptide replacement treatment, there was a statistically significant improvement in SCV for the patients receiving C-peptide, amounting to 0.48 ± 0.19 m/s assessed as peak velocities and 0.93 ± 0.29 m/s for the initial response reflecting the velocity in the fastest axon in the nerve. These changes were statistically significant within the group, but not so vs. the placebo-treated patients. The number of positive responders, defined as patients with an improvement in peak SCV >1 m/s, was greater in the group receiving C-peptide as compared to those on placebo (37 vs. 19%, resp., $p<0.03$). It is noteworthy, though, that among the included patients some had quite marked nerve conduction deficits at baseline, and with the treatment duration being relatively short (6 months), it is conceivable that the patients who were relative severely affected at baseline may have a limited potential for improvement within the time frame

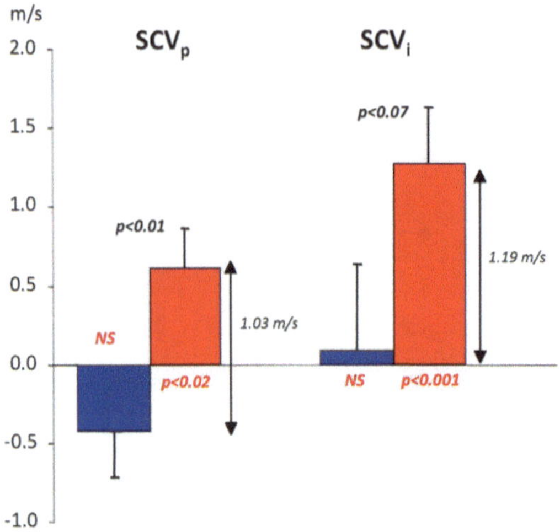

Fig. 12.3 Change in SCV (initial and peak values) from baseline to 6 months of C-peptide (*red columns*) or placebo administration (*blue columns*) in the patients who showed the least affected nerve conduction velocity at baseline ($n=70$). *p* Values in *red* indicated differences within the groups, values in *black* denote differences between the C-peptide and placebo groups. Data from ref. [20]

of the study. Therefore, a subgroup analysis was performed including the half of the patient population with the least affected SCV at baseline. In this group, i.e. the patients with an impairment of nerve function similar to that of the patients in the first trial, C-peptide administration for 6 months resulted in an improvement that in absolute terms was 1.03 m/s greater as compared to the change in the corresponding placebo-treated patients ($p<0.014$) (Fig. 12.3). Again, there were significantly more positive responders in this group compared to placebo ($p<0.004$). Accompanying these changes in sural NCV, there was an improvement within the C-peptide-treated patients with regard to vibration perception. There was also a trend towards an improvement in clinical neurological examination scores following C-peptide treatment (Fig. 12.4). When the findings for sural NCV from the two clinical trials described above are combined in a meta analysis, the average improvement in sural NCV is 1.5 m/s, documenting a clinically relevant change in the patients with mild-to-moderate DSPN in response to C-peptide treatment.

C-peptide was well tolerated by the patients in the C-peptide-treated groups in the 3- and 6-month trials and none reported any adverse events that could be related to C-peptide. Blood glucose levels were unchanged during the studies, but it was noted that patients on C-peptide in the 6-month trial tended to reduce their insulin dosage. All patients monitored their blood glucose levels several times daily, and on average, reduced their insulin doses by 15% [38]. The male patients responded to a sexual dysfunction questionnaire at baseline and at the end of the study period. Interestingly, it was found that 46% of the patients on C-peptide reported improved erectile function vs. 9% for patients on placebo (Fig. 12.5), a finding that requires further study but may be referable to the peptide's stimulatory effect on blood flow [27] and on autonomic, primarily vagal, nerve function [39].

In addition to the findings in DSPN, there is also evidence of beneficial effects of C-peptide administration on autonomic function in type 1 patients. Deficient autonomic nerve function may be evaluated in patients as reduced heart rate variability (HRV) during deep breathing, a measurement that, with a high degree of reproducibility, primarily reflects vagal function. In a short-term study, patients were studied on two occasions 7–10 days apart under normoglycemic conditions and during a 3-h period of intravenous infusion of either human C-peptide or saline in a double-blind fashion. At baseline, HRV was $13\pm1\%$ (normal reference value 24%) and during the C-peptide infusion, which restored plasma concentrations to physiological levels, HRV improved to $20\pm2\%$, while no significant change was seen after saline infusion ($p<0.001$) (Fig. 12.6) [39]. The heart rate brake index after a tilting maneuver was also improved after C-peptide for 3 h in the patients showing reduced index before the study. Autonomic nerve function was evaluated also in a study involving primarily C-peptide's effects on urinary albumin excretion in diabetic nephropathy [30]. At study onset, these patients had only a mildly reduced HRV ($18\pm2\%$), but at the end of the 3 month study period it had increased to $21\pm1\%$ ($p<0.03$), reflecting an improved cardiac autonomic nerve function after C-peptide administration.

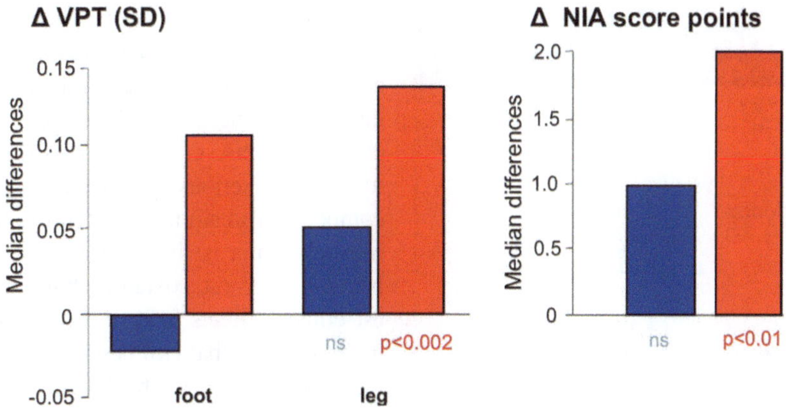

Fig. 12.4 Median changes in vibration perception threshold (VPT) and neuropathy assessment score (NIA) from baseline to 6 month of C-peptide (*red columns*) or placebo administration (*blue columns*). Data from ref. [20]

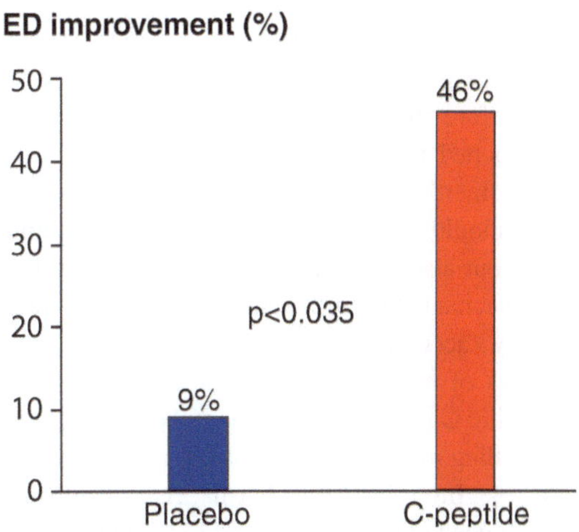

Fig. 12.5 Percent of patients reporting improved erectile function after 6 months of C-peptide therapy (*red column*) or placebo administration (*blue column*). Data from ref. [20]

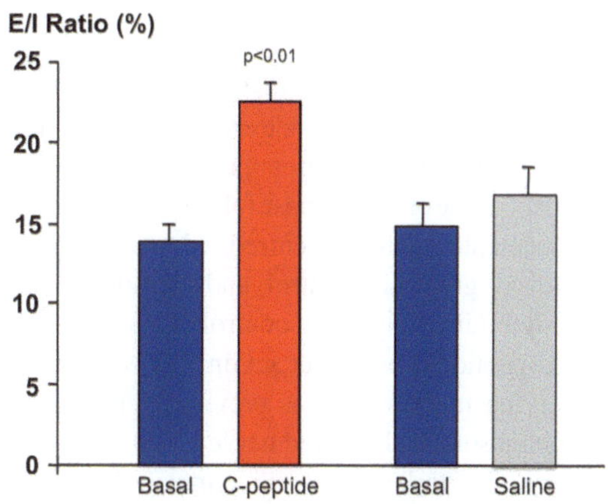

Fig. 12.6 Heart rate variability (%) during standardized deep breathing (E/I) in type 1 diabetes patients in the basal state (*blue columns*) and following i.v. infusion of C-peptide (*red column*) or saline (*gray column*) for 90 min. Modified from ref. [39]

Treatment of Diabetic Neuropathy

It is well established that the onset and progression of the diabetes-induced microvascular complications may be delayed by intensive insulin therapy and optimized glycemic control [20–22]. In the DCCT, the incidences of diabetes neuropathy were substantially lower in patients on intensive insulin treatment as compared to those on conventional insulin therapy [21]. For the patients in the DCCT secondary prevention group, with an average age of 28 years and a diabetes duration of 9 years, the 2% improvement in HbA1c seen following 5 years of intensified insulin treatment was accompanied by an improved SCV of 1.5 m/s, whereas patients with unchanged metabolic control in the conventional treatment group experienced a 2.2 m/s decrease in SCV. Interestingly, the patients in this group are directly comparable with regard to age and diabetes duration to those in the 3-month C-peptide intervention study described above (Fig. 12.7), in which

DCCT: secondary prevention group		C-peptide in early neuropathy patients	
- Age	28±7 yrs	- Age	29±1 yrs
- Diabetes	9±4 yrs	- Diabetes	10±1 yrs
- HbA_{1c}	9%	- HbA_{1c}	7%
5 yrs conventional:		**3 mo placebo:**	
- HbA_{1c}	-0.1%	- HbA_{1c}	-0.1%
- SCV	-2.2 m/s	- SCV	+0.6 m/s
5 yrs intensive:		**3 mo C-peptide:**	
- HbA_{1c}	-2.0%	- HbA_{1c}	-0.1%
- SCV	+1.5 m/s	- SCV	+2.7 m/s

Fig. 12.7 Comparison of C-peptide replacement therapy for 3 months vs. intensive insulin treatment for 5 years with regard to improvement in sensory nerve conduction velocity (SCV). Data from the DCCT study and ref. [19]

C-peptide replacement resulted in 2.7 m/s improvement in SCV. Yet, it should be noted that the patients in the C-peptide study were already on an intensive insulin treatment regimen [19]. The magnitude of the response following C-peptide replacement treatment occurred independently of improved glycemic control and on top of an already optimal glycemic control. This suggests that C-peptide does in fact act on DSPN disease-modifying mechanisms, as previously indicated in animal studies. Impaired nerve blood flow secondary to perturbed nitric oxide metabolism [34, 36] and reduced levels of nerve Na^+,K^+-ATPase activity [40, 41] are both factors that have been implicated in the pathogenesis of the DSPN [7]. The ability of C-peptide to improve endoneurial blood flow and Na^+,K^+-ATPase activity as well as its stimulation of neurotrophic factors as demonstrated in several animal models of type 1 diabetes [25, 35, 40] is thus likely to contribute to the positive effects of the peptide.

There is no effective pharmaceutical therapy available for DSPN today, but several therapeutic interventions (inhibitors of aldose reductase, PKCβ, and reactive oxygen species) have previously been evaluated for this indication. However, it should be noted that the vast majority of these have been directed towards correction of the adverse effects of hyperglycemia. One approach involves the reduction of nerve sorbitol accumulation by aldose reductase inhibitors (ARI). Although there have been beneficial effects on neuropathy for some ARIs [42–45], several clinical trials involving these compounds have been discontinued because of low effect size or unacceptable adverse effects, such as skin rash, renal toxicity, and serious hepatic effects [46]. Another compound also aiming to minimize the effects of hyperglycemia is the specific protein kinase C beta inhibitor, ruboxistaurin, but with only modest clinical effects [47]. It has become increasingly apparent that DSPN presents a clear unmet medical need, and the health authorities and representatives for patient associations have expressed concern [5]. Previously, the regulatory agencies have required relief of symptoms, healing of wounds, or diminished amputation frequency in order to accept a new drug application. However, it is now becoming increasingly recognized that treatment of DSPN should be started well before the deterioration of nerve function has reached the stage of severe symptoms and development of foot ulcers. Moreover, the treatment should not only be directed at symptom relief, but also to modifying the underlying disease mechanisms. In the case of peripheral neuropathy accompanying type 1 diabetes, the findings of beneficial effects on nerve function following C-peptide replacement therapy provide compelling evidence of a possible new treatment principle. Input from the pharmaceutical industry will be needed since costly and extended clinical trials will be needed to finally determine the usefulness of C-peptide in the treatment of DSPN.

References

1. Dyck PJ, Davies D, Wilson F, et al. Risk factors for severity of diabetic polyneuropathy: intensive longitudinal assessment of the Rochester Diabetic Neuropathy Study cohort. Diabetes Care. 1999;2(9):1479–86.
2. Sugimoto K, Murakawa Y, Sima AAF. Diabetic neuropathy – a continuing enigma. Diabetes Metab Res Rev. 2000;16(6):408–33.
3. Asbury AK, Porte Jr D, Genuth SM, et al. Report and recommendations of the San Antonio conference on diabetic neuropathy. Ann Neurol. 1988;24(1):99–104.
4. Ziegler D. Treatment of diabetic polyneuropathy. Ann N Y Acad Sci. 2006;1084:250–66.

5. Boulton A, Vinik A, Arezzo J, et al. Diabetic neuropathies. Diabetes Care. 2005;24(4):956–60.
6. Said G, Slama G, Selva J. Progressive centripetal degeneration of axons in small fibre diabetic polyneuropathy. Brain. 1983;106(4):791–807.
7. Thomas PK. Diabetic neuropathy: mechanisms and future treatment options. J Neurol Neurosurg Psychiatry. 1999;67(3):277–9.
8. Shaw J, Zimmet P, Gries F, Ziegler D. Epidemiology of diabetic neuropathy. In: Gries F, Cameron NE, Low P, Ziegler D, editors. Textbook of diabetic neuropathy. New York: Thieme; 2003. p. 64–82.
9. Coppini D, Bowtell P, Weng C, et al. Showing neuropathy is related to increased mortality in diabetic patients – a survival analysis using an accelerated failure time model. J Clin Epidemiol. 2000;53(5):519–23.
10. Forsblom CM, Sane T, Groop PH, et al. Risk factors for mortality in type II (non-insulin-dependent) diabetes: evidence of a role for neuropathy and a protective effect of HLA-DR4. Diabetologia. 1998;41(11):1253–62.
11. Brownlee M. The pathobiology of diabetic complications. Diabetes. 2005;54(6):1615–25.
12. Greene DA, Sima AAF, Stevens M, et al. Complications: neuropathy, pathogenic considerations. Diabetes Care. 1992;15(12):1902–25.
13. Low P, Nickander K, Scionti L. Role of hypoxia, oxidative stress, and excitatory neurotoxins in diabetic neuropathy. In: Dyck P, Thomas P, editors. Diabetic neuropathy. Philadelphia: W.B. Saunders; 1999. p. 317–29.
14. Cameron NE, Eaton EM, Cotter MA, Tesfaye S. Vascular factors and metabolic interactions in the pathogenesis of diabetic neuropathy. Diabetologia. 2001;44(11):1973–88.
15. Brismar T, Sima AAF, Greene DA. Reversible and irreversible nodal dysfunction in diabetic neuropathy. Ann Neurol. 1987;21(5):504–7.
16. Cherian VP, Kamijo M, Angelides KJ, Sima AAF. Nodal Na^{+}-channel displacement is associated with nerve-conduction slowing in the chronic diabetic BB/W rat: prevention by aldose reductase inhibition. J Diabet Complications. 1996;10(4):192–200.
17. Sima AAF, Nathaniel V, Bril V, et al. Histopathological heterogeneity of neuropathy in insulin-dependent and non-insulin-dependent diabetes, and demonstration of axo-glial dysjunction in human diabetic neuropathy. J Clin Invest. 1988;81(2):349–64.
18. Murakawa Y, Zhang W, Pierson CR, et al. Impaired glucose tolerance and insulinopenia in the GK-rat causes peripheral neuropathy. Diabetes Metab Res Rev. 2002;18(6):473–83.
19. Sima AAF. New insights into the metabolic and molecular basis for diabetic neuropathy. Cell Mol Life Sci. 2003;60(11):2445–64.
20. DCCT Research Group. The effect of intensive diabetes therapy on the development and progression of neuropathy. Ann Intern Med. 1995;122:561–8.
21. DCCT Research Group. Effect of intensive diabetes treatment on nerve conduction in the diabetes control and complications trial. Ann Neurol. 1995;38(6):869–80.
22. Reichard P, Nilsson BY, Rosenqvist U. The effect of long-term intensified insulin treatment on the development of microvascular complications of diabetes mellitus. N Engl J Med. 1993;329(5):304–9.
23. Rigler R, Pramanik A, Jonasson P, et al. Specific binding of proinsulin C-peptide to human cell membranes. Proc Natl Acad Sci U S A. 1999;96(23):13318–23.
24. Wahren E, Ekberg k, Jörnvall H. C-peptide is a bioactive peptide. Diabetologia. 2007;50(3):503–9.
25. Pierson CR, Zhang W, Sima AAF. Proinsulin C-peptide replacement in type 1 diabetic BB/Wor-rats prevents deficits in nerve fiber regeneration. J Neuropathol Exp Neurol. 2003;62(7):765–79.
26. Hansen A, Johansson BL, Wahren J, von Bibra H. C-peptide exerts beneficial effects on myocardial blood flow and function in patients with type 1 diabetes. Diabetes. 2002;51(10):3077–82.
27. Johansson BL, Linde B, Wahren J. Effects of C-peptide on blood flow, capillary diffusion capacity and glucose utilization in the exercising forearm of type 1 (insulin-dependent) diabetic patients. Diabetologia. 1992; 35(12):1151–8.
28. Johansson BL, Sjöberg S, Wahren J. The influence of human C-peptide on renal function and glucose utilization in type 1 (insulin-dependent) diabetic patients. Diabetologia. 1992;35(2):121–8.
29. Johansson BL, von Bibra A, Hansen A, Wahren J. Effects of C-peptide on regional myocardial function in patients with type 1 diabetes. Diabetes. 2001;50: A256.
30. Johansson BL, Borg K, Fernqvist-Forbes E, et al. Beneficial effects of C-peptide on incipient nephropathy and neuropathy in patients with type 1 diabetes mellitus. Diabet Med. 2000;17(3):181–9.
31. Sjöberg S, Gunnarsson R, Gjötterberg M, et al. Residual insulin production, glycemic control and prevalence of microvascular lesions and polyneuropathy in long-term type 1 (insulin-dependent) diabetes mellitus. Diabetologia. 1987;30(4):208–13.
32. Sjöberg S, Götterberg M, Berglund L, et al. Residual C-peptide excretion is associated with a better long-term glycemic control and slower progress of retinopathy in type I (insulin-dependent) diabetes mellitus. J Diabet Complications. 1991;5(1):18–22.
33. Zerbini G, Mangili R, Luzi L. Higher post-absorptive C-peptide levels in type 1 diabetic patients without renal complications. Diabet Med. 1999;16(12): 1048–9.
34. Cotter MA, Ekberg K, Wahren J, Cameron NE. Effects of proinsulin C-peptide in experimental diabetic neuropathy: vascular actions and modulation by nitric oxide synthase inhibition. Diabetes. 2003;52(7): 1812–7.
35. Sima AAF, Zhang W, Sugimoto K, et al. C-peptide prevents and improves chronic type I diabetic polyneuropathy in the BB/Wor rat. Diabetologia. 2001; 44(7):889–97.

36. Stevens M, Li F, Zhang W, Sima AAF. C-peptide corrects endoneurial blood flow but not effect oxidative stress in type 1 BB/Wor rats. Am J Physiol Endocrinol Metab. 2004;287:E497–505.
37. Ekberg K, Brismar T, Johansson BL, et al. Amelioration of sensory nerve dysfunction by C-peptide in patients with type 1 diabetes. Diabetes. 2003;52(2):536–41.
38. Ekberg K, Brismar T, Johansson BL, et al. C-peptide replacement therapy and sensory nerve function in type 1 diabetic neuropathy. Diabetes Care. 2007;30(1): 71–6.
39. Johansson BL, Borg K, Fernqvist-Forbes E, et al. C-peptide improves autonomic nerve function in IDDM patients. Diabetologia. 1996;39(6):687–95.
40. Ido Y, Vindigni A, Chang K, et al. Prevention of vascular and neural dysfunction in diabetic rats by C-peptide. Science. 1997;277(5325):563–6.
41. Stevens M, Dananberg J, Feldman E, et al. The linked roles of nitric oxide, aldose reductase and, (Na+, K+)-ATPase in the slowing of nerve conduction in the streptozotocin diabetic rat. J Clin Invest. 1994;94(2): 853–9.
42. Hotta N. New approaches for treatment in diabetes: aldose reductase inhibitors. Biomed Pharmacother. 1995;49(5):232–43.
43. Sima AAF, Bril V, Nathaniel V, et al. Regeneration and repair of myelinated fibers in sural-nerve biopsy specimens from patients with diabetic neuropathy treated with sorbinil. N Engl J Med. 1988;319(9):548–55.
44. Bril V, Buchanan R, AS-3201 Study Group. Aldose reductase inhibition by AS-3201 in sural nerve from patients with diabetic sensorimotor polyneuropathy. Diabetes Care. 2004;27(10):2369–75.
45. Bril V, Buchanan R, Ranirestat Study Group. Long-term effects of Ranirestat (AS-3201) on peripheral nerve function in patients with diabetic sensorimotor polyneuropathy. Diabetes Care. 2006;29:68–72.
46. Foppiano M, Lombardo G. Worldwide pharmacovigilance systems and tolrestat withdrawal. Lancet. 1997;349(9049):399–400.
47. Vinik A, Bril V, Kempler P, et al. Treatment of symptomatic diabetic peripheral neuropathy with the protein kinase C β-inhibitor ruboxistaurin mesylate during a 1-year, randomized, placebo-controlled, double-blind clinical trial. Clin Ther. 2005;27(8):1164–80.

Proatherogenic Effects of C-Peptide

13

Daniel Walcher and Nikolaus Marx

Keywords
C-peptide • Atherogenesis • Monocytes • T-cells • Smooth muscle cells

Introduction

Patients with diabetes and insulin resistance exhibit an increased propensity to develop arteriosclerosis with its sequelae acute myocardial infarction and stroke [1]. Advanced glycation end products (AGEs), formed by nonenzymatic glycation of reducing sugars with macromolecules, are crucially involved in atherogenesis in these patients. Binding of AGEs to the receptor for AGEs (RAGE) activates intracellular signaling processes, thus mediating proinflammatory AGE effects [2]. Given that RAGE expression is increased in the vessel wall in diabetic patients [3], this mechanism might potentially contribute to a vicious circle that promotes lesion development in these patients. Due to peripheral insulin resistance, these patients temporarily demonstrate also elevated levels of the proinsulin cleavage product C-peptide. For a long time, C-peptide has been considered to be a biological inert substance, without any physiological function. Recent work in kidney cells suggests that C-peptide can activate intracellular signaling pathways such as Na-K-ATPase [4]. In addition, C-peptide activates various signaling pathways in different cell types [5, 6], suggesting that C-peptide may be biologically active. Some groups have shown that C-peptide administration in type 1 diabetes mellitus results in amelioration of diabetes-induced renal and nerve dysfunction. For example, in patients with diabetes 1 C-peptide treatment for 6 months improves sensory nerve function [7, 8]. Furthermore, beneficial effects on renal function and structure in type 1 diabetes by C-peptide replacement were shown by other groups [9, 10]. In the kidney, C-peptide supplementation suppresses diabetes-induced abnormal renal eNOS expression. This down-regulation could be an explanation for C-peptides beneficial effects on diabetic nephropathy [10, 11].

The following review will focus on C-peptides proatherogenic effects in vascular cells and discuss the potential relevance of these effects on atherogenesis in patients with type 2 diabetes.

D. Walcher (✉)
Department of Internal Medicine II – Cardiology, University of Ulm, Ulm, Germany
e-mail: daniel.walcher@uniklinik-ulm.de

N. Marx
Department of Internal Medicine I – Cardiology, University of Aachen, Pauwelsstraße 30, 52074 Aachen, Germany

A.A.F. Sima (ed.), *Diabetes & C-Peptide: Scientific and Clinical Aspects*, Contemporary Diabetes, DOI 10.1007/978-1-61779-391-2_13, © Springer Science+Business Media, LLC 2012

Atherogenesis

Atherogenesis is currently understood as an inflammatory process in the vessel wall with different phases and stages [12]. The early phase of atherogenesis is characterized by endothelial dysfunction caused by various risk factors like smoking, diabetes, hypertension, or hypercholesterolemia. In addition, the endothelium is activated in this phase, releasing chemotactic proteins such as MCP-1, a monocyte chemoattractant, or RANTES and IP-10, both chemoattractants for lymphocytes. These chemokines attract inflammatory cells, mainly monocytes and CD4-positive lymphocytes, to adhere to endothelial adhesion molecules, with subsequent migration of these cells into the vessel wall. Monocytes, once migrated into the subendothelial space, become macrophages, expressing scavenger receptors on their surface, which mediate the uptake of lipoprotein particles such as oxidized low-density lipoprotein (LDL). Through lipid uptake, these cells differentiate to foam cells, the classic cellular substrate of arteriosclerotic lesions. These macrophage foam cells then express additional proinflammatory and proatherogenic mediators such as cytokines, matrix metalloproteinases, and reactive oxygen species, as well as procoagulant molecules such as tissue factor, which all act on other cells in the vessel wall, thus promoting lesion development [13, 14]. The second inflammatory cell type recruited during endothelial dysfunction is the CD4-positive lymphocyte. These cells enter the vessel wall as naïve TH0 cells [15]. In the subendothelial space, these cells then encounter antigens like oxidized LDL and differentiate towards TH1 cells which release proinflammatory cytokines such as IFNγ, TNFα, and IL-2. Some of these cytokines then enhance endothelial expression and release of T-cell specific chemokines, creating a vicious cycle of cell activation and cell recruitment [16]. In addition, these TH1 cytokines activate other cells in the vessel wall like macrophages and smooth muscle cells (SMCs), thus orchestrating the inflammatory response in the vessel wall. With increased recruitment of these inflammatory cells, fatty streaks develop and SMCs from the media start to proliferate and migrate into the intima. As lesion formation progresses, advanced and potentially complicated lesions are formed. These lesions may lead to a progressive narrowing of the vessel lumen, thus potentially creating stable angina if located in the coronary artery. Alternatively, these plaques may become vulnerable and upon rupture can cause an acute coronary syndrome [17].

C-Peptide Deposits in the Vascular Wall of Atherosclerotic Lesions

Patients with metabolic syndrome or type 2 diabetes mellitus exhibit an increased propensity for the development of a scattered and extensive pattern of arteriosclerosis [1]. Typically, these insulin-resistant patients demonstrate increased serum levels of insulin and C-peptide. C-peptide, a cleavage product of proinsulin, is released into the blood stream in amounts equimolar to those of insulin. The role of insulin in atherogenesis has been examined by various groups over the last decades. It has been suggested that insulin may promote lesion development, for example, by inducing proliferation of vascular SMCs [18], whereas others demonstrated that insulin exhibits anti-inflammatory and antiatherogenic properties in vascular cells such as monocytes [19, 20]. Overall, the role of insulin in atherogenesis remains unclear. Most important, currently, we are lacking both clinical as well as epidemiologic evidence that insulin may have harmful effects with respect to macrovascular events.

For a long time, C-peptide has been considered to be biologically inert, but recent data suggest that C-peptide binds to specific, yet unidentified, cell surface receptors. Recently, our group hypothesized that C-peptide might deposit in the vessel wall in these patients in early atherogenesis [21]. Immunohistochemical analyses of early arteriosclerotic lesions of patients with diabetes from the PDAY Study (Patho-biological Determinants of Atherosclerosis in Youth) revealed C-peptide deposition mainly in the subendothelial space and the intima. Some of the diabetic subjects also exhibited C-peptide deposition in the media. In contrast, very little C-peptide deposition has been found in early arteriosclerotic lesions of nondiabetic subjects. Computer-assisted analyses revealed significantly higher C-peptide deposition in lesions from diabetic individuals compared to lesions of age, sex, and risk factor-matched nondiabetic subjects. Interestingly, no deposition of insulin or proinsulin was detectable in diabetic or nondiabetic subjects.

C-Peptide Colocalizes with CD4-Positive Cells and Monocytes in the Vessel Wall

Staining of parallel sections as well as immunofluorescence techniques demonstrated colocalization of C-peptide with intimal monocyte/macrophages and CD4-positive lymphocytes in some of the diabetic individuals [21, 22]. In the studies cited above, C-peptide deposition has been found in 100% of the 21 diabetic individuals examined, while monocyte infiltration was only present in 77% and $CD4^+$ lymphocyte infiltration only in 57%. These data suggested that C-peptide deposition may precede monocyte and T-cell migration into the vessel wall. Based on this observation, the hypothesis was raised that C-peptide may deposit in the vessel wall during early atherogenesis and then – through chemotactic effects – promote the recruitment of monocytes and CD4-positive lymphocytes.

C-Peptide and its Chemotactic Activity

In vitro migration assays, employing a modified Boyden chamber, revealed that C-peptide induces the migration of both monocytes and $CD4^+$ lymphocytes. Interestingly, insulin did not have such an effect. Stimulation of monocytes with C-peptide induced cell migration in a concentration-dependent manner with a maximal augmentation of 2.3 ± 0.4 at 1 nmol/L. The extent of C-peptide-induced monocyte migration resembled the effect of the established monocyte chemokine MCP-1, which increased monocyte migration by 2.9 ± 0.2 fold. Stimulation of $CD4^+$ cells with C-peptide induced cell migration in a concentration-dependent manner with a maximal induction of 2.1 ± 0.5 at 10 nmol/L. The extent of C-peptide-induced $CD4^+$ cell migration was similar to the effect of an established T-cell chemokine, RANTES, which led to a 2.1 ± 0.6-fold increase in cell migration. It is interesting that combined stimulation of $CD4^+$ cells with C-peptide and RANTES did not have an additive migratory effect. In addition, checkerboard analyses showed that C-peptide induces chemotaxis rather than chemokinesis [21, 22]. Moreover, C-peptide did not induce the migration of human neutrophils, cells that are not present in arteriosclerotic lesions, underscoring the specificity of C-peptide's chemotactic effects on monocytes and lymphocytes.

C-Peptide Activates Intracellular Signaling Pathways in Inflammatory Cells

Inhibition migration assays in monocytes and CD4-positive lymphocytes as well as western blot analyses and activity assays demonstrated that C-peptide mediates its chemotactic activity through an as of yet unidentified pertussis toxin-sensitive G-protein-coupled receptor with subsequent downstream activation of PI3-kinase γ.

Previous work from other groups has shown that Src-kinase is involved in, e.g., IP-10 (interferon-gamma-inducible protein-10)-mediated chemotactic response of lymphocytes [23]. In our experiments, a specific inhibitor of Src-kinase, PP2, as well as transfection of Src siRNA, abolished C-peptide-induced T-cell migration, suggesting that C-peptide also signals through this pathway. Additional experiments demonstrated that PI3-Kinase activation leads to the involvement of small Rho-GTPases, like RhoA, Rac-1, and Cdc42 in these cells. Furthermore, C-peptide stimulated phosphorylation of PAK (p21 activated

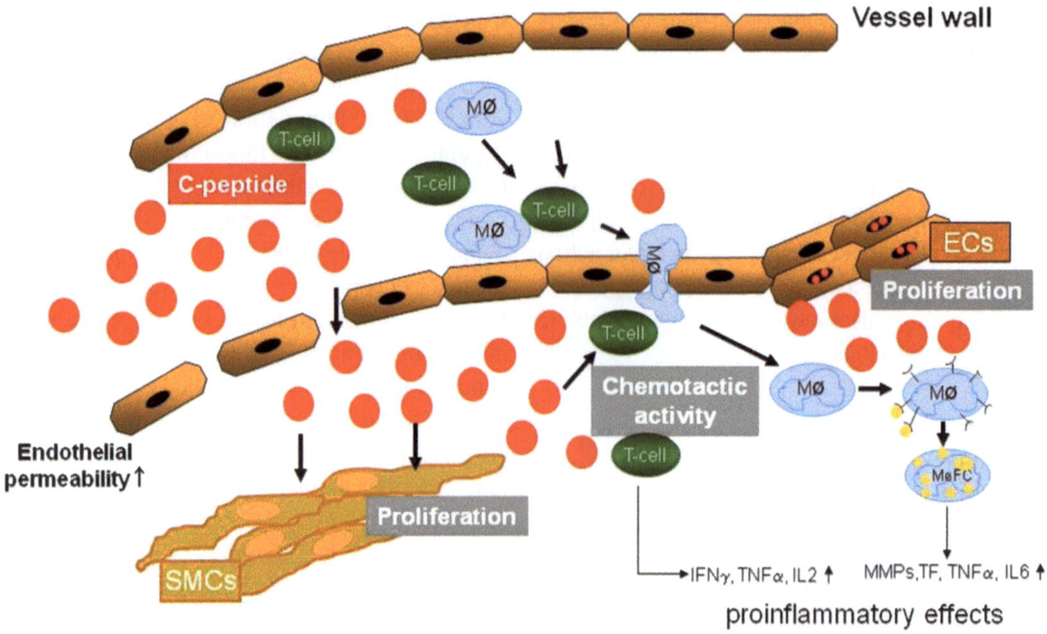

Fig. 13.1 Potential role of C-peptide in early atherogenesis in patients with insulin resistance and early type 2 diabetes mellitus. During endothelial dysfunction with increased endothelial permeability, C-peptide could deposit in the intima and through its chemotactic activity on monocytes and $CD4^+$ lymphocytes facilitate the recruitment of these inflammatory cells into the vessel wall and perpetuate the proinflammatory process. In addition, C-peptide promotes the differentiation of monocytes/macrophages. Furthermore, C-peptide can activate smooth muscle cell proliferation and endothelial cell proliferation. *EC* endothelial cell; *T-cell* CD4-positive lymphocytes; *Mo* monocytes/macrophages; *MoFC* macrophage foam cell

kinase), LIMK (LIM domain-containing protein kinase), and cofilin downstream of Rac-1 and Cdc42, leading to cofilin inactivation and actin filament stabilization. On the other hand, C-peptide activates ROCK (Rho kinase) and MLC (myosin light chain) phosphorylation downstream of RhoA, thereby stimulating myosin-mediated cell contraction [24]. These data supported an active role of C-peptide in chemotaxis of inflammatory cells.

In summary, these data suggest that – during endothelial dysfunction with increased endothelial permeability – C-peptide may deposit in the arterial intima in patients with insulin resistance and early type 2 diabetes mellitus and subsequently attract monocytes and CD4-positive lymphocytes into the vessel wall. Such mechanisms may promote lesion development and potentially explain why patients with diabetes develop such a diffuse and extensive pattern of arteriosclerosis at a very early timepoint (Fig. 13.1).

C-Peptide Promotes the Differentiation of Monocytes/Macrophages

In addition to the chemotactic effect, interesting data exists that in monocyte-like THP1 cells C-peptide increases the expression of the PPARgamma-regulated gene CD36, an important scavenger receptor for the macrophage uptake of oxidized LDL in arteriosclerotic lesions [25]. These data suggest that C-peptide may also promote the differentiation of monocyte/macrophages towards foam cells, thus representing another potential proatherogenic effect of C-peptide.

C-Peptides' Intracellular Localization

Recent reports have shown internalization of C-peptide in the cytoplasm of HEK-293 and Swiss 3T3 cells. In addition, Lindahl et al. [26]

demonstrated C-peptide transport into the nucleus using a labeled peptide. The internalization was followed at 37°C for up to 1 h and was reduced at 4°C and after preincubation with pertussis toxin. Hence, it is concluded that this internalization of C-peptide occurs via an energy-dependent, pertussis toxin-sensitive mechanism (see Chap. 2). More recently, C-peptide internalization has also been shown in vascular cells, like endothelial cells and vascular SMCs. C-peptide was detected as punctuate intracellular structures and these structures were identified as early endosomes. From these results, the authors concluded that endosomes could be a signaling station, through which C-peptide might achieve its cellular effects [27] (see Chap. 10). Similar results we found in monocytes and CD4-positive cells (unpublished data).

Recently, published data showed new functional properties of proinsulin C-peptide and its intracellular localization. C-peptide, upon cellular entry, is localized to the nucleoli, where it promotes transcription of genes encoding for ribosomal RNA. C-peptide binds to histones and enhances acetylation of lysine residue 16 of histone H4 at the promoter region of genes for ribosomal RNA. The regulation of ribosomal RNA provides a mechanism by which C-peptide can exert transcriptional effects and implies that the peptide has growth factor activity [28] (see Chap. 2).

Role of Smooth Muscle Cell Proliferation in Atherogenesis and Restenosis Formation

Vascular SMCs play a crucial role in the development of arteriosclerotic plaques by proliferating and subsequently moving from the media into early lesions and fatty streaks [12]. Furthermore, VSMCs are of critical importance in restenosis formation after coronary intervention. After vascular injury, these cells start to proliferate and then migrate into the developing neointima, thus becoming the major cellular substrate of the restenotic tissue [28]. Strategies to modulate VSMC proliferation after intervention, e.g., by the implantation of drug-eluting stents, reduce neointima formation and restenosis [29], underscoring the pathophysiological relevance of VSMC proliferation in these processes. Several mechanisms like PDGF release from activated platelets or the secretion of cytokines and growth factors from inflammatory cells have been shown to induce VSMC proliferation during atherogenesis and restenosis formation [12].

C-Peptide Colocalizes with Smooth Muscle Cells in the Media of Diabetic Subjects

In the PDAY-study mentioned above, C-peptide deposition has been found in intima in 100% of the 21 diabetic individuals examined, while deposition in media was found in 40%. Since C-peptide also colocalized with SMCs in early arteriosclerotic lesions in these eight diabetic subjects, it has been suggested that C-peptide could also exhibit biological activity in these cells [30]

C-Peptide: Role on Smooth Muscle Cell Proliferation

Conflicting data exist on the role of C-peptide in SMC proliferation. A recent report coming from Kobayashi et al. demonstrated an inhibition of rat SMC proliferation after 3 days of treatment with human C-peptide under high glucose concentrations [31]. These effects observed at high C-peptide concentrations (100 nmol/L) were mediated by an inhibition of PDGF-beta receptor expression as well as by a reduction in p42/p44 MAP-kinase phosphorylation.

Recently, published data from another group support a causative role for insulin in human SV neointima formation with a novel counter-regulatory effect of proinsulin C-peptide. The mitogenic effects of insulin can be prevented by coincubation with 10 nmol/L C-peptide. In their experiments, C-peptide did not affect insulin-induced Akt or extracellular signal-regulated kinase signaling, but array data and gene silencing implicated sterol regulatory element-binding transcription factor 1 as a target molecule [32].

These data are in contrast to results from our own group demonstrating an induction of SMC proliferation upon C-peptide stimulation [30]. In our experimental setting, human C-peptide induced the proliferation of human aortic SMCs, while rat C-peptide exhibited similar effects in rat aortic SMCs. Moreover, C-peptide stimulation of VSMCs activates Src- and PI-3 kinase and leads to downstream phosphorylation of the MAPK ERK1/2. Previous work has shown that Src-kinase is involved in LDL-induced VSMC proliferation [33]. Activation of PI-3 kinase by C-peptide has recently been demonstrated in various cell types including vascular cells like monocytes and CD4-positive lymphocytes, suggesting a critical role of this signaling molecule in C-peptide-induced cell activation in different cell types. The downstream control of VSMC proliferation by extracellular stimuli takes place in mid- to late G_1 phase of the cell cycle, where D-type cyclins promote G_1- to S-phase transition by leading to Rb phosphorylation [34, 35]. Our data, showing an increase in cyclin D1 expression as well as Rb phosphorylation, suggest that C-peptide acts via similar signaling pathways [30].

C-peptides' mitogenic effect was also found in other cell types, like endothelial cells, HEK293 cells, and in chondrocytes. When endothelial cells were exposed to C-peptide, a 40% significant increase in cell number was observed [32]. Others have found that C-peptide stimulates rRNA synthesis suggesting that the peptide can have proliferative effects and induces expression of 47S in HCS-2/8 chondrocytes derived from a human chondrosarcoma. After 72 h of exposure to C-peptide, cell counting under a phase contrast microscope and measurement with a cell proliferation kit and BrdUrd staining established that C-peptide exerts proliferative effects on chondrocytes [28].

In addition to its chemotactic effect on monocytes and CD4-positive lymphocytes, C-peptide could enhance VSMC proliferation in the vasculature, thus promoting both, the development of arteriosclerotic lesions as well as neointima formation after coronary intervention. Still, future studies in animal models have to evaluate the pathophysiological relevance of C-peptide-induced VSMC proliferation in atherogenesis and neointima formation in vivo.

C-Peptide: Why Do We Get Different Results in Type 1 and Type 2 Diabetes?

The majority of data described above suggest that C-peptide may promote lesion development in patients with type 2 diabetes mellitus and insulin resistance, while the application of C-peptide in type 1 diabetic patients who lack C-peptide has been shown to improve diabetic microvascular complications such as diabetic nephropathy and neuropathy (see Chaps. 4, 7, 8, and 12). The potential proatherogenic action of C-peptide is not in contrast to such clinical benefits of C-peptide treatment in patients with type 1 diabetes. From other clinical disorders, like hypo- and hyperthyroidism, we know that treatment with L-thyroxine in patients with hypothyroidism is beneficial, but elevated levels of L-thyroxine in those with hyperthyroidism can cause serious clinical manifestations. In comparison with this situation, supplementation of C-peptide in type 1 diabetic patients may be beneficial, while an increase in C-peptide levels in patients with insulin resistance and type 2 diabetes may be harmful.

Conclusions and Perspectives

Further studies in animal models of arteriosclerosis are warranted to examine whether the hypothesis of C-peptide's proatherogenic effects holds true in vivo. Moreover, additional work is needed to identify the C-peptide receptor. Such a receptor could be an interesting therapeutical target for both, patients with type 1 or type 2 diabetes. Activating such a receptor could be beneficial in type 1 diabetic patients, while blocking of C-peptide receptors in patients with insulin resistance and early type 2 diabetes may help to prevent vascular complications from early on.

Acknowledgment This work was supported by grants of the Deutsche Forschungsgemeinschaft (SFB 451, project B9 and B11, MA2047/4-1, WA2145/1-1) to Prof. Dr. Nikolaus Marx and to Prof. Dr. Daniel Walcher, as well as a grant from the Else-Kröner Fresenius Stiftung to Prof. Dr. Daniel Walcher.

References

1. Beckman JA, Creager MA, Libby P. Diabetes and atherosclerosis: epidemiology, pathophysiology, and management. JAMA. 2002;287:2570–81.
2. Schmidt AM, Yan SD, Wautier JL, Stern D. Activation of receptor for advanced glycation end products: a mechanism for chronic vascular dysfunction in diabetic vasculopathy and atherosclerosis. Circ Res. 1999;84:489–97.
3. Ritthaler U, Deng Y, Zhang Y, et al. Expression of receptors for advanced glycation end products in peripheral occlusive vascular disease. Am J Pathol. 1995;146:688–94.
4. Wahren J, Ekberg K, Johansson J, et al. Role of C-peptide in human physiology. Am J Physiol Endocrinol Metab. 2000;278:759–68.
5. Kitamura T, Kimura K, Jung BD, et al. Proinsulin C-peptide rapidly stimulates mitogen-activated protein kinases in Swiss 3T3 fibroblasts: requirement of protein kinase C, phosphoinositide 3-kinase and pertussis toxin-sensitive G-protein. Biochem J. 2001; 355:123–9.
6. Kitamura T, Kimura K, Jung BD, et al. Proinsulin C-peptide activates cAMP response element-binding proteins through the p38 mitogen-activated protein kinase pathway in mouse lung capillary endothelial cells. Biochem J. 2002;366:737–44.
7. Ekberg K, Brismar T, Johansson BL, et al. Amelioration of sensory nerve dysfunction by C-peptide in patients with type 1 diabetes. Diabetes. 2003;52:536–41.
8. Ekberg K, Brismar T, Johansson BL, et al. C-peptide replacement therapy and sensory nerve function in type 1 diabetic neuropathy. Diabetes Care. 2007;30: 71–6.
9. Samnegård B, Jacobson SH, Jaremko G, et al. C-peptide prevents glomerular hypertrophy and mesangial matrix expansion in diabetic rats. Nephrol Dial Transplant. 2005;20:532–8.
10. Sjöquist M, Huang W, Johansson BL. Effects of C-peptide on renal function at the early stage of experimental diabetes. Kidney Int. 1998;54:758–64.
11. Kamikawa A, Ishii T, Shimada K, et al. Proinsulin C-peptide abrogates type-1 diabetes-induced increase of renal endothelial nitric oxide synthase in rats. Diabetes Metab Res Rev. 2008;24:331–8.
12. Ross R. Atherosclerosis – an inflammatory disease. N Engl J Med. 1999;340:115–26.
13. Hansson GK. Inflammation, atherosclerosis, and coronary artery disease. N Engl J Med. 2005;352: 1685–95.
14. Libby P, Geng YJ, Aikawa M, et al. Macrophages and atherosclerotic plaque stability. Curr Opin Lipidol. 1996;7:330–5.
15. Robertson AK, Hansson GK. T cells in atherogenesis: for better or for worse? Arterioscler Thromb Vasc Biol. 2006;26:2421–32.
16. Marx N. Diabetes und Arteriosklerose. Diabetes Stoffwechsel. 2003;4:205–11.
17. Libby P, Simon DI. Inflammation and thrombosis: the clot thickens. Circulation. 2001;103:1718–20.
18. Trovati M, Anfossi G. Influence of insulin and of insulin resistance on platelet and vascular smooth muscle cell function. J Diabetes Complications. 2002;16:35–40.
19. Dandona P, Chaudhuri A, Ghanim H, Mohanty P. Anti-inflammatory effects of insulin and pro-inflammatory effects of glucose: relevance to the management of acute myocardial infarction and other acute coronary syndromes. Rev Cardiovasc Med. 2006;7:25–34.
20. Dandona P, Chaudhuri A, Mohanty P, Ghanim H. Anti-inflammatory effects of insulin. Curr Opin Clin Nutr Metab Care. 2007;10:511–7.
21. Marx N, Walcher D, Raichle C, et al. C-peptide colocalizes with macrophages in early arteriosclerotic lesions of diabetic subjects and induces monocyte chemotaxis in vitro. Arterioscler Thromb Vasc Biol. 2004;24:540–5.
22. Walcher D, Aleksic M, Jerg V, et al. C-peptide induces chemotaxis of human CD4-positive cells: involvement of pertussis toxin-sensitive G-proteins and phosphoinositide 3-kinase. Diabetes. 2004;53:1664–70.
23. Kukhtina NB, Arefieva TI, Krasnikova TL. Intracellular signal cascade in CD4+ T-lymphocyte migration stimulated by interferon-gamma-inducible protein-10. Biochemistry (Mosc). 2005;70:652–6.
24. Aleksic M, Walcher D, Giehl K, et al. Signalling processes involved in C-peptide-induced chemotaxis of CD4-positive lymphocytes. Cell Mol Life Sci. 2009;66:1974–84.
25. Al-Rasheed NM, Chana RS, Baines RJ, Willars GB, Brunskill NJ. Ligand-independent activation of peroxisome proliferator-activated receptor-gamma by insulin and C-peptide in kidney proximal tubular cells: dependent on phosphatidylinositol 3-kinase activity. J Biol Chem. 2004;279(48):49747–54.
26. Lindahl E, Nyman U, Melles E, et al. Cellular internalization of proinsulin C-peptide. Cell Mol Life Sci. 2007;64:479–86.
27. Luppi P, Geng X, Cifarelli V, Drain P, Trucco M. C-peptide is internalised in human endothelial and vascular smooth muscle cells via early endosomes. Diabetologia. 2009;52:2218–28.
28. Lindahl E, Nyman U, Zaman F, et al. Proinsulin C-peptide regulates ribosomal RNA expression. J Biol Chem. 2010;285:3462–9.
29. Bittl JA. Advances in coronary angioplasty. N Engl J Med. 1996;335:1290–302.
30. Walcher D, Babiak C, Poletek P, et al. C-Peptide induces vascular smooth muscle cell proliferation: involvement of SRC-kinase, phosphatidylinositol

3-kinase, and extracellular signal-regulated kinase 1/2. Circ Res. 2006;99(11):1181–7.
31. Kobayashi Y, Naruse K, Hamada Y, et al. Human proinsulin C-peptide prevents proliferation of rat aortic smooth muscle cells cultured in high-glucose conditions. Diabetologia. 2005;48:2396–401.
32. Mughal RS, Scragg JL, Lister P, et al. Cellular mechanisms by which proinsulin C-peptide prevents insulin-induced neointima formation in human saphenous vein. Diabetologia. 2010;53:1761–71.
33. Cho HM, Choi SH, Hwang KC, et al. The Src/PLC/PKC/MEK/ERK signaling pathway is involved in aortic smooth muscle cell proliferation induced by glycated LDL. Mol Cells. 2005;19(1):60–6.
34. Beijersbergen RL, Bernards R. Cell cycle regulation by the retinoblastoma family of growth inhibitory proteins. Biochim Biophys Acta. 1996;1287(2–3):103–20.
35. Harbour JW, Dean DC. Rb function in cell-cycle regulation and apoptosis. Nat Cell Biol. 2000;4:65–7.

Conclusions and Future Outlook 14

Anders A.F. Sima

It is indeed encouraging to see the rapid accumulation of new data on the pathophysiological role of C-peptide and the clinical benefits of its replacement in type 1 diabetic patients. It is also a pleasure to acknowledge an increasing number of investigators and clinicians joining the field.

Since its discovery in the late 1960s by Donald Steiner and collaborators, C-peptide was initially regarded as a biologically inactive byproduct of insulin synthesis. Only in the early 1990s was there a resurgence of the interest in C-peptide, after the Stockholm group demonstrated clinical effects of C-peptide replacement on early nephropathy, neuropathy, and on skin microcirculation in type 1 diabetic patients. Since these early encouraging observational data were published almost a decade and a half ago, a wealth of information has been gathered with respect to C-peptide's various signaling mechanisms, interactions with insulin, and its physiological effects in various cell types paramount to their specific functions.

The clinical effects were replicated and elucidation of underlying mechanisms was expanded upon using in vivo experimental animal models of type 1 diabetes and in vitro cellular systems. Systematic studies in the kidney have demonstrated normalizing effects on the intricate interplay between afferent and efferent vascular tone with effects on hyperfiltration and glomerular filtration rate and subsequent structural changes affecting tubular and glomerular components. Likewise, longitudinal studies in peripheral nerves have demonstrated beneficial effects on the early Na^+/K^+-ATPase-coupled nerve conduction defect, suppressed expression of neurotrophic factors, and its consequences as to structural and functional proteins eventually resulting in nodal degeneration, axonal atrophy, and loss. The recently recognized diabetic encephalopathy causing cognitive deficits in type 1 patients has been demonstrated to be largely preventable following C-peptide replacement in animal models. The role of C-peptide deficiency has been firmly established regarding the components of the microvasculopathy itself such as red cell deformability, capillary blood flow, and platelet function. Its anti-inflammatory effects have been well documented in the vascular endothelium and smooth muscle cells and in the cerebral cortex and white matter. Hence, such animal experiments have had a major impact on establishing proof of concept, thereby firmly establishing C-peptide deficiency as a major pathogenetic component in the development of the chronic complications in type 1 diabetes. At the same time, they have convincingly demonstrated the beneficial therapeutical effects of C-peptide replacement on these complications.

There is now clear evidence demonstrating that C-peptide binds to cell membranes with

A.A.F. Sima (✉)
Department of Pathology, Wayne State University and Detroit Medical Center, 540 E. Canfield Avenue, Detroit, MI 48201, USA

Department of Neurology, Wayne State University and Detroit Medical Center, Detroit, MI 48201, USA
e-mail: asima@med.wayne.edu

A.A.F. Sima (ed.), *Diabetes & C-Peptide: Scientific and Clinical Aspects*, Contemporary Diabetes, DOI 10.1007/978-1-61779-391-2_14,

intracellular signaling activities which can be prevented by pretreatment with pertussis toxin, in many but not all tissues, suggesting binding to a G-protein-coupled receptor. It exerts profound effects on major signaling pathways such as PI-3 kinase and MAPK signaling with downstream effects on Na^+/K^+-ATPase and eNOS activities in a variety of tissues. C-peptide enters into various cell types and accumulates in cytoplasmic endosomes and terminates in lysosomes. It attenuates protein tyrosine phosphatase activity with activation of the insulin receptor and signaling without interacting with the insulin receptor itself, hence providing a scaffolding effect. A variety of transcription factors are regulated by C-peptide with effects on gene and protein expression of functional and structural proteins in the kidney, peripheral, and central nervous systems, suggesting that C-peptide may interact with insulin-signaling activities, which in some systems can be abolished with Wortmannin. NF-κB is a transcription factor that is regulated by C-peptide with downstream effects on inflammatory activities as well as apoptosis in the central nervous system and vasculature. Therefore, C-peptide exerts anti-inflammatory and anti-apoptotic effects. In certain systems, C-peptide displays effects in the absence of insulin. C-peptide bound to Zn^{2+}-ions is taken up by red blood cells in which it exerts glycolytic effects and promotes ATP synthesis with effects on red blood cell deformability and promotes secondary effects on platelet and rheological functions. C-peptide also enters into cell nuclei with effects on ribosomal RNA synthesis with growth factor and gene-modulating effects.

Recently, it was demonstrated that C-peptide also has extracellular effects mediated by close interactions with insulin. Both insulin and C-peptide have self-associating properties. Insulin forms hexamers in vivo held together by zinc ions. C-peptide attracts and binds the zinc ions, thereby dehexamerizing insulin and liberating active monomeric insulin. Hence, it is obvious that C-peptide has several physiological functions, which may explain its diversified effects in various biological systems and the important role that C-peptide deficiency plays in the pathogenesis of the diverse chronic complications in type 1 diabetes.

Most research activities with respect to C-peptide have been focused on the secondary complications in type 1 diabetes. Only recently have effects of elevated or too much circulating C-peptide as in hyperinsulinemic type 2 diabetes been explored. Elevated C-peptide levels have been shown to have adverse effects on atherogenesis by promoting macrophage recruitment and smooth muscle cell proliferation in the macrovasculature. Taken together, these findings suggest that C-peptide exerts its normal physiological functions within a narrow concentration range. Hence, without any doubt, C-peptide deficiency plays a very prominent role in type 1 diabetes and its complications, while excessive C-peptide has detrimental effects on the macrovasculature.

It is therefore clear that C-peptide possesses several modes of action. It interacts with cell membranes, it has direct intracellular actions, and it interacts with insulin extracellularly. Despite the substantial progress that has been made, some key mechanisms remain to be clarified. The foremost question is its interaction with the cell membrane, or in other words, does a C-peptide receptor exist, which would explain its activation of major signaling pathways? Or is the membrane interaction nonchiral? Another area that has only started to be explored is the adverse effects of hyper-C-peptidemia in type 2 diabetes, like its involvement in atherosclerosis. For instance, is elevated C-peptide levels, like hyperinsulinemia, involved in the development of the clinical expressions associated with the metabolic syndrome or the heightened risk of Alzheimer's disease in type 2 diabetes?

In summary, therefore, it is obvious that type 1 diabetes is a two hormone deficiency disorder. We have now for almost 90 years substituted one of these hormones to control hyperglycemia. As has been repeatedly demonstrated in this volume of Contemporary Diabetes, there is more to type 1 diabetes and its complications than hyperglycemia. So why do we not replace also the second deficient hormone C-peptide, which with a large degree of certainty would have major impacts on the prevention and treatment of the debilitating complications accompanying type 1 diabetes? This becomes even more urgent when considering the explosive global increase in the incidence of type 1 diabetes. Based on the present data, we would urge patient organizations and interest groups, responsible national funding agencies and the patient conscience pharmaceutical industry to promote, initiate, and fund necessary large scale clinical trials to enable the clinical use of this second missing hormone. This realization would with all likelihood have major impacts on the quality of life of millions of type 1 diabetic patients. Not only that, it would also undoubtedly have economic impacts on the escalating health care costs for a rapidly increasing patient group.

Index

A.A.F. Sima (ed.), *Diabetes & C-Peptide: Scientific and Clinical Aspects*, Contemporary Diabetes,
DOI 10.1007/978-1-61779-391-2, © Springer Science+Business Media, LLC 2012

N

O

P

R

MIX
Papier aus verantwortungsvollen Quellen
Paper from responsible sources
FSC® C105338

If you have any concerns about our products,
you can contact us on
ProductSafety@springernature.com

In case Publisher is established outside the EU,
the EU authorized representative is:
Springer Nature Customer Service Center GmbH
Europaplatz 3, 69115 Heidelberg, Germany

Printed by Libri Plureos GmbH
in Hamburg, Germany